Pandemic Providers

Charles R. Figley • Lenore E. A. Walker
Ilene A. Serlin
Editors

Pandemic Providers

Psychologists Respond to Covid

Springer

Editors
Charles R. Figley
School of Social Work
Tulane University
New Orleans, LA, USA

Ilene A. Serlin
Independent Practice
San Francisco, CA, USA

Serlin Institute of the Healing Arts
San Francisco, CA, USA

Lenore E. A. Walker
College of Psychology
Nova Southeastern University
Fort Lauderdale, FL, USA

Walker & Associates, LLC
Fort Lauderdale, FL, USA

ISBN 978-3-031-27579-1 ISBN 978-3-031-27580-7 (eBook)
https://doi.org/10.1007/978-3-031-27580-7

This Springer imprint is published by the registered company Springer Nature Switzerland AG
The registered company address is: Gewerbestrasse 11, 6330 Cham, Switzerland

Preface

In December 2019, the first human cases of COVID-19 were identified in China, and the World Health Organization declared a public health emergency of international concern on January 30, 2020, and a pandemic on March 11, 2020. Therapists and mental health providers were stunned by the overwhelming anxiety and fears brought to them. People were confused, afraid to touch or be touched, angry, isolated, and in despair. The authors of this book echoed the primary question from the practitioners: What do we do?

There was no handbook about how to help mental health providers navigate this new and unknown threat. In March, therefore, a group of trauma psychologists began to meet online to share experiences and resources. They were joined online with social workers, private practitioners, well-known scholars, and professors. But most of us were practitioners during those dark days.

We met weekly at noon Fridays. We quickly discovered that our group was among very few behaving collectively as practitioners to help practitioners. We were psychologists, social workers, counselors, lawyers, nurses, and other mental health specialists and experts who quickly became active in healing the nation and the world, in our own way. Although we came together under the APA rubric initially, we were on our own mission as a Task Force. Like the pandemic, the mission was emerging gradually.

Within a few months, our Task Force was gaining traction as well as members within the American Psychological Association and other related professional groups. Our focus was first on APA as an organization of fellow psychologists. Soon other divisions within APA joined the Task Force in support of our mission.

This book is the story of our journey through the darker times of the COVID-19 pandemic as an editorial team and as active members of the APA Interdivisional Task Force on the Pandemic. While living under pandemic fears and restrictions ourselves, to deliver the services and resources we discovered. These services and resources took form as this book. We hope, through these services and resources, to help current and future mental health providers with a roadmap for working with current and future pandemics, and to support our fellow pandemic providers.

New Orleans, LA, USA — Charles R. Figley
Fort Lauderdale, FL, USA — Lenore E. A. Walker
San Francisco, CA, USA — Ilene A. Serlin

Endorsements

Pandemic Providers *could not be more timely, given the Covid-19 pandemic and those yet to come. The book's editors and chapter authors are skilled professionals who had to work their way through uncharted territories, creating a roadmap for the intrepid practitioners who are dealing not only with the current health crisis but also for those who will deal with pandemics yet to come. It is written in a lively, reader-friendly manner that allows its insights to be put to immediate use.*

Stanley Krippner, Ph.D., Affiliated Distinguished Faculty, California Institute of Integral Studies. Co-author *Post-traumatic Stress Disorder: Biography of a Disease*

The sudden onset of the pandemic left many psychologists unprepared for the traumas caused by complex and new challenges. This group of psychologists, led by experts from the trauma division of the American Psychological Association, grew into a multidisciplinary group of volunteers who dedicated themselves to learning to address these challenges and to document their learning so that other healthcare providers could benefit. The result is a valuable record of those challenges and lessons learned from multiple perspectives, international affiliates, and creative new methods. The world needs caregivers who can meet the rapidly changing challenges, and this book can help teach and train others to do so. I highly recommend it for graduate students, volunteers, and healthcare providers.

Philip G. Zimbardo, Ph.D., Professor Emeritus Psychology Stanford University, Past President APA and WPA, William James Book of the Year Award

In the true spirit of the practitioner-scholar model, this timely compendium based on the work of notable psychologists from around the world offers fresh perspectives to practitioners and researchers to address the consequences of the COVID pandemic and to help them prepare for future ones.

V. K. Kumar, Ph.D., Professor Emeritus, West Chester University of Pennsylvania

An outstanding compilation of visionary accomplishments during the Pandemic by extraordinary leaders in the profession. Addressing the unique challenges and opportunities across the life span, the Lessons Learned hold great promise for the future. Interprofessional collaboration, technological innovations, and the importance of therapeutic empathy remain critical.

Pat DeLeon, former APA President

Pandemic Providers *is a much-needed book at this time due to the global pandemic. Following the worst of the pandemic, there is a tremendous need for psychologists and other health care providers for supportive information and skills to enable them to help the thousands of people suffering physically and psychologically from dealing with the pandemic. Many people are highly anxious, afraid, depressed, grieving, suffering, and traumatized by the ordeal we have all suffered. The trauma and vicarious trauma that many have suffered cry for the psychological skills and tools covered in* Pandemic Providers. *It is comprehensive and heartfelt coverage that members of APA and others have ably provided readers with the materials we need now and for some years to come. It will take that amount of time to recover from what we have gone through globally.* Pandemic Providers *is a companion for that recovery.*

Eleanor Criswell Hanna, Ed.D., Professor emeritus psychology, Sonoma State University

Introduction

The appearance of the new coronavirus, named COVID-19, thrust everyone in the helping professions out of their typical comfort zones, and we all had to learn to adapt quickly. *Pandemic Providers* is the story of our colleagues in psychology, counseling, social work, family therapy, psychiatry, nursing, and other professions who worked and continue to work under extraordinary circumstances, including their own pandemic conditions. This book is about and by these pandemic providers of mental health services who report on what it was like for them during the pandemic, and how their experiences have taught them about how they see human services evolving in today's world. As we write this book, we are toward the end of the third year of this pandemic. It has changed over this time from the unknown, out-of-control but deadly threat to a somewhat tamed but still serious health threat that we continue to live with in what might be called a post-pandemic world. It has morphed from a pandemic to a systemic to an endemic, merging with threats of climate and political change. It has, in many ways, destabilized our world and we are learning to live with its impact. It has changed the way we communicate, the way we work, and it is affecting our authors and their students, family members, and the rest of us. And we, as mental health providers, had to pivot to learn how to navigate the new world as we try to take care of ourselves and others. What are we observing about how the pandemic is affecting each of us, and what can we learn and share with others that help deal with psychological impacts from the pandemic.

Our mission in this book, therefore, is to provide guidance to all who want to learn our lessons. This includes mental health professionals, no matter their stage of development, to learn about how to manage new, unfamiliar, and sometimes frightening new forms of service delivery. This means just-in-time training in universities, hospital settings, private practice, and, of course, online for those needing continuing education.

This book may also be useful for historians, economists, and political scientists. Our government did not rely on science initially to help figure out how to deal with the pandemic. By the time they did seek out vaccines to reduce the health threat, millions of lives had been lost and too many others hesitated to accept the vaccine fearing its safety. Conflicting advice by political leaders caused huge numbers of people to refuse to follow the simple steps of mask-wearing and social distancing that might have slowed down the contagion and mutations. Our task force members spent time trying to help people understand why these methods could protect them swimming upstream against a tide of political disbelievers and developed tools and outreach projects to reach communities in need.

We write in this book about the challenges faced and lessons learned that may help other providers mobilize, collaborate, and provide effective and compassionate services. We describe how we and those we worked with dealt with the total shut down of the world during that first frightening year. We are still trying to understand the consequences of having to homeschool children while trying to work from home. Some gave up trying and quit jobs while others volunteered to help first responders. Computers, smart phones, and the internet supplanted paper and pens. People died alone without family but with janitors holding their hands in over-crowded and understaffed hospitals. Parents formed small groups and tried to live more normally. Others survived by locking their doors and not emerging for several years, ordering food and basic needs to be delivered. We pandemic providers ourselves experienced tremendous fear, distrust of others, fear of being touched, and loneliness. We saw and felt it in our communities and wanted to help. This is the collective concern that brings us all together in this book: We must apply the lessons learned to the inevitable future pandemics.

Origins

Here we briefly note the origins of the collaborative group that we formed through the leadership of the American Psychological Association's Division of members who specialize in trauma psychology, Division 56. Ninety-five people joined initially searching for ways to help others deal with trauma. When asked what motivated them, almost all stated they felt helpless in the face of the unknown; working with others gave them hope and purpose. Not all continued to work with the task force throughout the 3 years; some of those who didn't stay on stated their workload increased so much that they could not afford the time to donate to the task force. Nonetheless, those who responded to our survey unequivocally found the work rewarding and satisfying. This book shares some of those successes especially in the second part.

Task Force

The APA Interdivisional Task Force on the Pandemic was created spontaneously at the outbreak of COVID-19 in the United States. The mission of the Task Force was, and continues to be, to gather, generate, and share innovative resources to address the complex traumas resulting from the pandemic. The Task Force constitutes an unusual collaborative effort among APA divisions and generations. Two divisions took the lead in advertising for anyone who wanted to work with the task force and quickly 14 divisions joined. This is unusual within APA as it did not come from the governance, which usually sets up task forces, but from the division members themselves. Charles Figley was appointed as chair. He announced a zoom meeting and almost 100 members from these different divisions jumped on. Within a short time, some volunteered to chair a working group, set up meeting time, and the groups began to meet separately but monthly together with Dr. Figley and the larger task force. A listserv was formed to make communication easier and each working group shared what they were doing with the larger task force. Others joined the working groups and didn't attend task force meetings. The loose structure worked well during the initial year; those who wanted the support of the larger group were able to get it while others who just wanted to do the work could do that, too.

By year two, the idea of keeping a record of what we were doing became a reality with the formation of a publication working group along with the others. Not all the working groups were able to document their work for various reasons. For some, the pandemic itself created a huge strain on their psychic energy. Others were ill or had other family and life crises. Still others became involved in other activities that demanded their attention. Students finished their training or graduated and went on to other work. One thing was certain in year two when the world began to open up, everyone became busier. We also understood that traumatic events are not easy to talk about, and without talking they won't get processed or remembered.

In year three, several of the groups no longer were working in the same way. The IPV group, for example, stopped the innovative weekly roundtables as they became too time consuming although continued posting resources on the various social media. The professional psychology groups found similar time constraints although they did spend some time working with the Ukrainian psychologists deal with the trauma from the war with Russia. The working group on immigration were unable to document the work they did with helping understand trauma from both refugee and immigrant status. The crisis intervention group tried to develop a new theory of responding to crises and disasters but were unable to test it out. Hopefully, they will continue to work on their creative approaches even though it didn't make it into the book this time.

Clinical practitioners, researchers, and students from the Task Force share lessons they have learned. These lessons are drawn from, and broadly reflect, the experience of other American or international clinical practitioners providing psychotherapy or other resources during the pandemic. This is consistent with the mission of the Task Force: to *enable psychologists and other practitioners to share knowledge and resources about the psychological impact of trauma and the pandemic.*

New Orleans, LA, USA — Charles R. Figley
Fort Lauderdale, FL, USA — Lenore E. A. Walker
San Francisco, CA, USA — Ilene A. Serlin

Contents

Editors

Editors Figley, Walker, and Serlin first assembled a collection of colleagues that turned into a set of a dozen or so work groups during the early weeks of the pandemic. They began to meet apart from the Task Force (Figley, 2020) and focused on worthy work at the time. Each work group noted their scope of work and areas of expertise and set out to find other members and work collectively to help improve our near environment. These groups formed into Work Groups that focused on either a particular issue (e.g., domestic violence), population (e.g., students), or modality (e.g., creative arts). The contributors to this volume all represent one of these Work Groups, although not all Work Groups have written chapters. They introduce an array mental health resources and services that emerged during the pandemic to address the critical needs of recipients. They included both clinical and instructional materials that were needed at the time and will again as our worlds shift and change. The book is both a collection of resources that can be shared online and within the book. We introduce this book and the editorial team:

Charles Ray Figley is the Henry Kurzweg, MD Chair and professor in Disaster Mental Health at Tulane University where he heads the University's Trauma Institute. He is author of more than 200 journal articles and 29 books.

Lenore E. A. Walker is professor emerita at Nova Southeastern University College of Psychology and author and editor of special issues, books, and articles with a specialty in understanding (and championing) and describing gender violence, domestic violence, and trauma. In addition to her editorial and clinical knowledge is her collaborative leadership style. Before a pandemic was declared she stepped forward (March 2020) to join what was to soon become the Interdivisional Task Force on the Pandemic. She worked with many of the authors and provided guidance as co-editor. She co-authored Chap. 3 and wrote Chap. 9.

Ilene A. Serlin is associated distinguished professor at the California Institute of Integral Studies and in independent practice of psychology in Marin county. She is also a dance therapist and uses the creative arts to assist in healing from trauma, training internationally through the Serlin Institute of the Healing Arts. She is the past president of the San Francisco Psychological Association, a Fellow of the American Psychological Association, Past President of the Division of Humanistic Psychology and recipient of its Rollo May award. She has edited several books, numerous articles, chapters, and magazine pieces on trauma, psychotherapy, creativity, and human thriving.

Reference

Figley, C. R. (2020). Trauma and the Human Costs of Humane Caring. A Webinar by the Tulane University School of Medicine: COVID-19 and Healthcare Professionals – Recognizing and Responding to Stress in Adults and Children, September 24.

Part I
Analyzing, Planning, and Delivering

The book is divided into three parts. Part I: Analyzing, Planning, and Delivering does just that, we call on our fellow practitioners to join our Task Force and the cause it represents: Stepping up to volunteer our time to help others in this growing hostile environment from many sources and through many forces. The call to action comes at a time of growing political and ideological conflict. The action is about retaining a sense of safety and coherence in our delivery of useful mental health services during a time that divides us from our common values and historic social ties.

Part I contains two chapters. The first chapter is an overall introduction to the book: How and why it is we created this book. Our common frame of reference was the growing recognition that this worldwide illness was like no other for a century. The SARS epidemic in 2004 was a warning that a virus could force people to curtain their lives to avoid becoming ill. But, few people took it seriously after SARS was contained. It was noted back in March 2020 that the last time the world was forced to cope with such a virulent illness as COVID-19 was in 1918, nearly 100 years ago. The pandemic of 1918. Chapter 2 provides an important starting point in our efforts in this book to provide a sense of reference and direction in more fully understanding and applying the lessons learned from past pandemics with special interest in the psychosocial consequences that shape how best to recover and respond with greater confidence and caring. Often called "the forgotten pandemic," the 1918 experience had some similarities with the political situation and ineffective leadership by the government. At that time, President Wilson was more interested in World War I than in protecting people. Fair to say, however, medicine was in its infancy concerning contagion and infectious diseases. Most important to psychology, no one knew that to heal from trauma a person must process it verbally – talk about it, mourn the losses, and then move on with life.

Chapter 1
In the Beginning

Charles R. Figley, Lenore E. A. Walker, and Ilene A. Serlin

This book is about our future both as people and as a profession. This book is about and by pandemic providers of mental health services who report on what they do, with whom, and under pandemic circumstances. What is it like for providers of mental health services who are impacted themselves? How do they see human services evolving in a post-pandemic world? Their reports in this book about challenges faced and lessons learned can help other pandemic providers mobilize, collaborate, and provide effective and compassionate services for inevitable future pandemics. The COVID-19 pandemic thrust everyone in the helping professions out of their typical comfort zones. We were in shock and disoriented and had to learn to adapt quickly.

We formed the Interdivisional Task Force on the Pandemic for the purpose of doing what we could with what we had for the most people. As editors, we immediately recognized the power and importance of the personal stories provided by different members of the Task Force as we met weekly. In those early weeks of the pandemic, we urged our fellow Task Force members to keep a written record of our experiences given the uncharted territory we were feeling our way through. We all felt like we wanted to help but were unsure of how to do it. The stress of grabbing the crisis as it morphed helped dissolve the old barriers to working together. There were few hierarchies; we needed the skills of our young members who could help us use new technologies to deliver the resources and treatment services more experienced psychologists could provide.

C. R. Figley (✉)
School of Social Work, Tulane University, New Orleans, LA, USA
e-mail: Figley@tulane.edu

L. E. A. Walker
College of Psychology, Nova Southeastern University, Fort Lauderdale, FL, USA

I. A. Serlin
Independent Practice, San Francisco, CA, USA

C. R. Figley et al. (eds.), *Pandemic Providers*,
https://doi.org/10.1007/978-3-031-27580-7_1

We were amazed at how well the members of the group learned to work with each other, relying on our various skills. Adopting new technologies such as social media put us in rapid touch with colleagues around the world, all dealing with similar if not identical problems. How do we motivate people to give up some personal freedom for the good of the entire planet? Although we were warned of a second wave coming, most were oblivious to it, just wanting to get through the first one.

Our mission in this book, therefore, is to provide guidance to all mental health professionals, no matter their stage of development, to learn about how best to manage new, unfamiliar, and sometimes frightening forms of service delivery and the context of its delivery. This means we intend this book to be read by all mental health professionals, such as but not limited to psychologists, counselors, social workers, nurses, physicians, marriage and family therapists, and those in training in universities, hospital settings, private independent practice, and those needing continuing education.

We write this book with the intention of making a difference through our stories, services, and contributions here. Among the questions we will ask and answer here are these five questions. They provide a kind of roadmap for guiding our discussions. Here we pose the critical questions, and in our last chapter we provide the answers as part of a summary set of statements about this book:

1. *What happened to the world and the USA during the first 3 years of the pandemic?*
2. *What were mental health professional during the pandemic?*
3. *What were the innovations and breakthroughs in pandemic-related mental health assessment and services?*
4. *What did we learn about gender, race, healthcare inequities, human relations, and helping our fellow humans?*
5. *How can we play forward what we have learned toward increased social services and greater care for others as well as ourselves?*

The Crisis Emerges: The Task Force Is Born

In this first chapter we briefly note the origins of the collaborative group that we formed, called the APA Interdivisional Task Force on the Pandemic Task Force, and describe the book we set out to write. We include descriptions of our experiences and insights working in the pandemic as we collaborated as a Task Force.

Our initial efforts in late March in 2020 emerged spontaneously at the outbreak of COVID-19 in the USA. Membership on the Interdivisional Task Force included practitioners with trauma expertise who can deal with the enormous waves of suffering that became apparent from the start of the pandemic. Other professionals in human services were also invited to join if they also had some clinical experience with trauma – especially collective trauma, disasters, and major events. These specializations frequently include crisis management, grief reactions, disasters response and mitigation, violence management, and related areas.

Clinical practitioners, researchers, and students from the Task Force will share lessons we have learned. These lessons are drawn from, and broadly reflect, the experience of other American or international clinical practitioners providing psychotherapy or other resources during the pandemic. This is consistent with the mission of the Task Force: to *enable psychologists and other practitioners to share knowledge and resources about the psychological impact of the pandemic.* The mission also notes that the Task Force seeks and shares guidance on *how we can cope with pandemic-related challenges as practitioners and as people, and how we can minimize psychological trauma and other deleterious impacts.*

As knowledge builds, human resources will be more available to help other psychologists, first-line responders, caregivers, families, and children who are impacted by this trauma now and in future pandemics. These new resources are being tracked, archived, and disseminated by members of the Task Force. Collectively, Task Force members working in one or more work groups continue to meet regularly to create new resources and amalgamate existing ones. These relevant resources include reading and reference materials, video productions, and links to services and training. The Task Force members disseminate their resources to other partner divisions and organizations through regularly scheduled meetings, roundtables, webinars, social media, blogs, APA presentations, and print.

This book will describe how a group of about 100 psychologists, many of whom did not know each other before, answered a call to join a proposed Task Force to help other mental health professionals deal with the new COVID-19 pandemic. As cascading waves of pandemics, known as "syndemics," continued to present new issues, we quickly came to understand that we needed to find new methods and collaborations. We also understood that we were learning as we were going and that documentation would help future mental health professionals deal with such complex traumatic issues that unfold over lengthy periods of time.

In April of 2020, just 2 weeks before the pandemic started to shut down the entire USA and the world, the Task Force held its first meeting. Charles Figley was invited to lead the Task Force. Soon after, colleagues from all over the world came together online. We were all eager to do something to help and quickly found collaborative soulmates among those who joined the Task Force in its early weeks. Creativity and resilience abounded even though there was uncertainty about everything in our lives. No one knew what the virus really was, except that it was causing serious illness and death to large numbers of people daily.

Led initially by trauma psychologists, the Task Force membership grew, as did its diversity. Within the first month psychologists from 13 other APA specialty divisions joined together with the trauma psychologists to explore new ways to help ourselves, other mental health professionals, and the general public cope with this pandemic. We began to meet weekly as a Task Force and formed working groups to disseminate information as quickly as we could learn it. Weekly attendance varied, but core Task Force members remained and provided a sense of support and collaboration for the rest. Divisional support, as noted in Appendix A, remained strong, and the number of divisions supporting the Task Force grew steadily to 14, led by Division 56 (Psychological Trauma). New divisions continued to join, the most recent being Division 35, The Society for Women, which joined when the news broadcasts told of the devastation to the careers women had fought so hard to achieve.

Who Are We and Why Did We Join the TF?

You will learn more about the different members of each working group in the subsequent chapters. But, here let us tell you a little about why some said they joined together, how it impacted them, and what they learned. We asked Task Force members to tell us this in their own words:

1. **What were your first thoughts when you decided to join the COVID Interdisciplinary Task Force?**

   Opportunity to make a difference, join colleagues in meaningful work to tackle the impact, and do something in a frustrating situation that is impacting the world.

   My family lives all over the world (Ireland, Germany, UK, Dubai, Canada, Florida) and I live in Puerto Rico. I supervise an online campus of more than 12 programs in psychology and related health fields. Maintaining personal and professional connections, keeping up with regional and international news, and going between the personal and professional perspectives on the issues is quite the challenge.

   The pandemic has had a significant impact on children's lives, and I wanted to bring more attention to them as a group. Although they are not as likely to suffer health consequences, they are more vulnerable to long-lasting mental health effects given the increased risk of maltreatment, seclusion, and lost educational opportunities.

   As the Arizona Psychological Association's disaster resource network chair, I knew it was my responsibility to participate in this Task Force to ensure that our state professional organization was participating in and receiving the most up-to-date information on the pandemic. I joined in April.

   I joined the Task Force in mid-August 2020. As an early-career researcher, my initial thoughts about the Interdisciplinary Task Force were that of hope and excitement that my colleagues were taking leadership and initiative on this key issue affecting us all, and, as a former analyst trainee at an international organization on matters of public mental health after technological disasters, I felt a sense of purpose that my unique training, interdisciplinary expertise, or contribution(s) might be prove useful in some way to the team.

   I joined in maybe May 2020, and my hope was to contribute based on my work with APA Practice on treatment and assessment guidelines for patients and for healthcare workers that APA Practice published.

   I wanted to find a way to help and contribute however I could. Part of my professional life is working with healthcare facilities, including nursing homes, helping with staff training, and my partner works in healthcare policy for older adults in nursing homes and assisted living facilities, so I was acutely aware of the trauma occurring.

My initial thoughts when joining in May were what a wonderful opportunity to try and positively contribute to the efforts to aid in these global public health and psychological health crises.

I was thinking that COVID presents a unique opportunity for psychologists to lend their expertise given the current and projected trauma and mental duress impact it has on both clinicians as well as patients. Joining the COVID ID Task Force was an excellent way to brainstorm how best to address this problem.

2. **Did it meet your expectations?**

The Task Force has exceeded my expectations in terms of meeting colleagues nationally and internationally with expertise on trauma and social justice.

It exceeded my expectations. Not only did this group produce valuable projects, but it also provided friendship, understanding, and support during a time of uncertainty and high emotions. Unexpected was the high level of collegiality, openness, and collaboration among members. Also unexpected was the respect and sharing among divisions and age groups.

It has been so helpful to be part of this wonderful and caring community of psychologists. Together we've grappled with this new normal and supported one another. While in some ways I'd hoped we could do more, it has been good to provide support to others in the professional collaborative drop-in groups. I'm just sorry that more people consistently didn't take advantage of the drop-in groups. It's not clear to me that it's due to their not being a need. Some facilitators have even dropped out due to difficulty setting aside times when no one shows. It seems that with the increase in COVID the numbers may be increasing again. Overall, the camaraderie of the TF is greatly appreciated.

This experience more than met my expectations. Through sharing experiences and hearing about the trials and tribulations that people experienced throughout the USA and around the world, the idea of forming an interdivisional Task Force became a very serious mission.

3. **Did you develop new relationships working on the Task Force and subgroups?**

In my time as a graduate student researching the process of radiation disaster recovery in Japan, I came across the construct of intolerance of uncertainty, recently tagged as a possible transdiagnostic indicator of anxiety, which I originally read was a variable to look out for in lessons on the H1N1 outbreak. My research on theories of anxiety since then have continued to rate it highly as a useful source of hypothesis formation. I have learned that our current pandemic bears similarities to former pandemics, and if a new one should come, we might be able to leverage the lessons of history (especially as it relates to the evergreen problem of uncertainty) and our experiences to generate resilience in our institutions, namely, with a list of clear risk factors and mental health and psychosocial support programs that have demonstrated usefulness and fidelity in implementation. As an outcome of the Task Force, I feel this could continue to take the form of identifying and clarifying the profiles and risk factors of those who become psychologically vulnerable under these circumstances and programs that provided observable benefits despite the duress of constraint satisfaction.

Most defiinitely there were benefits. I was recently speaking with my family about how I'm less in touch with friends outside the field these days given the not socializing. And yet I don't feel deprived. I attribute it to my new friends on this TF.

There is not one individual who hasn't been affected by this pandemic. Everyone has been having difficulties dealing with emotional reactions and physical "space." This is natural and "normal." It is important to be aware and accepting of our negative reactions and difficulties and to be open in admitting these difficulties, and to discussing them. It is important for individuals – especially those who live on their own to reach out to family, friends, and neighbors both to aid and to request help when needed. Therapists should be open to admitting and discussing that worldwide – this is unknown situation, and that there are no prescribed answers. We are learning more as we cope with the unknown. As therapists, we have to be flexible in responding to those reaching out to us. If we are unable to help with their requests, we should make every effort to help the requester get to the appropriate "address." We have to be open to admitting when we don't know the answers and to be able to work together, learning how to deal with these situations.

It was reassuring and validating to meet clinicians who had the same concerns and interests. It is wonderful to work with our group of committed members who are intelligent and good team workers.

The relationships that were developed as part of professional support for psychologists WG have been an unexpected outcome. As a group, we have hosted Clinician Support Collaborative meetings in which mental health clinicians come together and provide mutual support. Ironically, it seems that there has been a parallel process of mutual support within our working group which has been an unexpected outcome.

4. **What have you learned so far should we have a new pandemic at some point in your life?**

   Our communities have very different ways of reacting and responding, based on different ways of communicating and problem-solving. Those who do not feel that their voices are heard or understood can sabotage an entire public health plan. They need to be more informed and involved. Transparency and buy-in are essential in public health plans.

   We need to start early and most importantly, the power of prevention. We have a very reactive response to crises – we could be better prepared for future crises with more of a prevention mindset.

   The importance of being proactive professionally, personally, and politically in advocating for others without a voice and the importance of honest and clear communication on all level of society. The field of psychology needs to be more proactive politically in terms of the impact of misinformation, healthcare disparities, racism, and prejudice.

We could cope with any pandemic as long as we have the will and make the collaborative efforts, with meaning in and of life.

Yes, because pandemics are not immediately considered as a potential disaster scenario, more time spent preparing would alleviate a lot of issues.

Unexpectedly, through the shared resources and updates, my eyes were opened to sources of entire research programs and ongoing projects to address issues being experienced by the disenfranchised. Especially with regard to the possible effects of the pandemic on the homeless and minority groups, I began to see the mission of the Task Force as awareness-raising in this light. I was also newly informed about implementation science efforts like "Battle Buddies," a peer support program for veterans, which struck me in my review of the shared documents as a worthy approach that has gone underreported in my spheres, especially in Japan.

In my time as a graduate student researching the process of radiation disaster recovery in Japan, I came across the construct of intolerance of uncertainty. This was recently tagged as a possible transdiagnostic indicator of anxiety. Anxiety, we learned, was a variable to look out for in lessons on the H1N1 outbreak. My research on theories of anxiety since then have continued to rate it highly as a useful source of hypothesis formation. I have learned that our current pandemic bears similarities to former pandemics, and if a new one should come, we might be able to leverage the lessons of history (especially as it relates to the evergreen problem of uncertainty) and our experiences to generate resilience in our institutions, namely, with a list of clear risk factors and mental health and psychosocial support programs that have demonstrated usefulness and fidelity in implementation. As an outcome of the Task Force, I feel this could continue to take the form of identifying and clarifying the profiles and risk factors of those who become psychologically vulnerable under these circumstances and programs that provided observable benefits despite the duress of constraint satisfaction.

I think that the work of the Task Force shows that barriers in the form of "within" as opposed to "across" discipline thinking can be overcome with passionate and strategic organization and networking demonstrated by our peers in their response to this pandemic, and a willingness to communicate and espouse a reflective attitude for those on the receiving and feedback end. It is this open attitude to consider work and camaraderie, demonstrated by this effort, that indicates to me that we might be able to overcome the "guild" barrier, or ivory tower(s), that sometimes comes to typify academic dilettantism, when we opt not for an organization of ignorance that says and justifies "this is for another division" but an organization of ways to identify and address our shared ignorance by saying, "this is a key point in the coalition of all divisions."

Getting to know so many great folks, the chance to disseminate my practice's "tips" for COVID sheets, and learning about so many things from the international perspective.

Flexibility and resiliency are key, as are helping however and wherever you can.

Thinking outside of the box and not just doing things the same way.

I've learned about the importance of communal help when coping with stress, trauma, and tragedy. It is something that has been striking for many communities of faith recently as they can't physically congregate the way they did. But from the experience with the TF work, this pandemic, one thing is clear: When events like this occur one can't go it alone. It is important to reach out particularly to those more isolated. It's something that those who've attended the clinician collaborative groups have spoken about.

It's important to document, which we hope a book from the group can provide. We are clearly not the first generation to live through a pandemic and yet from researching the 1918 one, there was so little documentation and hence so little memory of it. We are now affected by that lack of memory or awareness. It's as if we are living through something unprecedented, a word commonly used, and yet it was precedented. A little over 100 years ago. When reading some of the personal reports, as some of those exist, it uncannily sounds like reports that might have been written now.

I believe our Interdisciplinary Task Force is an important support for this group. The section that is open to practitioners has been doing outreach to therapists throughout the world. This group should be widened and strengthened. A directory of therapists who would be willing to give support through Zoom, WhatsApp, and Google Groups could be made available online. It is important to indicate that this is a support effort and not supervision – because of insurance and liability problems.

The importance of collaboration, organizing effectively, and not duplicating efforts to preserve resources. We strongly need more supports for families working without childcare who have young children. Babies and toddlers do not just easily get on a zoom.

5. **In what ways were you personally impacted by COVID?**

Complete change in my professional and personal life due to the lack of travel (I usually traveled once a month, in the USA and internationally). My whole schedule and engagement with colleagues and family was disrupted.

My colleagues were quite sick – most were not hospitalized but they were out sick for 10–14 days and severely ill. I was afraid that they might die and realized how fragile life is and how important relationships and connections are. My desire to get involved in the impact on mental health increased with the experience.

One extremely close member has since recovered. However, another very close friend is currently hospitalized (trying to remain optimistic). Akin to an earthquake, it feels like the ground crumbling beneath your feet.

During COVID I had 22 deaths, including my Mother at 97, only 5 from COVID.

Among my clients, the pandemic hit many hard, especially those who had previous traumas that were impacted by the isolation, political aggression, or intensification of their family issues. It was sometimes hard to keep my own balance, especially holding the emotions of clients and family members. After the recent election, the extent of relief I felt showed me how much stress I was carrying for myself and others.

My work had taken me to China and other countries. Having to work starting in February on Zoom with Chinese in lock-down taught me a great deal about human similarities and cultural difference and helped us all share common experiences.

I was ill and unable to work for almost 2 weeks, although the case would be considered mild since I had no lung involvement. I had a wretched fever, a terrible headache, and could not sleep. The nights were the worst, with not just discomfort and pain, but chills and sweats, and cognitions of despair. The nights feel remarkably isolating and very (severely) depressing. As I listened to my thoughts, I was shocked at my level of despair and emptiness. I related it to CNS inflammation likely causing the headaches.

Several friends and colleagues have contracted the illness as well as my 92-year-old mother living in South Africa. Most of my younger colleagues as well as several students contracted the virus and recuperated easily. Several friends of my vintage (age) died from COVID-19. My 92-year-old mother was on oxygen for 6 weeks in the hospital in South Africa, miraculously survived, and with her dementia does not remember that she was ill. It was difficult to be so far away from my mother when she contracted the virus; however the whole country in South Africa was in lockdown then as well as her assisted living facility being closed to family making it impossible to have seen her even if I was there.

While it has been scary to know others who have tested positive, my main focus remains maintaining the health of my elderly parents and husband who has a sensitive immune system. It has at times been a challenge, maintaining the things that I find fulfilling and worrying about those around me. It has been a challenge to be unable to go visit my 98-year-old grandmother due to the pandemic. It remains a challenge, given how integral my family is to my life.

6. **Were there other experiences with COVID that impacted your life?**

Concerns about misinformation and differences of opinion around risk, spread, and civic duty vs *civil liberties.*

As with many Americans, it has impacted my professional plans (work) and personal life. But I am grateful and humbled by those who have lost so much.

It left me with a keen appreciation of how invalidating using approaches like mindfulness would seem to patients. I am skilled at mindfulness and CBT, and I was overwhelmed. It left me convinced and empathy and a sense of connection to another would be more useful than any CBT technique. When a colleague sent me a fruit basket and reached out, it did more for my mood and adjustment than any effort at relaxation or mindful attention redeployment.

Having a 2-year-old whose daycare closed temporarily, luckily, while having two working parents was eye-opening, as many of my students (I am a full-time lecturer at a community college) work, go to school full-time, and have childcare duties. COVID also forced me to slow down, not having to commute as much (I was on the road for 15 hours a week on average) and allowed me to spend more time with my daughter.

My daughter was to be married to her British fiancé in June. They have yet to have their real wedding, although after much effort he is now in the USA. I've had to reduce my visits to my elderly father (age 96) and constantly weigh the benefits of human contact and our visits with the very real risks to him. My physician husband goes every day to the hospital. While he's not on the very frontline, it poses a risk to us, which for the most part we try to ignore.

As I mentioned, being over 80, the Israeli government restricted this age group (in particular to lockdown: to remain at home, to go no more than 100 meters from one's home, to avoid shopping, not to socialize). Volunteers would call, having been informed of my age, asking me how they could help, without even asking if I need help and – what help I might need. As a physically active person who drives a car, does Pilates with a trainer three times a week, walks between 5000 and 1000 steps away, and meets friends for coffee, lunch, and dinner, this was a very constricting situation – especially when adding the fear of becoming effected with COVID-19. I was glued to the TV and became concerned as to what I might endure should I become infected with COVID. I decide to leave instructions regarding my medical treatment should I be infected and not able to consent to or refuse treatment. I meet with my physician and fill out a detailed list of medical instructions including do not resuscitate, requested my son and a friend to accept power of attorney should I be in a state that I was unable to indicate my requirements for treatment. These forms have been filed with the Israel Ministry of Health. Should I be hospitalized, these forms will be made available to any place I would be hospitalized, so that my wishes for treatment or its suspension will be honored. Having done this resulted in a feeling of relief and control. I began exercising with two zoom groups at least once and often twice a day. I took my dog out for walks 3–4 times daily, and was able to meet and converse with other dog walkers (socially distancing and with masks). I continued to do grocery shopping. I joined zoom webinars and lectures, discussions, and meetings. I have returned to my individual Pilates sessions and meet with friends for takeout meals and coffee. As the lockdown has been lifted, a significant part of my weekly activities is participating in the Task Force meetings.

I have been without childcare for about 5 months of the pandemic. I have a newly turned 3-year-old and a baby. This has been really, really challenging. I have been really dismayed and disappointed by the general lack of support for women without childcare (not in the Task Force). My husband and I have experienced significant salary cuts but are fortunate to have jobs.

This is probably universal – I have been working virtually for almost a year. That has caused to dial in to the affective/interpersonal aspects of the work even more.

On the personal side, I walk miles every day as a way to feel alive and present.

I was on a round the world journey starting in December 2019 visiting several Asian countries and expecting to travel for a full year within Africa, the Middle East, and Europe. I was stationed in South Africa from January 2020, on a Fulbright Senior Scholar award to develop a dance therapy program at the University of the Witwatersrand and expecting to be there for 6 months. Within

2 days in mid-March 2020, all the Fulbright scholars worldwide were recalled, the South African government closed the border and withdrew all visas, and we unexpectedly found ourselves back in the USA where we have been pretty much socially isolating since that time.

The pandemic and resulting syndemic series of events have created a roller coaster of diversity, equity, and inclusion (DEI) and US political disturbances of horrendous proportion. I remain in close contact with family, friends, and colleagues around the world, and the worldwide impact of all this is profound. As a creative arts therapist and educator I feel that our skills and contributions have never been more important than now – as we move through this pandemic and learn to deal with the present as well as the aftermath.

The Challenge: Figuring Out What We Could Do

Shortly after its formation, the Task Force began to focus on areas requiring attention, and leaders quickly volunteered to lead break-out groups called "work groups" which permitted trauma specialists to join in smaller numbers with a more specific focus in an important area of their choice. The weekly meetings of the larger Task Force provided a home base for all its members to check in and share their findings. The real work happened within the work groups. Each of them focused on their areas of interest including special populations of service providers and recipients. Over the summer it became obvious that each member of each group had stories to tell. We needed a book to help frame the stories about members' particular experiences. At the same time, the larger group was needed to share these experiences and develop ways to publicize our work through a variety of channels. The supportive tone in these meetings stimulated more creativity and innovation that then was transferred to those working in the smaller groups. Some of the groups also collaborated with each other, producing original joint projects such as the Intimate Partner Violence group with the International Whole Person group while others invited other members to join, such as the Hospital Workers and Addictions group, adding new perspectives to their work. Thus, the stories in this book document the organic nature of our formation.

First the pandemic affected the elderly, but then it started to infect younger, healthier people, and fear gripped the world. Who would be next? Was transmission airborne, or just from direct contact? Would wearing masks help? People started fearing closeness and being touched by others. Distrust of each other and the government grew. Everyone was forced to stay indoors, businesses were shuttered, and children sent home from school. Technology, in the form of a computer or smart phone in every home, became essential to communicate with others. Instructions on how to deal with the pandemic were inconsistent, causing more fear and uncertainty. Psychological care was critically necessary for the healthy as well as the vulnerable. But we could no longer deliver our services in the usual way: face-to-face with our patients. We all had to learn to become more computer savvy and use telehealth or other digital therapeutics while remaining at home and not in the office. One of the unique features about this book's development is the easy collaboration of students together with long-term practitioners working to add their expertise to the work. For example, students were the experts who taught the experienced clinicians how to deliver services using new technology, while the more experienced clinicians taught the students tips on mental health treatment. Rarely do we find this lack of hierarchical relationships except in crisis situations.

Each chapter was written by one or more Task Force members well-oriented to the focus and interconnections among the other group members. Most focus on populations, especially since the pandemic impact was so different on, for example, vibrant older adults than those in blue-collar jobs. Each chapter covers different perspectives on that population, integrating research studies, clinical approaches, and personal experiences. They all deal with trauma across different cultures internationally although one of the work groups does focus exclusively on diverse approaches to working with trauma, and some of the members cross cultures internationally. Bringing multiple perspectives to problems – as well as the breadth of populations and cultures covered – became a strength of our approach and, we think, one of the strengths of this book. At the same time, the book provides good clinical material for students in graduate programs. The suggestions for practice focus not only on the welfare of the recipients of mental health services, but also and especially on the professionals who deliver these services. It became clear that professionals and students were themselves highly stressed and in need of self-care. The Task Force also functioned as an important support group for members and a credible model for self-care. One of the work groups focuses on the underserved population of graduate students, for example, some of whom went through traumas connected with political, immigration, and family issues, as well as the new educational challenges. The current list of chapters emerged from those early days.

Chapter Content

Chapter 2, *Lessons Learned from the 1918 "Forgotten Flu,"* is about learning from history to help us prepare for inevitable future pandemics. Focusing on the 1918 pandemic, the authors consider the history, similarities, and differences between the two pandemics. They reflect on these differences and ask what lessons can be learned. One major lesson learned is that we need to *apply our new understandings of the role of trauma in a pandemic* and discover what approaches can reduce suffering. We want to remember and to mourn to avoid repeating mistakes.

We now turn to Chap. 3, *The COVID Interpersonal Violence (IPV) Work Group.* They note, among other things that interpersonal violence, especially domestic violence, increased at least three times during the first 2 years into the pandemic. Most psychologists were not trained to work with battered women and other trauma victim/survivors. In this chapter we describe some of the innovative ways we provided the necessary support and taught new skills using social media.

In Chap. 4, *Parenting During a Pandemic: Challenges and Lessons Learned from the Children and Families Workgroup*, the work group's overarching aim is to help support children, caregivers, and families who have been impacted by the COVID-19 pandemic, as well as professionals working with these groups. This chapter described their collective efforts to aid children, caregivers, families, and professionals working with children and families during the pandemic, including dissemination of resources.

In Chap. 5, *Vibrant Older Adults* (VOAWG), the group has focused on the experiences of active older adults, whom we termed *vibrant older adults*, during the COVID-19 pandemic. The VOAWG group had an additional focus of exploring of the impact of the trauma of the Holocaust on the reactions of Holocaust survivors. The chapter concludes with insights and actionable suggestions gleaned from the different interventions and offers a public health perspective for continued coping with the uncertainty associated with waves of the pandemic, better preparedness for future crises, and improved services for active older adults during the pandemic and beyond.

In Chap. 6, *The Hospital, Health and Addiction Workers, Patients and Families Working Group*, the mission of the work group is to reduce and, when possible, prevent COVID-19-related psychological trauma and to facilitate developing resiliency and post-traumatic growth by focusing on an extraordinary range of clinical issues especially for hospital staff and patients. Through reflections, this chapter highlights four major areas of the members' clinical work, including trauma, international and national leadership roles, the national impact of the pandemic and policy implications for at-risk populations, and dissemination of clinical interventions.

Chapter 7, *Supporting Mental Health Clinicians in Navigating Pandemic-Related Challenges Through the Professional Support for Psychologists Working Group*, focuses on us as practitioners with a need for personal and interpersonal understanding and support. Therefore, the APA COVID-19 Interdivisional Task Force established a work group dedicated to providing professional support to mental health clinicians with symptoms that include compassion fatigue/burnout, isolation, managing boundaries, and work-related concerns.

In Chap. 8, *International Somatic and Creative Arts Whole Person Approaches Working Group*, the members of this group are psychologists, artists, clinicians, researchers, and scientists. Together, this group has focused on experiential and practical ways of supporting grief and trauma recovery in the face of the pandemic. These methodologies can become models for future Tool Kits that could be sustainable for future pandemics or emergencies.

Chapter 9, *The Higher Education Working Group*, provides an inspirational overview of student concerns during this dynamic and stressful period. The group is composed of student leaders in psychology graduate programs across the world, dedicated to building on the strengths and resiliency of the student and trainee community, and to provide resources and support during and following the COVID-19 pandemic.

Chapter 10, *Telepsychology and Digital Technologies During COVID* The pandemic with its stay-at-home mandates fostered the growth of a new model for psychological assessment, diagnosis, and psychotherapy that was conducted totally on the Internet using a variety of digital platforms including audio and video adapted for telepsychology. This chapter discusses some history of telepsychology prior to the pandemic and describes modifications to laws, rules, and regulations and ethical practice to accommodate the digital practice.

In Chap. 11, *International Advancements on Covid-19 Scholarship: Research Initiatives Working Group*, the mission statement of the group is to compile a collection of the currently available knowledge base on the psychological impact of COVID-19 from a multidisciplinary and international perspective. The goal is to inform students, researchers, policymakers, practitioners, stakeholders, professionals, and relevant scholarship on the multidimensional impact of COVID-19 and related psychological treatment, prevention, and intervention resources.

Why Write This Book Now?

Although we are not yet out of the pandemic, we have a sense of urgency and do not want to wait until it's over to relay what we've learned. Most agree that, as of this writing, we are into a third wave with openings and lockdowns continuing to occur as different countries try to avert even more devastation. We don't want to lose what has been successful, what worked, and why, as happened after the 1918 influenza pandemic. We also understand that we may never go back to the "old normal"; many of these changes will continue. In addition, variants of the virus will still be present, and we will face new crises. How can we prepare for these unknowns?

We think the best way to prepare for the future is to document this historic phase as researched and experienced by professionals who, in turn, share *the resources necessary for other pandemic providers to deliver excellent and targeted mental health services.* To achieve this purpose, the book includes the above-cited chapters written by and for pandemic practitioners about their clinical population of clients. The reader will be guided by a set of clinical guidelines and case notes specific to their practice population, and useful to both practitioner professionals and their clients. *Matched to the particular population's circumstances and requirements*, the resources include addressing, measuring, managing, and monitoring psychological trauma.

The Focus on Practitioners

The editors agree that this book focuses on best practices in organizing and carrying out emergency human services for a population of people in critical need. These critical best practices are a feature of all work groups, and by extension the chapters contained herein. From the beginning we elected to focus on *providers of mental health services* and these providers' policies and practices during the pandemic. This includes licensed mental health practitioners, but also psychology students and trainees and others in direct practice, teaching practitioners, scholar educators, and/or supervisors. In focusing on many kinds of mental health service providers, each work group had broad access to various professional groups and their resources. We understood that crisis necessitated getting out of our own professional siloes and working cooperatively across disciplines.

The book is by and for practitioners *not only* in the USA, but also throughout the world. To our surprise, many international colleagues joined our work groups as the pandemic dragged on, collecting other crises, including racial tension, political upheaval, and climate change disruptions not limited to the USA.

We editors hope that the book will be useful to professionals at all levels of training, including undergraduate, graduate, and continuing education. We also see it as useful for healthcare policymakers so that they may provide trauma-informed services for whenever another pandemic may occur. We hope that the lessons learned and resources gathered during the pandemic will help future generations face and cope with traumas arising from future pandemics.

Author Note The authors thank the American Psychological Association's Interdivisional Task Force on the Pandemic for the framework, divisional collaboration, and extraordinary membership that made this book possible.

Chapter 2
Lessons Learned from the 1918 "Forgotten Flu"

Judith L. Alpert, Arlene (Lu) Steinberg, and Benjamin A. Laddis

Introduction

As we write this chapter, COVID continues to afflict. It is our third year living in a world with COVID. While vaccines and boosters exist, they are not available to everyone. In addition, not everyone wants them. These are tough times. Many of us are sad, lonely, isolated, grief-stricken, and frightened. There have been other pandemics in the past. We can learn from them.

One of these pandemics is the 1918 pandemic, called "the forgotten flu" (Crosby, 1989). We believe that it was not actually forgotten. We think that it was too painful to remember and was therefore, dissociated, cut off from our awareness and memory. Dissociation is an understandable collective or cultural coping mechanism that helps us deal with the unimaginable death and horror of a devastating trauma. Therefore, a decision is sometimes made at the unconscious level, by both individuals and society, to forget the painful memories. We believe that the feelings of helplessness, pain, suffering, loneliness, and other unbearable emotional reactions resulting from the 1918 pandemic were replaced with manic exuberance as the Roaring Twenties followed the 1918 flu. Manic exuberance (for ex., excessive entertainment, additions) is another coping mechanism people sometimes use to deny pain. We believe that the memories of loss and loneliness from the 1918

J. L. Alpert (✉)
Department of Applied Psychology, New York University and Postdoctoral Program in Psychoanalysis and Psychotherapy, New York University, New York, NY, USA
e-mail: judie.alpert@nyu.edu

A. Steinberg
Ferkauf Graduate School, Yeshiva University, New York, NY, USA

B. A. Laddis
Tufts University, Medford, MA, USA
e-mail: Benjamin.laddis@tufts.edu

C. R. Figley et al. (eds.), *Pandemic Providers*,
https://doi.org/10.1007/978-3-031-27580-7_2

pandemic were not really forgotten. While they were never spoken about, they lived on.

There is one significant difference between the 1918 flu and the present pandemic. We now have a developed understanding of trauma. We understand the emotional impact of the devastation resulting from pandemics. We know it is important to acknowledge trauma, grieve both invisible and visible losses caused by the flu, and tell and re-tell our pandemic stories. We know that trauma impacts people differently and that certain populations are especially vulnerable. We know that trauma involves shame and stigmatization, issues surrounding racial disparity, tragic economic consequences, as well as other shattering losses. We can anticipate and recognize psychological expressions of trauma, including anxiety and depression, domestic violence, and addictions. We know that trauma impacts people differently and that certain populations are especially vulnerable. We want to bear full witness to the gravity and meaning of catastrophic trauma. Given this, we encourage the development of memorials in order to remember, and monuments in order to provide places to grieve and rituals in order to continue to remember.

Trauma brings loss. Grieving, while difficult to do, plays an important role in healing after loss. It frees up energy and enables us, in time, to reinvest the energy and emotional reserve. If we don't grieve, we remain tied to the past. We must reclaim the ability to feel the full range of emotions. Grief is what we think and feel on the inside and includes panic, pain, emptiness, fear, and loneliness. It is the internal meaning we give to the experience of loss. Mourning, on the other hand, is the outward expression of our grief. If it is delayed or incomplete, there is a missing presence of what had been transpired and endured. It means that we have not fully witnessed the gravity and meaning of the trauma. Only through mourning can we rediscover our inner life and go on. Stories of catastrophic trauma need to be told, as they have the capacity to regulate, modulate, organize, soothe, and ultimately make meaning of the experience (Alpert, 2015; Grand & Salberg, 2016; Steinberg, 2014). Humans need a narrative. Stories must be told as they can serve an important function in active mourning and mourning helps us remember and integrate trauma as well as learn from it. We do not want the present pandemic to be the next forgotten flu.

Grieving is essential to process the emotional impact of trauma, yet the need to grieve often clashes with the terror of appearing pathetic or weak. Emotions from the conflict press for representation. Incomplete grief results in denouncing tender feelings. Unshed tears ead to eyes closing and inability to see, integrate, and learn from the past or impact the future. There was so much trauma to confront after the 1918 pandemic ended. World War I, causing 40 million deaths and casualties, ended about 8 months (November 1918) after the pandemic dissipated. The subsequent events, including the Russian Revolution, the Great Depression, and WWII, all needed psychological processing. There was simply too much to process and little time to do this psychological work.

There is much work to be done now, at and following COVID. We need to identify the mental health and physical disparities among groups of people with respect to service delivery, and we need to find better ways to reach people. There needs to be mass recognition. There needs to be societal mourning of the trauma caused by COVID. This book provides one way to help remember, memorialize, and address the psychological impact of COVID. Each of the chapters in the book suggests ways that grieving, mourning, loneliness, fear, and anguish may be conceptualized, confronted, and contained, and specific populations that COVID affected. We share what we are learning from this COVID pandemic that might help people cope with the psychological effects of COVID.

By means of this volume, the Interdivisional Task Force on the Pandemic, under Charles Figley's leadership, provides resources and support to children, families, students, older adults and their caregivers, hospital workers, other healthcare and essential workers, and mental health professionals. By creatively addressing the needs of these vulnerable groups and providing resources and support to caregivers and healthcare workers and then documenting it in the form of a book, future generations of mental health professionals will have a resource for the next pandemic. Thus, the existence of this volume provides some promise that COVID-19 will not be forgotten. In this chapter there will be additional consideration about how we can work to keep the memory of the present pandemic alive on a cultural level.

Comparison of 1918 Flu and COVID-19

We understood the need to document our challenges faced and lessons learned from COVID, especially in light of the fact that so little information about the 1918 pandemic had been volunteered or memorialized. The father of one of the authors, for example, grew up in Boston, among the cities hit hardest by the 1918 pandemic. Boston was also one of the last cities to close its schools. Judie Alpert's father was 14 years old in 1918, and most likely among the school children who would stand in the streets and watch the child-size caskets being transported. Yet he, like many others, never spoke about the pandemic to anyone. Interestingly, there is a striking contrast between the lack of rituals, memorials, and monuments from the 1918 flu with other catastrophic traumas. For example, the 9/11 terrorist attacks resulted in the death of 3000 people. There were numerous containers for the 9–11 terrorist events, including memorials, museums, and annual rituals. On the other hand, the 1918 pandemic that infected about one-third of the world population (500 million people) and killed 675,000 Americans and 50 million people worldwide was not memorialized.

We wanted to learn more about what was told to generations that followed the 1918 pandemic. Therefore, we posted a simple request on several mental health professional list serves. The request was: "Please let us know what you were told about the 1918 pandemic." While many people wrote that they had never heard of it, we did receive some responses that reveal a colossal impact from one of the world's deadliest disease outbreaks. Some of the comments we heard are written verbatim throughout this chapter, with disguised names (use of initials) and deletion of some extraneous details.

We also want to provide a context for our history of the 1918 pandemic by first considering the state of medicine and mental health around that time. We consider some of the political and health inequities and racial issues from 1918, and then again during COVID. We look at other similarities and differences between the 1918 pandemic and COVID, and end by emphasizing the importance of addressing the psychological issues from Covid.

As with the present pandemic, the severity of impact of the 1918 pandemic varied by location and time, also varying by state, country, and phase of illness. However, no place was exempt from exposure. For example, about a century ago, influenza struck sailors aboard a ship in Boston's Commonwealth Pier and spread quickly to nearby naval installations and shipyards. By mid-September, it had infected over 20,0000 sailors stationed in the Boston area, and a make-shift hospital-tent had to be erected for the growing number of influenza patients. In time, more temporary emergency hospitals were constructed. Despite attempts to contain the 1918 flu, it spread rapidly to the civilian population, with thousands of cases and many deaths; at the same time there were few medical personnel available due to their engagement in military service. To combat influenza, within 2 months public gatherings were limited and many public places such as saloons, bowling alleys, and theaters were closed. People were urged to avoid unnecessary travel. When it appeared that the peak of the epidemic had passed, Boston's closure orders were removed, and Bostonians flocked to theaters, cafes, and hotels in search of release and relief. Not surprisingly, the number of cases and deaths again rose. The epidemic lasted for several years. Various agencies were blamed for the increases in deaths and illness. In the end, Boston was one of the worst hit cities in the USA; the death rate was over 710 per 1000,000 residents (Barry, 2004; Crosby, 1989).

The flu can be very dangerous, as Bill Gates reported. In a 2015 TED talk, he warned that if anything were to kill over ten million people over the next decade, it would most likely be the influenza virus. After reviewing the damage from Ebola and the 1918 pandemic as well as other epidemics, Gates noted that the USA was concentrating on the wrong killer, focusing on missiles rather than microbes. He went further and recommended some broad areas to help prepare for the next epidemic, such as building strong health systems in poor countries and developing medical response corps. He also recommended simulations and advanced R and D that focus on vaccines and diagnostics. Yet his warning and recommendations were not heeded. Why not? Perhaps it was because the 1918 pandemic was not processed adequately. It is our belief that the 1918 pandemic was not sufficiently encoded in societal memory, resulting in collective dissociation. Clearly, society needed to forget before it could remember.

Another parallel between the former pandemic and the present one includes a failure at the macro level to prevent, control, or treat everyday illness. For example, in 1918 the government failed by putting money toward the war effort instead of toward public health. A similar case could be made for the present pandemic, during which time public health did not receive needed funds.

1918 Pandemic: The State of Medicine and Mental Health Treatment

The state of medicine was rudimentary prior to the twentieth century. There was little medical knowledge and doctors had limited training. They graduated from medical school without working in a laboratory, dissecting a cadaver, or seeing a patient. Fortunately, there were medical advances prior to the 1918 influenza epidemic. The use of quarantining and the understanding of contagion allowed for the use of measures similar to today's "social-distancing." Measures to control the 1918 influenza spread included closing borders, partitioning hospital wards, and closing schools and non-essential businesses. In fear of a meningitis or pneumonia outbreak, public health experts inspected camps, advised military officials to avoid overcrowding, and created partitioned wards for sick patients to isolate for 10–14 days. There were attempts to contact-trace and isolate potential exposures from the source. Gauze masks were introduced at the peak of the flu, and it did slow the spread of the virus. However, the infrastructure was not there to support it in 1918, and the gauze supply ran out shortly after distribution. In addition, many of the doctors were involved in military activity and therefore doctors were in short supply. And, of course, vaccines did not exist for influenza in 1918. Influenza proved too explosive to contain.

Once the outbreak spread to the public, some public health officials tried to warn people to avoid crowds. However, the public was misled by President Woodrow Wilson who wanted the focus to be on winning the war. He did not want distractions from this focus, and he suppressed the press (Barry, 2004). It soon became clear that the 1918 influenza was unlike anything seen before. Instead of killing the old and the weak, it disproportionately preyed on strong, healthy young adults. In Chicago, the deaths among those aged 20–40 were unprecedented: nearly five times as high as the deaths of those aged 41–60 (Barry, 2004). Scientists at the time recognized that disease tended to spread quickly during the winter months, when everyone huddled together for warmth. Medical experts urged generals to minimize overcrowding in barracks, encouraged better training of medical personnel, and attempted to publicize the need for social distancing. Yet those in positions of power did not prepare or educate the public adequately. In August 1918, many politicians and media outlets declared that the pandemic was over and underestimated its continued destructive capabilities. Unaware of the concept of mutation, these officials came to a rude awakening when the second wave came in full-force and proved more deadly than the first.

Like the state of medicine, the state of psychology in 1918 was in its infancy. When WW I broke out in 1914, it was a turning point for academic psychology in Germany. Psychologists helped make the German war effort more scientific, rational, and modern. For example, Max Wertheimer, who later became identified with Gestalt therapy, created a device to help soldiers locate enemy artillery over long distances. Research on combat motivation was being investigated as well. The focus of psychology and psychiatry in the USA and in England and France in 1918 was also war-related. In the USA those who worked in industry were useful to the military. Psychological testing was developed to help the military eliminate some vulnerable recruits. Aptitude tests were being used to select pilots, truck drivers, and other military specialists. Also, around this time, US psychologists were engaged in the IQ wars.

World War I first brought a new understanding of psychological trauma as a real event. As Herman (1992) reports, some soldiers, even those who had not been exposed to any physical trauma, began to act like "hysterical women." At that time, asylum doctors believed that mental illness was entirely hereditary and so neurologists were perplexed by what was called "shell shock" or combat neurosis. While some viewed the soldiers with this condition as "moral invalids," others were beginning to recognize it as a psychiatric condition which could occur even in soldiers who had good moral character. In any case, the goal of treatment was to return the soldier to combat. While the efficacy of the talking cure was recognized by a few at this time, it was only much later that the mental health field came to identify and use the diagnostic term "post-traumatic stress disorder" and even use the word "trauma" (Herman, 1992). Thus, at the time of the 1918 pandemic, there was little understanding of psychological trauma as a phenomenon, and without an appreciation of psychological trauma, it was difficult to encode its traumatic experience. Clearly, psychologists were not prepared to help people cope with the devastation brought on by the pandemic or the war. Given the two horrific events of the 1918 flu and World War I, people were dealing with death, social isolation, anxiety, loss, shutdowns, depression, job and income losses, family instability, parental stress, poverty, suicide, and breakdowns. Very young children and young adults were dying. Families were losing many children within a short period of time. And a war was waging. In addition to the general populace, healthcare professionals had to be suffering a great deal from, among other triggers, secondary traumatic stress or compassion fatigue (Figley, 2015). The psychological trauma had to be massive, as the following vignettes indicate.

> One side of our family had 18 children. Five children died within 2 years due to the 1918–1919 flu. I can only imagine the grief of the poor mother. This family lived in the northern suburbs. (LB)

> I had a great aunt and uncle who lost three children within a few months in 1918. (T.R.)

> My mother told me she was 8 years old and very ill with the Spanish Flu, almost died, no real treatment except symptomatic. Living in the Bronx, NY with her parents and two older brothers. She didn't speak of the child-sized coffins on the sidewalks that I have since heard of.

> My mother was quite young-9 years old. She had vivid memories of being led with classmates to line up on the sidewalk to watch a procession of little coffins go by on the street, her classmates. This was in Montclair, New Jersey. (E.B.)

> My grandfather came to America in 1917, at age 17 after Mount Etna erupted and destroyed his town of Santa Flavia, Sicily and the caponata factory where he was employed. He came

to America and opened a barber shop in East New York, Brooklyn. Shortly after opening it, the 1918 pandemic began. In those days, barbers acted as makeshift doctors, stitching up cuts and performing other medical procedures. My grandfather told us that as the pandemic began to claim more people, he was approached by the mayor's office and asked to store bodies in the back room of his barber shop since the morgues were full. He said the streets of Brooklyn were noticeably less crowded and became more and more empty as the pandemic progressed. (R.F)

Politics and Health Inequity and Racial Issues

There are a number of issues common to both epidemics that deserve consideration and have implications for future pandemics. We consider two below: (1) politics and (2) health inequity and racial issues.

The first important lesson from 1918 is the importance of telling the truth (Barry, 2004). In 1918 President Woodrow Wilson misled the public and did not tell the public how dangerous the flu was, nor did national or local government officials. One national public health leader, for example, referred to the 1918 flu as "ordinary influenza by another name" (Barry, 2004). Basically, the public was told that there was no cause for alarm, when of course there was. This deception not only resulted in the public distrusting Wilson, it also led to more deaths.

Why did the news media report falsely? The Sedition Act of 1918 was an Act of the United States Congress that covered a broad range of offenses, including speech that cast the government or the war effort in a negative light. The Act made it punishable by 20 years in jail to "utter print, write, or publish any disloyal, profane, scurrilous or abusive language about the government of the United States." After the Supreme Court ruled the sedition act constitutional, it determined that negative news could be interpreted as an offense that hurt morale (Barry, 2004). An example of the effect of this ruling is the case of Philadelphia's Liberty Loan parade. Medical experts urged that the parade be canceled. Likely due to concern based on pressure from Wilson's Sedition Act, the parade occurred as scheduled. Within 2 days of the parade, the incubation period of influenza, the city's hospitals had to turn away patients due to the influx of influenza cases. The death toll climbed exponentially every day. Five days after the parade, virtually all public institutions and gatherings were banned. If the public had been warned, the disastrous consequences of this "super-spreader event" could have been avoided.

During the present pandemic, the public was also deceived by President Trump and the right-wing media who minimized the seriousness of COVID. Although the President knew that the coronavirus was deadly and worse than the flu, as he later admitted to Bob Woodward in February 2021 (Woodward & Costa (2021), he nevertheless misled Americans. He said that COVID-19 would dissipate with the arrival of warmer weather, much like the seasonal flu. He continued to downplay the impact of the virus, stating that it was under control and would disappear, and that nothing should shut down. In January 2020, according to *The New York Times*, the national Security Council office responsible for tracking pandemics predicted the spread of the virus to the USA. At that time, Trump was advised to shut down large cities and suggest that American stay home from work. He had been warned that there could be as many as half a million deaths and trillions of dollars in economic losses. Instead of focusing on social distancing or staying at home measures, he focused on the economy and keeping the country open. After Dr. Deborah Birx, the Trump administration's coronavirus response coordinator, left the administration, she revealed what was actually happening. She told a congressional committee investigating the federal pandemic response that in the mid to late 2020, White House officials demanded that information be withheld and misinformation given. Also, the Trump White House did not release some documents which provided information about both the spread and containment of the virus (Weiland, 2022). Thus, in the present epidemic as in the 1918 pandemic, the government tried to create a belief that we were not dealing with a serious epidemic. What we know now is that, with early intervention, truth telling and the imposing of restrictions, there is less illness.

In both pandemics, trust in authority disintegrated along with the misinformation. People did not know who or what to believe, and trust between people eroded as well. Life as it had been prior to the flu changed. School, church, and social life were all different. People were afraid to kiss and hug. Human beings were viewed as dangerous to each other. Every person was a potential death threat to every other. People experienced isolation and alienation. They experienced death and dying. In both pandemics, there was massive anxiety, with misinformation only increasing that anxiety.

Stigmatization occurred in many ways to both pandemics as well. Both pandemics were named wrongly after a country. While many countries suppressed news of the 1918 flu, Spain, which remained neutral during WWI, was free to report in full detail. Since Spain was the country which first reported the existence of the flu, the incorrect assumption was that the pandemic began there. It did not. Similarly, COVID-19 has been called the "China Virus" and "Wuhan Virus." This name appears to have been given by government officials under the Trump administration. As a result, Asian-Americans and Asians around the world have been the object of attack and faced discrimination. Assigning blame feeds stigma and undermines empathy. It can also exacerbate the virus' impact, as stigmatized individuals may be afraid to report to hospitals to receive medical treatment. We now understand that blaming or stigmatizing is often a psychological response to a traumatic event. For example, there were overt acts of racism during and after 9/11 with both Muslims and Jews targeted (Alpert & Nguyen-Feng, 2020). Why does blame follow? Sometimes people unconsciously choose to express anger rather than fear, as anger is a more active response, leaving one with more of a feeling of being in control. It may be that "choosing" anger is a way of fighting back. It is easier to think about "us versus them" than to admit that the virus (or terrorist event) threatens all and cannot be controlled. In both pandemics, immigrants and those who had fewer resources suffered the most. There was clear inequality then as there is now. Those at greater risk were the poorest and most vulnerable, with the least access to healthcare and often living in crowded conditions.

The vignettes which follow illustrate some of these psychological issues and were the response from several division list serves when we asked for their stories. The initials of the story narrators follow each entry.

> My paternal grandfather died in the epidemic. Not much was said about it as my grandmother eventually remarried and was forbidden to talk about him. Certainly, there is a story, but I don't know it. I do know that my father was the youngest of four and he was six months old when his father died. My grandmother was very depressed. No money, four young children etc. They were evicted from their apartment when my father was in elementary school. Came home to find all the furniture in the street and his mother hysterically crying. That eviction shadowed my father until he died. When I was about 30 years old (and my father had died about seven years before), my father's first cousin told me that his mother (my grandmother) wanted to put the three youngest children in an orphanage as she didn't know how she would cope. The family somehow stopped her, but things were horrible. She was eventually set up with a widower and they lived a long, silent, loveless, quite barren life together. The fallout from that 1918 death was enormous. I think I felt it without knowing what it was for most of my childhood. (Z.S.)

> My grandfather came from Ireland at about age 20 in 1900. He married in 1908, and his wife died giving birth to their only son the next year. He re-married within a year, needing someone to care for the child. His second wife had four children. My father, the youngest, was born in August, 1918. His second wife died from the flu in November 1918. My grandfather, now with 5 children, sent a telegram to his late wife's sister in Ireland asking her to come with her youngest sister to help. She arrived within a few months, married him a year later and went on to have four children. Her sister lived with the family, never married and helped raise the family. My grandfather died in 1927 from a heart attack and the two women kept the family together. The urgency to remarry both times was driven by the fact that social service agencies looked very closely at immigrant families and would place children in orphanages. They were sent next to orphan trains, where children were transported to the West to be adopted by families. Many Catholic and Jewish social agencies emerged at that time to keep their own children in the community. There was also quite a bit of anti-Catholic and anti-Semitic activity at the time and rumors that both Catholics and Jews were kidnapping children when actually the opposite was true. (D.T.)

Health inequities and racial issues were numerous. Clearly, the way medical research was being conducted around 1900 was unjust. For example, vaccine trials on mentally ill patients, orphans, and the incarcerated were standard with little or no oversight. No common protocols for clinical trials existed. Additionally, little attention was given to racial and socioeconomic disparities. Black Americans were victims of this immoral system. W.E.B. Du Bois' analysis of a 1900 census revealed that African-American death rates were two to three times higher than for Caucasians for diseases such as tuberculosis, pneumonia, and diarrheal disease. However, the causes and potential solutions of this disparity were not researched. Instead, research focused on helping white society. People of Color, including African-American and indigenous populations, experienced the epidemic from positions of disadvantage, both economically and medically. Further complicated by racial prejudice, their experience was either neglected in health records, seen as problematic, or sometimes blamed for the disease course. However, mobilization within the community in response to the dearth of resources led to the creation of makeshift hospitals and clinics. Also, Black nurses and doctors, who were barred from service during WW1, provided care to both white and Black communities (Barry, 2004). Medical providers treating American Indian populations stated that deaths might have been avoided if these communities had better access to medical advice. Instead, they were sometimes blamed for their intransigence and commitment to traditional healing practices. The lack of government support to indigenous peoples was also seen in Alaska. At that time, Alaska was a territory and not yet a US state. Some regions in Alaska fared better than others, with disease course being dependent upon the ferocity of the wave to which they were exposed, as well as the availability of nearby healthcare resources. In addition, many of those indigenous communities that were hit the hardest also lost their means of sustaining themselves as individuals were no longer able to continue their livelihood (Crosby, 1989).

Racial tensions, exacerbated by the traumatic impact of the flu, reached a high point in 1919, leading to race riots (Bristow, 2012), much like the recent riots that followed the murder of George Floyd. During the 1919 pandemic, murder of a young Black man led to riots that began in Chicago and spread to other US cities. Eugene Williams was murdered in Chicago by a group of white youth, who stoned him after he reportedly crossed the unofficial barrier separating the "Black" and "White" beaches and the police officers refused to arrest the white youths. This time period also coincided with the great migration of African-Americans from the South to escape racism. Many white people and returning white veterans experienced financial insecurity as they felt that southern Blacks and immigrants were taking their jobs. Returning Black veterans, who just risked their lives fighting for their country and democracy, found themselves denied basic rights in the same nation for which they fought. Race riots occurred in the summer of 1919 in Washington, DC, Knoxville, Tennessee, and in Texas, Arkansas, Nebraska, and the south side of Chicago. President Woodrow Wilson blamed white people for instigating the riots in Chicago and DC and introduced efforts to encourage racial harmony. 1919 also may have marked a beginning of Black people fighting through protest for their rights in the face of racism and injustice. Today, as well, we see strong protest by Blacks in response to racism and injustice.

The Two Pandemics: Some Similarities and Differences

There were many other similarities between the two pandemics. One important similarity is that, while travel was more limited in 1918, both pandemics migrated. Then as now, the urban population was affected first and then it spread to rural areas. Another similarity concerns nonpharmaceutical treatments. Despite developments and advancements in medicine, the same nonpharmaceutical treatments (e.g., quarantine, social distancing, closures of schools and other institutions, masks, staying home when sick, hygienic practices such as washing hands and coughing into elbow) that are utilized with COVID were also used in 1918. Another similarity is that doctors and nurses and other healthcare professionals were traumatized then and now. In both times, people were isolated, and they viewed one another as dangerous. While isolation was a problem in 1918, it may be a lesser problem now as social media and technology enable people to see and communicate with one another and to work from home. And, most important, the danger is less now given the existence of vaccines and medication.

There are some other striking differences between the 1918 pandemic and the pandemic which began about 100 years later. As of this writing, COVID continues. We cannot predict when it will end or what it will be like in the future. What we can say is that the present pandemic has a longer duration than the 1918 flu and continues to mutate and infect. There were three distinct waves with the 1918 pandemic, whereas as of this writing (July 2022) we have already experienced five. The 1918 influenza pandemic killed at least 50 million people, twenty per cent of the world's population, across the world, including about 675,000 people in the USA. More people died by the 1918 pandemic than in World War I. In contrast, as of this writing (July 2022), there have been approximately 550 million cases of COVID and 6.34 million deaths. The USA has had the most cases of COVID-19 (87 million cases and 1.02 million deaths). India has had the second most, with 43.5 million cases and 525 thousand deaths. These numbers continue to change. However, without question, the COVID-19 pandemic is the deadliest disease event in American history.

In terms of target age, the 1918 pandemic targeted young adults and was cruel to young men, the elderly, and young children. In contrast, the elderly and minorities have been the hardest hit in the present pandemic. The incubation period differed, also. The Spanish flu lasted 1–4 days, while COVID-19 lasts longer (2–14 days). With the 1918 flu, it was not unusual for people to wake up feeling sick and then be dead by dinner time; people got very sick quickly and died very quickly. We heard many stories about these early deaths and about the horrific hardships that followed a death of an immigrant family member. Some of the following vignettes are illustrative.

> A small recollection-my mother's father was a streetcar conductor in St. Paul, MN. He came home from work, felt sick, and was dead within hours. He had immigrated to the U.S. by himself, so my grandmother then had to rely on her sisters to care for my mother and my aunt (eight and five year-old) while my grandmother got settled and eventually ran a boarding house. (P.A.)

> While researching the life of Clara Thompson, I was intrigued by the fact that she was in medical school during the pandemic of 1918. She graduated in 1920, so she was right in the middle of it during her training. Unlike the wave of the 2020 virus, in 1918 the virus was most fatal to perfectly healthy adults in their 20s and 30s. Her cohort. People would wake up feeling mildly ill and be dead by evening. Baltimore, where Thompson was at John Hopkins, closed all the schools and businesses except for drug stores. Funerals were prohibited, people were not allowed to gather in groups, and masks were mandatory. It was the same strategy as today. It must have been frightening and have taken a toll on those young physicians like Thompson, yet I've found no discussion of it in her papers or correspondence. What happened to all those feelings, losses, and fears? How were they metabolized? Were there lessons learned that can help us now? (A.D.)

There were other differences as well. Since July 1946, the USA has had the Communicable Disease Center (CDC). During COVID-19, Dr. Anthony Fauci,

Director of the National Institute of Allergy and Infectious Diseases at the National Institute of Health, updated the public regarding current epidemic and recommended steps. The main game changer came in December 2020 with the first coronavirus vaccine available in New York to those 16 years of age and older. In May 2021, it was available to 12- to15-year-olds. As of this writing (June 2022), it is available to everyone in the USA older than 6 months. There are also booster shots and anti-viral medication for those infected. There is, however, less availability in other countries. The existence of more advanced technology was another major difference between the two time periods. Although isolation has been a problem with COVID-19, technology tempered the isolation and enabled people to work from home, and vaccines have led to safer socializing.

There were many similarities between the two pandemics, including noticeable acts of kindness. For example, if whole families were sick in 1918, neighbors would leave food at their door. During COVID-19, Cornell technology students on Roosevelt Island offered remote technology support to older New Yorkers (Alpert & Nguyen-Feng, 2020); young and healthy New Yorkers shopped for older neighbors and donated meals to hospital workers; film location scouts helped locate needed hospital space; ordinary citizens made and donated masks and raised funds for hospitals. Acts of kindness continue now as the epidemic marches on.

However, in other ways we seem to be making some of the same errors as monkey pox is striking this country. At this time (Summer, 2020), a stable infrastructure and public healthcare investment seems to be inaccessible. Specifically, there have been vaccine and testing delays for monkey pox, echoing failures we experienced with COVID, and there are problems with the New York City monkey pox vaccine website. The vaccine rollout seems designed to reach the privileged and the process to access medication unequal.

Finale

In this final section we will briefly review the political, medical, social, and psychological motivations for suppressing the 1918 flu. We will conclude by pointing out ways that we can help society, institutions, and individuals remember, mourn, assimilate, and memorialize the current epidemic. There was failure at the macro level to prevent, control, or treat an everyday illness. The government failed and has not been held accountable. The press followed governmental dictate. There was a political motive to forget. Science and medicine and public health also failed. No one knew how to treat this disease and its course was not understood. The poor, many of whom were immigrants, were living in highly crowded conditions which were a flu-haven of sorts. Black people were deprived of necessary medical treatment. Sometimes they were not admitted to hospitals or admitted to the basement of hospitals where care was inferior. It may have been easier for science and medicine and public health to suppress the 1918 epidemic than to face failure and experience shame.

There is almost nothing written about mental health and the 1918 pandemic. The 1918 flu had a long-term impact as the vignettes indicate. It changed people's lives. People dealt with such events as death, poverty, loss of the breadwinner, movement to orphanages, isolation, and terror. In 1918, the casualties of World War I seemed to eclipse an awareness of the even greater deaths from disease. Although the 1918 flu disappeared from popular memory for more than 60 years, emotional traumas produced by the influenza of 1918 had long-term impact.

In summary, there was an unconscious decision to opt for amnesia. It was simply too painful for the institutions, the fields, or the people to acknowledge the degree of failure that was committed and the tragedy that was endured. As there was no or little grieving or mourning, loss was not integrated into their lives.

We cannot afford to *not* know any longer about the 1918 epidemic or the present epidemic, as there is much to learn. But the focus now needs to be on processing what we have been through, as well as mourning our losses. We can look to examples of societal mourning around 9–11 and to slavery for some wisdom. We know, for example, that there are numerous 9–11 memorials, monuments, parks, books, rituals, and statutes. We know that there are global memorials which trace the international impact of slavery, as well as memorials which honor the victims of slavery. Texts, images, and performances, for example, honor what one is unable to capture otherwise. There needs to be mass recognition and we need to tell stories that have the capacity to regulate, modulate, organize, soothe, and make meaning of the experience. The internal work of deep healing needs to be done. Testimonies can undo the silencing enforced by trauma. Wounds need to be healed and the disintegrative effects of trauma need to be dealt with. Human suffering needs to be confronted in order to expand our psychic world and our relational resources. As Herman points out (1992), when we deny the wounds of history, we experience episodic amnesia and trauma is then reproduced and visited on the next generation. We cannot integrate what we have been through without mourning. Memorials are needed. The present book is one such "memorial."

Author Note The authors thank Dr. Ilene Serlin for her meticulous editorial assistance.

References

Alpert, J. L. (2015). Enduring mothers, enduring knowledge: On rape and history. *Contemporary Psychoanalysis, 51*(2), 296–311.

Alpert, J. L., & Nguyen-Feng, V. N. (2020). COVID in New York City, the epicenter: A New York University perspective and COVID in Duluth, the bold north: A University of Minnesota perspective. *Psychological Trauma: Theory, Research, Practice, and Policy, 12*(5), 524–528.

Barry, J. M. (2004). *The great influenza: The story of the deadliest pandemic in history*. Penguin Books.

Bristow, N. (2012). *American pandemic: The lost worlds of the 1918 influenza epidemic*. Oxford University Press.

Crosby, A. W. (1989). *America's forgotten pandemic: The influenza of 1918*. Cambridge University Press.

Figley, C. R. (2015). *Compassion fatigue: Coping with secondary traumatic stress disorder in those who treat the traumatized*. Routledge.

Gates, B. (2015). The next outbreak? We're not ready. Ted Conferences. https://www.ted.com/talks/bill_gates_the_next_outbreak

Grand, S., & Salberg, J. (Eds.). (2016). *Transgenerational trauma and the other: Dialogues across history and difference*. Routledge.

Herman, J. (1992). *Trauma and recovery*. Basic Book.

Steinberg, A. (2014). Reclaiming Holocaust history: The past lives within us, *Clio's Psyche*, (Special Issue on Psychology and the Holocaust).

Weiland, N. (2022, June 24). Deborah Birx says Trump White House asked her to weaken Covid guidance. *New York Times*, A13.

Woodward, B., & Costa, R. (2021). *The Woodward triology: Fear, rage, peril*. Simon and Schuster.

Part II
Experiences in the Work Groups

The second part of this book depicts some of the ways that the trauma from COVID affected different groups of people and how they found ways to relieve their psychological suffering. From our review of the 1918 Spanish flu in Chap. 2, we learned that the psychological dimensions of trauma were as real then as they have been during this current COVID pandemic. Moreover, when psychological experiences are not addressed, more people get sick and die. Our job during the COVID task force was to assist the various populations we worked with to identify and develop positive coping mechanisms they could use to deal with trauma. Interestingly, at the same time, the psychologists working with these groups were trying to identify and develop their own positive coping mechanisms. Some of the negative coping strategies identified during the past pandemic included forgetting, denial, projection, somatization, and manic defenses. In reviewing what happened during the 1918 flu, we realized that these coping strategies, especially forgetting the pain of what happened, prevented people from being prepared for the current pandemic.

The psychological impact of such a catastrophic period was also affected by the social and medical realities of the time, and that affects different groups in different ways. Hesitation to wear a mask, socially distance from others, or accept the vaccine made the difference between life and death for many groups. Overcoming such hesitation was important to assist people who were rightfully confused by different messages given out by government leaders. The enormity of the change in people's lifestyles needed to be acknowledged and losses suffered grieved. One of the most important positive coping strategy was the use of verbal and nonverbal support groups to help with grieving and memorializing these losses.

In Chap. 3, we describe how we helped people deal with one of the psychological expressions of trauma, increased frustration and rage, and how this resulted in increased interpersonal violence, especially during the lockdown with courts closed. In fact, the U.S. Centers for Disease Control (CDC) found that domestic violence increased to three times what it had been before. Child abuse resulting in death or serious injury also increased as seen by hospital reports. However, with children locked in homes and not in school, we are only learning now the impact of psychological child abuse, especially on teens. Confounding the trauma felt by people from interpersonal violence were the race riots during the first year of the pandemic following the police killing of George Floyd and other Black citizens and the climate trauma resulting from hurricanes, floods, and earthquakes. The pandemic became a syndemic also exposing the inequities in the healthcare system so that people of color were more likely to die during COVID. Here we describe the use of social media to reach people across the world learning new techniques to reduce anxiety and increase wellness.

Chapter 4 focuses on the special stresses quarantine had on working families and children home from school. When working fathers and mothers had to also be their children's teachers, the attempt to keep children learning their curriculum via the internet during the pandemic failed miserably. The burden fell more harshly on mothers whose jobs outside the family conflicted with their role in managing how the family survived. This working group dealt with questions such as whether a 5-year-old child should get vaccinated, should a mother have to give up her seniority in a company if she takes time off to deal with family crises, or how to help teenagers continue the developmental pattern without direct contact with peers. One of the chairs of this group had a premature baby during this time and other members helped take on some of her responsibilities so she could attend to her own family crisis.

Older adults and caregivers were the focus of Chap. 5. This group decided to look at a very vulnerable part of the older adult population; those who were vibrant and lived a full life prior to the pandemic. They documented how when this group had to go into lockdown and slow down, it became difficult to regain their former strength once they could go out again. The psychologists who worked with this group had to deal with their own vulnerabilities in addition to others. A special group of holocaust survivors now going through the pandemic was used to illustrate the possibility of epigenetic trauma that passes down from one generation to another.

First-line responders who worked in the hospital and addiction are the focus of Chap. 6. Here the working group got off to a slow start until they decided that they wanted to focus on the first-line workers in the hospital unprepared to deal with so much illness and death; janitors, dieticians, cooks, and others rather than the nurses and doctors. These workers and their families were being exposed to the deadly virus on a daily basis. They were the ones holding the hands of those dying, unprepared to do anything other than simply being a compassionate person. Those suffering from addictions were also in a precarious position with supplies on the streets being even more dangerous. With doctors not seeing patients in person, getting opioid pills also became more difficult in some places and easier with other doctors prescribing online. This working group developed a blog on a magazine, *Psychology Today*, that was able to broadcast their message on a regular basis.

In Chap. 7, members of the work group share how they formed a support group for psychologists with secondary or vicarious trauma. During the height of the lockdown, there were different groups meeting daily. The schedules were advertised and people could drop in when their schedules permitted. Therapists who were unused to working virtually on the internet with patients were able to share their experiences with each other. This included use of technology as well as adapting therapy techniques for the virtual environment. There was lots of informal sharing of coping strategies including ways to relieve the reported exhaustion from sitting at the computer all day long. During the second year of the pandemic, as the world began to open up in the United States, other countries such as India were facing lockdowns, and the groups expanded to assisting psychologists there also.

Chapter 8 uses somatic and creative arts-based modalities to reach nonverbal individuals and whole communities. This working group helped other mental health workers learn how to use the creative arts to help heal trauma. Song and dance from different countries demonstrated how healing trauma can occur using the creative arts from their own culture. This working group also joined the roundtables with the IPV group and shared presentations with the international following that had developed.

Finally, graduate students in psychology investigated and documented the unique stresses and coping mechanisms of COVID on students in Chap. 9. Part of the training for psychologists occurs in practicum settings working with real live people. However, all these practicum sites were closed and students had to work virtually. Those who joined our task force were invaluable in helping us set up social media sites so that we could distribute resources as quickly as possible to graduate students so their learning would not be interrupted. Having the students working with those of us "old-timers" in the other working groups also helped us begin to use social media as they were so much more knowledgeable than others.

Chapter 3
Interpersonal Violence During COVID

Lenore E. A. Walker, Marilyn Safir, Giselle Gaviria, Michaela Mendelsohn, Patricia Villavicencio, Rita Rivera, and Lori Gill

In the Beginning

Lenore, Fort Lauderdale, Florida

I don't remember what day of the week it was when I woke up to the news that the world as I knew it was about to change in such unfathomable ways, even I, a psychologist and fiction writer could not have imagined. I first heard a commentator on the television questioning an announcement from the government; the coronavirus was now here in the USA, and we were ordered to shut down all our activities and quarantine until the threat left. Unthinkable. "Could our lives really be put on hold?" I asked myself. "Was an unseen-by-the-naked-eye virus capable of changing

L. E. A. Walker (✉)
Nova Southeastern University College of Psychology, Fort Lauderdale, FL, USA

Walker & Associates, LLC, Fort Lauderdale, FL, USA
e-mail: walkerle@nova.edu; lw@drlenoreewalker.com

M. Safir
University of Haifa, Haifa, Israel

G. Gaviria
Walker & Associates, LLC, Fort Lauderdale, FL, USA

M. Mendelsohn
Independent Practice, Boston, MA, USA

P. Villavicencio
Hospital Clinico San Carlos de Madrid, Madrid, Spain

R. Rivera
Carlos Albizo University, Miami, FL, USA

L. Gill
Attachment and Trauma Treatment Centre for Healing, St. Catharines, ON, Canada

C. R. Figley et al. (eds.), *Pandemic Providers*,
https://doi.org/10.1007/978-3-031-27580-7_3

everything? Would a lockdown really protect us?" I held up my hand and swished at the air wondering if the red spiked balls illustrating the virus on television had invaded my bedroom, yet.

Those were immediate questions I had, not expecting any answers. I understood that I was in a high-risk group given my age and medical conditions, but I also was in a privileged group. I lived in a large apartment with my husband, equipped with Internet that mostly worked, surrounded by loving friends and family, with access to many resources including competent medical providers. As a psychologist and professor emeritus from the nearby Nova Southeast University, I had nearby colleagues and students. My research already had moved from the university to my home office overlooking the beautiful beach and ocean. I could order anything I needed to be delivered to my door. I remember thinking, "I can get through this." but I had no idea just how long or how difficult it would be.

Our entire lives were about to be changed in ways that could not have been imagined. The unspeakable losses and depth of grief, the new skills to learn to survive, the overcoming of old resistances, and adopting new routines in everyday life were enormous. But, on the other hand, the new connections and friends that I was about to make were also unimaginable at that time. As an avid APA listserv junkie, I retreated to my computer, and began to communicate with other trauma providers, understanding that we would be called upon to assist those who had difficulty surviving the new reality of life. I especially understood that the battered women and survivors of other forms of gender violence would be in that group, especially if they were required to quarantine with their abusive partners. But I had no idea that the known rates of intimate partner violence (IPV) would at least triple during this period and once schools shut down and children remained home, their abuse would also increase at unknown rates since there would be no one outside their home who could see the bruises.

Within a short time, I joined with 95 other trauma psychologists answering the call to form a COVID Task Force to assist in dealing with the trauma from this deadly threat. I knew Charles Figley for many years, first as author of the most important early work on trauma including its impact on those who experience it vicariously like families of military soldiers who survived with PTSD. Later we worked together on the APA Council of Representatives, often agreeing on many social justice initiatives. When he was appointed chair of this new task force, I was thrilled to be a part of whatever solace it might bring to our professional community.

Marilyn, Haifa, Israel

When I read Charles Figley's call to members of Division 56 to join a Zoom meeting to discuss a Covid Task Force, I immediately joined despite the time difference in Israel where I now lived full time as a psychologist and professor emeritus from the University of Haifa. From the earliest meetings, we considered and discussed the needs of both professionals and lay folks resulting from the disruptions in daily life due to the COVID-19 pandemic. This experience more than met my expectations. Through sharing experiences and hearing about the trials and tribulations that people experienced throughout the USA and around the world, the idea of forming an interdivisional task force became a very serious mission.

I became much more aware of the effects of living on my own, having been recently widowed. Suddenly, I became part of a group that was seen as endangered and fragile being over 80 years old. This conflicted with my self-evaluation as independent, competent, achieving, and in-control person. I joined Irit Felsen who researched and worked with seniors and called attention to folks like me, who were able to care for themselves and to contribute, as to how we could reach out to other older adults of a wider range of lifestyles and activities that hadn't yet been addressed.

Having been retired, I reestablished contact with some former professional contacts in particular, Lenore Walker, with whom I had been in contact with from the early days of identifying and focusing on violence towards women. By joining the IPV and Vibrant Older Adult taskforces, I established new friendships with individual from different age groups and geographical areas. I have become more active and involved professionally and this has positively affected my daily life. I think that as an interdivisional task force of APA, by taping our roundtables, webinars, the various research projects, and future publications, we are preparing the ground work for recommendations and the development guidelines for that can serve as "roadmaps" for providing measures and methods for more appropriate and efficient means of dealing with future predicted pandemics.

Michaela, Boston, Massachusetts

As the COVID-19 lockdown continued, I became increasingly aware of how much the pandemic was impacting the mental health of my patients as a psychologist in independent practice working primarily with adult traumas survivors. I was especially concerned about those individuals who were living with volatile partners or were in otherwise unsafe relationships because their options for respite or escape were so limited. I read news reports indicating that rates of interpersonal violence appeared to be increasing and that children in particular were at high risk because of lack of contact with schools, health professionals, and others who are usually able to identify abuse and engage families with appropriate services. Personally, I was finding my work doing back-to-back remote sessions with individual patients very isolating and exhausting. Even though I had been exclusively in private practice for a number of years, I had always made a point of seeing and connecting with colleagues, through participating in shared trainings or peer supervision, or even just briefly greeting fellow clinicians in the hallway of our office suite between patients. I was eager for collegial contact, especially with others who cared deeply about the problem of interpersonal violence and its escalation during COVID-19. I wanted to learn more about how others were dealing with this issue in their clinical work and think together about ways of alleviating suffering in the midst of this unprecedented situation. It was these factors that lead me to join the APA COVID-19 Interpersonal Violence Task Force.

It was uplifting and enlivening to meet and connect with colleagues at various points of their careers in the USA and abroad, and work together to develop the weekly roundtables and social media posts. I learned from other practitioners about approaches and techniques that they implement with patients (e.g., body-oriented interventions and therapy using creative arts) and I was able to apply some of these in work with my own patients. I developed more familiarity with the use of social media platforms such as Facebook, Twitter, and Instagram in promoting mental health and wellness. I was also able to share psychoeducation and coping skills that I teach in my practice and feel like they had a larger impact than when I work with patients individually. It was especially meaningful to hear about the circumstances and work of colleagues in diverse countries (such as Spain, Israel, and Uganda) as it broadened my perspective while also making the world feel smaller and more connected. I found that being part of something creative that promoted resilience and recovery and enabled me to join with like-minded professionals and students was very helpful in mitigating the burnout that I was experiencing as a result of the heavy load of virtual clinical work during the pandemic.

Patricia, Madrid, Spain

A few days after the COVID-19 lockdown in Spain – March 13, 2020 – I started to be very active recording and downloading videos in my YouTube channel since I realized that many of my patients needed some sense of connection with their psychotherapist especially during the confinement. They also needed some visual guidance to understand the recommendations I was giving them – including parents of children and teenagers – via phone calling and/or e-mails. It is also well known that written information usually is hardly comprehensive and understood under stressful conditions, and COVID-19 lockdown has been and still is very stressful. In some cases it is also very traumatic. Therefore Lenore's invitation made me feel enthusiastic and gave me the sense of not being alone in my quest of sharing resources to cope with this pandemic. Being part of an APA Task Force assured me to go beyond Spanish-speaking countries and help also the people of the communities I support through Spain's EMDR association in Uganda. This task force initiative was something greater that went beyond my personal solidarity and motivation.

This Task Force has met all my expectations and beyond. Being part in such remarkable group of professionals has given me the sense of togetherness and global support as a mental health professional. All of the members have shared very valuable knowledge, tools, resources, and above all a profound cohesion and respect within our group and collective solidarity with the community-at-large.

I learned about the Hospitals First Responders subgroup that seemed very interested in reaching out to the Spanish-speaking communities in the USA. There I developed new relationships that directly impacted my job as a psychologist and first responder in a Madrid hospital. The Task Force against violence in my hospital in Madrid was very interested in finding ways to collaborate with other similar hospital groups in the USA so this was a perfect opportunity to get to know others. I have learned that working in a group as international as COVID IPV helps to reduce the stress impact of the pandemic not only to the community at large, but especially to each one of its members including colleagues who follow us in our weekly Zoom and roundtable meetings and social media publications. It has definitely made me feel emotionally and professionally supported.

Giselle, Boca Raton, Florida

I joined the COVID IPV GROUP initially because I knew there was a need to communicate with others through social media to get information out to help survivors and victims of Intimate Partner Violence. I wanted to help individuals who were experiencing difficulties within their relationships as well as to be able to communicate with other professionals around the world. I really enjoyed being able to learn from other professionals in our group. What I did not realize was that eventually they would become more like a support system for me as well. During the tapings of our roundtable videos to help others, I suddenly lost my mother. I turned to the group for support and received much more than I expected. The group provided a community even though I was not able to have physical contact with them. I am grateful for the lessons learned about trauma, grieving, coping skills, and safe spaces to aid others in life.

Lori, Ontario, Canada

As the Founder and Clinical Director of a trauma-specific treatment center (www.attchniagara.com) and trauma training organization (www.attch.org) at the onset of the pandemic, we immediately started adapting our model to allow our therapists as well as those using our model worldwide to offer our Integrative Trauma and Attachment Treatment Model (ITATM)® in an online format. I also recognized that there would be many people sheltering at home who would require additional resources and support, and I was quite concerned for their well-being. As a result, our non-profit ATTCH Niagara created an online Facebook platform ATTCH Niagara Caring Community Connections which provided regular guided practices, strategies, weekly wellness hours, and psychoeducation resources to help people reduce stress and increase a sense of connection during this time of isolation. We also offered a series of free groups for caregivers and their children: children, teens, and caregivers. We were fortunate to start this quite quickly, and we had excellent participation, especially during the initial lockdown period when there were few resources available. We gradually decreased posts on this site as we found the need for individual therapy was too great and needed to focus our attention there but have created a solid foundation of resources that people can continue to use. It has been incredible to observe how professionals all over the world have collaborated to share resources and provide support during this time.

When I read the call for members of the APA Division 56 Interdivisional Task Force on COVID-19 in March, I was immediately drawn to become involved. With all the uncertainty happening worldwide, I anticipated an increase in overwhelm, helplessness, anxiety, and fear resulting for many and as such wanted to assist in providing support where possible. Joining this task force seemed like a great way to do so. Although I was drawn to many of the working groups as we work with all ages and traumas at our center, I worried that the uncertainty and fear that there would be an increase in violence and felt concerned for those sheltering in place in unsafe situations which is what led me to initially join the COVID IPV working group. Sadly, rates of violence are reported to have increased worldwide and on many levels. This is so unfortunate and at the same time has further validated that work of this working group as quite timely and essential. Through collaborative efforts we have created social media platforms focused on providing information and resources aimed at reducing stress, increasing safety as best as possible given the circumstances, and teaching skills to help promote overall well-being. Our following and resources continue to grow each week. It has truly been an honor to be involved in this process and to work alongside other like-minded trauma experts.

Rita M. Rivera, Honduras/United States

As a psychology trainee and early career professional, one of my goals has been to advocate for issues pertaining to minority mental health. During the COVID-19 pandemic, I was pursuing my doctorate in clinical psychology in Florida, USA. As an international student from Honduras, I also served as a psychotherapist in my home country. The pandemic led me to seek collaborative opportunities to improve my clinical skills further and connect with like-minded professionals interested in serving traditionally marginalized populations. I learned of the APA COVID-19 Interdivisional Taskforce through emails from APA divisions I continue to hold membership. After participating in the initial meeting, I was interested in collaborating with the IPV Task Force to help promote increased global awareness of the novel challenges impacting this population. I wholeheartedly believe the work conducted by this working group has been significant in fostering a solid network of support for mental health clinicians and researchers and educational material for the public. The resources and educational programming created and disseminated by the WG continue to be accessible to individuals worldwide. Moreover, members of the WG have developed partnerships and alliances, further highlighting the value of interdisciplinary collaboration facilitated through the Task Force. I am personally grateful for the opportunity to be part of such a supportive, qualified group of professionals who continue to inspire me to promote psychology's advancement through advocacy, research, and clinical practice.

The Origin of the IPV Work Group

The COVID IPV Work Group coalesced in April 2020, about 1 month after the COVID Task Force suggested breaking into smaller groups designed to assist mental health workers in dealing with transforming their practices to help others deal with the pandemic. Ten members joined the first Zoom call, each sitting in our own little box on the computer screen. I knew a few from prior IPV work together, but some became new professional friends and colleagues. We were a diverse group from the beginning; nine women and one man, three students and three over the age of 70, English, Spanish, and Hebrew speakers, and one woman with an Indian heritage. All had expertise in helping people heal from interpersonal trauma, especially women who were physically, sexually, and psychologically abused. Later many more joined our group and once we began disseminating knowledge through social media; others were invited to join for specific presentations. We quickly set to work in creating our mission statement which became:

> To find, create, and disseminate resources to assist those people who are in danger of experiencing and/or perpetuating physical, sexual, and/or psychological abuse during the pandemic. We will promote the use of tools for emotional regulation to help manage overwhelming emotions arising from the pandemic and to enhance safety.

We easily agreed upon our mission, and all also agreed to focus on interpersonal violence with a strong emphasis on Intimate Partner Violence (IPV). It was understood that many people face multiple victimization, especially women who are more likely to experience domestic violence, child abuse, and sexual abuse including rape, harassment, and exploitation by those in powerful places. It didn't take long for our focus to broaden to decrying police violence especially against people of color. Riots broke out in cities during the early phases of the pandemic, climate change creating floods and fires ravaged across the USA, and trauma seemed to be everywhere. The APA Chief Executive Director, Arthur Evans, named it the season of the "syndemic" including all these cataclysmic forces impacting us around the world.

Daily reports brought more uncertainty than solace as governments, including the USA, began politicizing the pandemic and posting confusing and erroneous information. The US President refused to accept that we were in a crisis period and refused advice from the best health scientists we had. Instead, he kept blaming China for creating the virus that caused the pandemic which resulted in our unpreparedness. In fact, as the confusion expanded, it became obvious the problems were magnified by his having disbanded the government's emergency health team and disbursed all the supplies needed to cope with the pandemic. The scientists at the Centers for Disease Control (CDC) said to wear masks and socially distance in order to control the disease. Then the government said it was not necessary when they realized there were not enough masks available.

Hospital workers went without adequate protection from COVID as there just were not enough gear available. People were dying in the hospitals while others securely locked in their homes banged on pots and pans nightly at 7 pm, supporting the hardworking first responders and essential workers. Make-shift hospitals and morgues were created in parking lots especially when bodies began piling up in nursing homes. Life as we knew it had been totally transformed by this virus that no one seemed to know how to stop. Countries with totalitarian governments were able to enforce strict rules but even that did not seem to slow down the virus, its mutations, and its death toll. In the USA no one was really sure what was the best way to survive except to stay locked in our homes, whenever possible. The diverse communities, many of whom had low-paying but essential jobs, experienced the hardest impact. African Americans were dying at more rapid rates, perhaps due to more chronic illnesses like hypertension and diabetes and poorer access to good medical care. Dr. Fauci, the kindly 80-year-old chief of the US CDC infectious unit became the face on television broadcasting these conflicting messages. This chaotic situation impacted mental health workers and the people we served, especially since we were all going through the same uncertainty and stressors that they were experiencing.

Some workers began using the Internet to substitute for in-person conferencing and communication. Children were kept home from school and required to attend lessons on the Internet. Teachers and parents were experimenting with how to help children develop and learn without contact with friends for social skill learning. Schools in many communities delivered tablets and other digital devices to connect as many homes as possible to the Internet. Smart phones were as necessary as were "chickens-in-the-pot" during the last century's depression. Mental health professionals needed to quickly adapt their approaches to provide support to clients and others who were overwhelmed around the world, while also experiencing the same uncertainty as everyone else. It truly was a shared experience, and for many it was the first time a therapist shared the experience of extreme stress with their patients. At the same time, families needed to be supported financially. Governments began to transfer funds to people if they could not go out to work. Stores began to develop ways to deliver food and other supplies to those quarantined in homes. Some supplies became scarce, like toilet paper. No one really knew why something like toilet paper became scarce but it piled up in people's homes when they were lucky to obtain some whenever it became available. Perhaps there was something psychological about such behavior, but no one really knew. Restaurants closed or opened with take-out or outside seating during the summer months. Alcohol sales soared. Courts were closed and some alleged criminals were released from jails that became COVID super-spreaders. Civil cases and divorces were postponed. Violence on the streets went down once the race riots stopped since no one was out on the streets. But, inside the homes, violence rates were soaring. This was the perfect recipe for the increase in domestic violence given the tensions over the uncertainty of the future.

There was no escape from either COVID or the batterer for battered women. Adult children could not go to visit their parents as the elderly were the most vulnerable to succumb to the virus. Those who had financial resources could not go to hotels as they were either closed or barely opening a few rooms that needed to be sterilized. Until vaccinations became available, sometime the following year, in February 2021, battered women were stuck: die from COVID or die from the abuser's escalating violence in the home. Against this backdrop, our COVID IPV group began to search for ways to help these women and their families.

Accomplishments Using Social Media

Our younger members suggested using social media as additional outlets for fast worldwide distribution of new ways for women to protect themselves. The senior members had almost no familiarity with media such as Instagram, Twitter, and TikTok, although some were on Linked-In and Facebook. Before we closed that first Zoom meeting, the younger members had established the COVID IPV Facebook group and #COVIDIPV accounts on Instagram and Twitter. We immediately began posting resources, first in English but then Spanish as well to reach our many Spanish-speaking colleagues. As new members around the world joined our programs, we began posting in their language, too. Our goal was to assist other mental health professionals who were not trained in working with trauma by sharing practical ways to help their patients as well as themselves. As we were using public social media, we believed the general public, including patients, would be able to follow our work, so we created materials that could be understood by non-psychologists, too. As of today, we have reached hundreds of people in over 30 countries by using the social media available.

- We posted messages daily on social media to help deal with topics of interest like:
  - Locked in homes with an abusive partner
  - Revising domestic violence protocols during the pandemic
  - Lowering anxiety and tension at home to avoid violence
  - New safety plans for battered women in lockdown with their abuser
  - Preventing youth suicide
  - Love, sex, and relationships during COVID
  - Avoiding Zoom fatigue
  - The healing power of creative arts
  - Tips for Telehealth with BW
  - Eye Zoom fatigue
  - Nutrition
  - Conducting Zoom groups

We held weekly roundtable discussions live on Zoom and Facebook to present new ways to survive and thrive during the pandemic and to re-enter life during the end of the second year. You can find copies of 30 of our roundtables posted on our YouTube Channel: https://youtube.com/channel/UCKc6tlpmfVomAkwlFaHUEoA

- We collaborated with the *International Whole Person Approach* to present roundtables.
- We presented on social justice issues around climate change and racial injustice.
- We learned about apps that could be used as therapy adjuncts or stand alone.
- We engaged in regular webinars on trauma topics.
- We invited speakers from other groups to present a roundtable.
- We searched for innovative ways to deal with IPV.

The first few months dealt with violence in the community as well as in people's homes, as George Floyd's murder by a Minneapolis police officer prompted riots across the US cities and around the world. It wasn't clear if the explosion that occurred had any relationship to the growing fear from COVID, or if everyone had enough of Black people being unfairly targeted by some police officers just because of the color of their skin. Such protests had happened before. But this time seemed different; white people marched alongside people of color demanding justice. Some members of our group were involved in dealing with the aftereffects of this community solidarity in many different places. Rohini led the march in Denver while Larry worked with police officers attempting to help them find better ways of doing their job. During this time Larry was elected president of the International Division in APA and was less able to spend weekly time with our group but continued to join in some roundtables and worked behind the scenes sharing new ways to keep stress, conflict, and violence low.

We participated with APA as other groups began to unravel the long history of health care inequities, particularly against people of color, who were less able to access or utilize psychological services. Our multicultural group supported those efforts and joined in where we could. Perhaps the common experience of living through the unknown during the worst of the pandemic initially gave those of us living with privilege insight into how meaningless privilege in one world can be when the world suddenly changes. All of us felt vulnerable to this virus that invaded our world.

Roundtables

We discovered the use of *roundtables* as a unique way to deliver our messages quickly and competently after about 2 months of weekly meetings with our group members on hour-long Zoom calls. The riots quieted down and the reality of the changes in dealing with domestic violence settled in. Women could not develop safety plans to escape their homes. Anxiety kept rising, tensions built up, and the explosions outdoors moved into people's homes. We had the tools to teach battered women how to reduce their tension and accompanying anxiety to better protect themselves from angry and abusive men inside their homes. But we couldn't wait to write papers or books to help non-trauma mental health clinicians learn how to teach these techniques; we had to act quickly. Again, our younger members, more familiar with social media suggested pairing Facebook together with Zoom and using our weekly hour to teach ourselves and others new trauma-specific techniques. And so we began 1-hour weekly roundtables that were broadcast both on Zoom for our group and on Facebook simultaneously on Thursdays at noon ET for all those watching. Our audience grew from just a few who tuned in initially to over 600 people from 30 different countries over the year that we produced the roundtables.

The roundtable had a particular format. We began with two volunteers from our group to discuss a particular concept, skill, or technique for about 5 to 10 minutes after we introduced everyone visible in the Zoom boxes. Then everyone else on that day's meeting discussed what had been presented. We differed from webinars or lectures in that we were informal and tried to discuss the issues with each other or others who tuned in via Facebook. Sometimes the discussions went off topic, especially if there was something special in the news. Primarily we focused on ways to recognize growing tensions and anxiety and how to change that energy. We stressed safety planning during the pandemic, preventing serious depression, grief reactions, keeping children interested in schoolwork, calming down angry children, and dealing with other daily activities that could lead to an abusive incident. Lori often demonstrated new techniques that her clinic in Canada was using to reduce anxiety in trauma survivors. Several of us practiced many of the exercises and found they were helpful for our own relaxation as we had been unaware that we were tense or anxious. We developed new safety plans as women couldn't leave their homes when the batterer became menacing. Instead, we helped them designate a safe place in their home, even if it was a chair or corner on the floor.

We also found that discussions among our members on Zoom that were posted on Facebook were getting a lot of attention, particularly those that attempted to provide scientific information about COVID and how to stay safe as the available information was changing. Research demonstrated the effectiveness of wearing masks and social distancing, especially for those who were most vulnerable to serious illness. Sometimes there were big surprises that occurred such as the day that Harriett Adong, the Director of Programs for Children at the Foundation for Integrated Rural Development (FIRD) in Uganda, joined us on Facebook. We gave her the Zoom link, and she quickly appeared in a Zoom box along with the others of our group on that day. She informed us how Ugandans were dealing with the pandemic using natural methods to boost their immune system as the vaccine was unavailable or too expensive for them. Thus, they drank plenty of lemon juice for its Vitamin C and socially distanced since they didn't have masks either. Harriett became a valuable member of our group and was able to appear when the Internet service in the city was available. When Harriett went into the rural areas, we couldn't reach her, but she came back filled with stories of their survival. Patricia, who had visited Harriett in Uganda, showed us videos of helping the children heal from trauma using song and dance. Amy, a dance therapist from Ilene's group, showed her videos of helping women suffering from cancer and trauma, and were joined by others who used dance, music, and art projects to help traumatized people heal. We knew that talking therapy worked; we learned how the creative arts can help heal from trauma, too.

Marilyn became our go-to person for the latest media information. She was able to review newspapers and other reports from all over the world and disseminated anything that she thought would interest us, especially dealing with PTSD, domestic violence, and trauma during COVID. Rado, from the research group, would also send information on the latest research that we could use to follow up in areas our group was discussing at any particular time. The breadth of knowledge of the people in our group became an important way of keeping up with the volumes of information that kept being published. During the first year, Charles had meetings of the large group several times a month where we got to hear what other working groups were doing. Much exciting work was going on.

Giselle became interested in the apps that could be used on smartphones to help trauma survivors heal. Some are used as an adjunct to psychotherapy especially those that were developed by the US Department of Veteran's Affairs to help those experiencing PTSD from war and sexual assaults, while others were commercially produced and could be used by themselves to help reduce anxiety or even to get a good night's sleep. Psychologist Skip Rizzo shared his work on virtual reality (VR), using psychological techniques from exposure therapy to help heal trauma effects. His videos demonstrating virtual immersion back into the traumatic experience were exciting, as newer technologies are being used to help get those unstuck in their fear and grief responses. We had a presentation from one of the London group of women psychologists who were studying the negative impact of COVID on women's advancement in the workplace. They presented us with the results of their study, showing that some women were losing jobs and others their seniority status, even before they gave formal presentations or wrote papers. Larry began posting weekly stories of random acts of kindness from people all over the world. He gave optimism to the hope that life would return to some semblance of normal one-day.

As the vaccinations became more available, about a year into the pandemic, we noted two major responses; people either fought to be in the first group that received the vaccine, or they hesitated and refused to be vaccinated. As psychologists, we used our knowledge about human behavior, to provide scientific information to encourage groups to become vaccinated, hoping that the more people who were protected, the sooner the pandemic would be over. It is difficult to say whether we persuaded anyone with our presentations, as many US politicians had politicized the medical information causing some people to believe it would harm them rather than help. It was disappointing to see how little trust the anti-vaxxers had in either science or the government despite the record-speed with which the vaccines were produced. Although this COVID pandemic was new to the world, scientists had been studying ways to create safe vaccines during other periods of similar illnesses such as SARS, EBOLA, and the common FLU that had new variants each year against which most people did accept the vaccine.

As mentioned above, when Ilene Serlin's Whole Person International Creative Arts group joined us in producing roundtables, we expanded our repertoire of ways to deal with rising emotions using the creative arts. We also expanded our outreach to new countries and providers as they had a greater presence in non-English or Spanish-speaking countries. While some group members were discussing the issues of the day, others were responding to notes entered on our Facebook page, COVIDIPV. Still others responded to Instagram posts or Tweets on Twitter. We were reaching out to people who primarily used social media with important information as we were utilizing it in our own practices. Most important, we were having fun learning from each other, especially celebrating holidays with dance parties. Although Facebook kept the videos of our hour-long presentations on our page for weeks afterwards, we decided to go the next step and develop a YouTube Channel that permitted people to download the session separately.

Other IPV Presentations

During year two the world began to open again albeit very slowly. Psychology meetings where information was often exchanged among participants went hybrid, and our IPV Task Force created short Zoom videos to insert in presentations at the American Psychological Association (APA) annual meeting that was held online. We were excited by the opportunity to share our work with the rest of the APA. The group from NSU also continued working on our assessment tool, the *Battered Woman Syndrome Questionnaire (BWSQ)*, with other professors from Nova Southeastern University, preparing it for commercial use. With a grant from the Department of Justice to Endolor Publishing LLC, Lenore and Giselle among others began to adapt the *Survivor Therapy Empowerment Program (STEP)* for use in the US Bureau of Prisons for Women to help battered women heal from the trauma they experienced. We began to see a future even though the COVID virus remains present, albeit in less dangerous variants. Vulnerable people are still wearing masks and socially distancing at this time but others are back at work and travel. Many psychologists have not gone back to offices, preferring to work using telepsychology from their home. Courts have reopened and domestic violence victims are better able to receive justice and help. Despite our efforts, the CDC reports that intimate partner violence was at an all-time high, with at least 3 times increase than prior to the pandemic.

Future Plans

We continued our weekly roundtable conversations inviting different experts on a particular topic aimed at reducing interpersonal violence well into year two but discontinued them when the students, who were integral to maintain our social media presence, graduated and the demand for 1:1 therapy became too great for therapists to volunteer their time on a weekly schedule. The demand for psychological treatment is at an unprecedented level with therapists worldwide carrying wait-lists, or even being closed to new referrals. With this in mind, we continue to post on Facebook and Instagram. As the world re-opens, we shall continue to post messages about how to deal with staying safe. As we learn of resources for dealing with domestic violence, sexual assaults, child abuse, and other forms of interpersonal violence, we will post them on our social media pages. We will continue to collaborate with our colleagues as we all go back to our regular jobs knowing that the friendships we've made here are lasting ones.

Chapter 4
Parenting During a Pandemic

Rachel Wamser-Nanney, Christina M. Rodriguez, Lauren Mizock, and Laura Nabors

The American Psychological Association (APA) COVID-19 Support for Children and Families workgroup's overarching aim is to help support children, caregivers, and families who have been impacted by the COVID-19 pandemic, as well as professionals working with these groups. Toward this end, we have worked to compile and disseminate COVID-19-related resources to support professionals who are working with children, caregivers, and families affected by the pandemic. This chapter describes our collective efforts to aid children, caregivers, families, and professionals working with children and families during the pandemic, including dissemination of resources. We also discuss key areas of concern we identified during the pandemic that professionals should consider in times of future crises, spotlight groups who were particularly vulnerable, and describe our successes, challenges, and lessons learned.

R. Wamser-Nanney (✉)
Department of Psychological Sciences, University of Missouri-St. Louis, St. Louis, MO, USA
e-mail: WamserR@umsystem.edu

C. M. Rodriguez
Department of Psychology, Old Dominion University, Norfolk, VA, USA
e-mail: crodriguez@odu.edu

L. Mizock
Department of Psychology, Fielding Graduate University, Santa Barbara, CA, USA

L. Nabors
School of Human Services, University of Cincinnati, Cincinnati, OH, USA
e-mail: naborsla@ucmail.uc.edu

C. R. Figley et al. (eds.), *Pandemic Providers*,
https://doi.org/10.1007/978-3-031-27580-7_4

Hardships Faced by Families During COVID-19

Disruptions to Daily Life

It is a gross understatement to state that the lives of children, caregivers, and families changed with the onset of the pandemic. The onset of COVID-19 resulted in changes that were often abrupt, unprecedented, and large in magnitude. For many caregivers, these radical shifts in daily living and resources were difficult to bear and overwhelming, particularly as it was apparent to many that there was no end in sight or near hopes for a return to normalcy. Caregivers are often instructed to take care of themselves and that they were "unable to pour from an empty cup." There is truth in this, but the pandemic often robbed caregivers of their typical access to "liquid": access to basic resources, childcare, social support, parenting-related supports, and self-care activities. The pandemic also taxed caregivers, many who were now expected to miraculously care for their children, even small children who require constant supervision, and work remotely, as well as serve as educators for children participating in remote learning. This is no easy, or even possible, feat for many. Dr. Wamser-Nanney can attest to the challenges of this as a mother of three young girls, two of which were born during the pandemic. Her two-year-old and newborn would not sit quietly all day while attending Zoom meetings or when she was lecturing, let alone allow her to engage in cognitively intensive research and other academic activities, or clinical work. Nap time is by no means sufficient to complete work requirements for full, or even part-time employees. And Dr. Wamser-Nanney is extremely privileged in several regards. She is white, married to a supportive partner, and has a Ph.D. She also has an occupation that allows her to work remotely – a considerable advantage not afforded for a sizable number of jobs. There is no way to work virtually and provide childcare if you are working a register at a grocery store, or stocking shelves, or are a first responder, nurse, or many other healthcare professionals.

Among the significant disruptions and negative impacts on families was the immediate financial impact given the collapse of the global economy, with obvious and devastating effects on children and families (Gassman-Pines & Gennetian, 2020). Within weeks of the pandemic onset and related restrictions, millions filed for unemployment benefits in the USA (Lambert, 2020). Similar employment losses were observed worldwide (International Labor Organization, 2021). Indeed, unemployment and economic turmoil rose to levels not seen since the Great Depression of the 1930s (Kochnar, 2020). Gender effects were also noted. Mothers who were able to work from home had a significant reduction in work hours compared to fathers who encountered little change (Landivar et al., 2020; Petts et al., 2021). Just prior to the pandemic, unemployment rates in the USA were equivalent for both women and men (4.4%), with the gap widening to 16.2% of women and 13.5% of men in April 2020 (U.S. Bureau of Labor Statistics, 2020). The current gap has diminished in 2022 (women 3.9%; men 3.8%), although the gender disparity remains significant.

The economic disarray was exacerbated when one of the core bedrocks of the economy was shattered: the sudden closure of in-person schools and childcare facilities (Donohue & Miller, 2020). Informal sources of childcare that families had relied upon, such as playdates and child activity facilities, also became unavailable during the initial stages and surges in the pandemic (Petts et al., 2021). The systemic closure represented an abrupt and fatal hit to the routine and structural infrastructure most working parents relied upon to be able to maintain employment. Childcare is the critical lynchpin for most parents to be able to attend work. Instead, parents became responsible for the childcare and homeschooling of their children. This has negative effects on not only the economic functioning of the family, but on the psychological functioning of these parents, who lost their non-parenting roles that may be key aspects of their identity.

Large droves of caregivers, particularly women, were immediately forced out of the workforce. It is not a new phenomenon that mothers tend to incur more negative employment outcomes during national disasters (U.S. Bureau of Labor Statistics, 2020). This phenomenon is contributed to by the traditional gender roles upheld in domestic labor, with women taking on more of the childcare, cleaning, and cooking (Miller, 2020; Petts et al., 2021). Women conduct approximately double the domestic labor as men weekly, on top of their work outside the home (Livingston & Parker, 2019; Petts et al., 2021). Among the theories for why this gender disparity occurs includes the cultural pressures of "intensive mothering," along with the "motherhood penalty" in paid labor, where domestic labor competes with paid labor opportunities and gets absorbed more by women (Petts et al., 2021; Correll et al., 2007). Loss of childcare is a consistent risk to job loss and reduced work hours for mothers in pre-pandemic times, because fathers tend to take on less responsibility for the childcare within the home (Petts et al., 2021). Among heterosexual parents, mothers risked unemployment during this time more than fathers, as mothers were more likely to assume the responsibility of childcare and homeschooling (Petts et al., 2021). Further, mothers who had to homeschool their children had triple the rates of job loss or reduced work hours, without this same occurrence for fathers. This study did report that when fathers became more involved in childcare during the pandemic, this served as a protective factor against mothers' negative employment outcomes, such as reduced work hours, forced labor exits, and unemployment.

Unfortunately, this situation may also negatively impact mothers' mental health. Mothers during COVID-19 have reported increased levels of maternal guilt and the moral distress of a "bad mom" identity from the challenges of replicating the quality of childcare and services their children received pre-pandemic (Smith, 2021). Women attempt to manage the mental load and a "triple burden" of paid work, unpaid care of their children, and domestic labor. Furthermore, some research suggests that when men prioritize or publicize their family responsibilities over work, they are seen as more competent than their female counterparts who do the same thing, representing a double standard in gender at work that couples the aforementioned "motherhood penalty" with the "fatherhood bonus" (Kmec, 2011). Clearly, the pandemic exacerbated these gender disparities in unpaid domestic labor and paid employment. While the gap in unemployment rates appear to be rapidly diminishing as shown in the statistics noted above (U.S. Bureau of Labor Statistics, 2020), the less visible negative effects of the pandemic appear in women's career advancement, promotions, and other employment goals (Kashen et al., 2020). Greater awareness and correction of these gender disparities in the home are necessary to adjust the balance in domestic labor inequities and prevent the undoing of 25 years of progress for women in the workforce.

Instead of, or in addition to, their work responsibilities (which were not necessarily reduced), many parents were thrust into full-time caregiving roles while overseeing the education of children overnight. Many parents had little preparation, expertise, or even the physical resources (i.e., access to the Internet, electronic devices) to engage in this educational mission (Thorell et al., 2021). E-learning during the pandemic has been fraught with complications and has exacerbated frightening public health disparities among children and adolescents at greater risk: children of color, those from lower incomes, and those with educational delays, diagnoses, and psychological challenges. Critically, it is apparent that these children are unlikely to "catch up," either quickly or ever. Caregivers serving as educators may not have had the ability or skill set to educate their children, particularly those with autism spectrum disorder (ASD), developmental delays, or learning challenges. Educators quickly discovered that nearly a third of students did not have reliable access to technology to allow for remote learning (Francom et al., 2021), with children of color more likely to have received little or no contact with educators in the first months of pandemic (Dorn et al., 2020). Recommended practices for enhancing the delivery and supervision of remote learning were not disseminated until several months into the pandemic – some of which rely on broader access to the Internet or televised educational programming as well as utilizing smartphone apps and similar outreach to more consistently communicate with children and families to track learning (Conto et al., 2020). Parents who felt less prepared to provide home schooling were more stressed, with many resorting to online materials outside of the official school system to provide their children structured activities (Adams et al., 2021; Lee et al., 2021a; Thorell et al., 2021).

Children, like all humans, tend to have reactions to sudden and seismic shifts in their lives. From their perspective, their lives had been turned upside down and continually shaken around like a snow globe as well. Children benefit from structure and routine and from school and socialization opportunities, but instead were similarly confined to their residences, electronic devices, and cut off from their peer support networks. Children also experience "Zoom fatigue." Yet, despite their developmental immaturity, children were expected to maintain attention and investment in their learning, overseen by parents and caregivers who were often simultaneously distracted by juggling work inside or (for workers considered "essential") outside the home. Children were expected to sustain their educational progress despite less structured environments that demanded greater focus and initiative to connect with typically virtual, less-engaging environments (Scarpellini et al., 2021). Many students increasingly disengaged with online learning over time (Spitzer et al., 2021). "Remote learning" became the new standard, but this sudden forced experiment with home schooling revealed that children's academic achievement soon lagged behind across subject areas, particularly for younger children, children who were struggling academically pre-pandemic, and children in lower-income families (Engzelli et al., 2021; Hammerstein et al., 2021).

The requirements for social distancing and fluctuating lockdowns dealt additional blows to caregivers and children. Although needed, these public health measures contributed to parents' social isolation as well as their inability to obtain respite from childcare as they lost access to babysitters and kinship care even beyond school and childcare center closures. These sudden alterations to children's school routines and seclusion at home prompted more mental health issues for children, particularly for older children, children of color, and children in lower-income families (Hawrilenko et al., 2021). Evidence has emerged that the pandemic heralded increased reports of behavior challenges and mental health problems among children and adolescents (Lee et al., 2021a; Patrick et al., 2020; Schmidt et al., 2021). The effects on children's behavior problems were magnified for adolescents and children with pre-pandemic mental health issues (Nearchou et al., 2020), indicating those who are already struggling with behavioral challenges need more immediate attention (Wong et al., 2020) when similar crises occur.

As the pandemic persisted through 2020 and into 2022, the waves of different COVID-19 strains rose and abated, and many parents were unsure how to engage in either short-term or long-term planning for their children, whether schools were safe, and whether they could or should return to work. Some systems have yet to return to pre-pandemic levels. For example, access to childcare remains problematic given the 9% decrease in childcare centers by 2022 in the USA alone (Leonhardt, 2022), which contributed to a disproportional drop in employment of formerly working mothers (Petts et al., 2021). Nations that do not provide parents access to reliable, affordable childcare will likely continue to experience economic impacts from forced closures in times of crisis.

Pregnancy, Delivery, and Fetal Risks

A key set of stressors for mothers in the pandemic have been the risks to pregnancy, delivery, and fetal development. The information and guidelines in these areas are still in development as research is accumulating, although a number of consistent findings have emerged (Subbaraman, 2022). Several large studies have found COVID-19-infected pregnant women had a more than 60% rate of intensive care unit (ICU) admission and a nearly 90% higher need for invasive ventilation than for their non-pregnant, same-age counterparts (Allotey et al., 2020; Zambrano et al., 2020). Pregnant women with COVID-19 also have a three times greater risk of preterm delivery, which can lead to infant health problems later on (Allotey et al., 2020). Persons of color may, unfortunately, be at greater risk for negative pregnancy outcomes, consistent with other health disparity research (Subbaraman, 2022). Pregnant women's mental health is known to be critically important and psychological difficulties among pregnant women are related to increased risk for preeclampsia, depression, preterm labor, low birth weight, and low APGAR scores (Ponti & Smorti, 2019; Smorti et al., 2019). The mental health of postpartum mothers is particularly vulnerable, given the challenges of adapting to sleep disruptions, new roles, and tasks involved in infant newborn care (Coates et al., 2014). The isolation and stress of the pandemic have only intensified these challenges for mothers. Further, pregnant women during the pandemic have unique challenges for their birth plans and recovery given the significant restrictions to the labor and delivery process, such as limitations on family visitors, birthing partners, and other support persons (Fernandes et al., 2021a). In February 2021, Dr. Wamser-Nanney gave birth very unexpectedly to her daughter Julia at 23 weeks, who, thankfully, survived. She can personally attest to the hardships of the COVID-19 restrictions for her labor and delivery experience, along with the ongoing pandemic restrictions during Julia's 5-month stay in the NICU (and then several additional months in the PICU in the Fall and Winter of 2021). The most difficult restriction was the intense isolation. Her other two daughters, parents, sisters, and grandparents were not even able to meet Julia until she was five months old and came home. These necessary restrictions have a very detrimental effect on pregnant women and new mothers, given the critical loss of social support.

Thankfully, there are some positive findings regarding COVID-19 and pregnancy. COVID-19 does not appear to lead to elevated incidence of stillbirth or slowed fetal development (Subbaraman, 2022). Vertical transmission of COVID-19 from mother to fetus also seems to be rare, which is protective against additional sickness and death among newborns (Edlow et al., 2020). Infants of mothers with active COVID-19 infections appear to be generally healthy at birth and in the following 6–8 weeks post-partum (Flaherman et al., 2021). Antibodies in the umbilical-cord blood of COVID positive mothers may even play a protective role for the newborn, although more research is needed in this area (Atyeo et al., 2021; Flannery et al., 2021). Vaccination of pregnant mothers against COVID-19 is also currently recommended, given that it appears to be a valuable protection of the mother and infant (Subbaraman, 2022).

Parental Mental Health

Given the enormity of the often adverse impacts of the pandemic, it is clear that humans worldwide are experiencing increases in psychological difficulties. Parents are, unsurprisingly, not exempt from this. The significant shifts in daily living and childcare outages and loss of parental supports have naturally led to increased psychological difficulties. Caregivers divorced from their support systems, and often faced with economic uncertainties, were struggling with social isolation and heightened stress levels (Perry et al., 2022). With elevated levels of adult depression and anxiety observed during the pandemic (Twenge & Joiner, 2021), parents reported substantial increases in their stress (Adams et al., 2021; Patrick et al., 2020) and numerous mental health concerns (Calvano et al., 2021; Lee et al., 2021a;

Wamser-Nanney et al., 2021). These psychological difficulties included an increase in sleep disturbances (Lin et al., 2021), eating disturbances (Avena et al., 2021; Linardon et al., 2022), and substance use problems (Avena et al., 2021; Gadermann et al., 2021). Parents have also reported lower levels of self-compassion, emotional awareness, and mindfulness in parenting behavior (Fernandes et al., 2021b). Given the death toll incurred by the pandemic (Verdery et al., 2020), many parents were also grieving the loss of loved ones. These challenges may also negatively impact parent-infant bonding and the parent-child relationship (Fernandes et al., 2021a; Viera et al., 2020).

To date, much of the research regarding parental mental health has been specific to mothers; however, fathers also likely negatively impacted. Mothers, however, may be at greatest risk: over one third of mothers of 0–18-month-old children met criteria for depression and anxiety during the first year of the pandemic alone (Cameron et al., 2020). Other research has found that clinical levels of stress, anxiety, and depressive symptoms have risen to over 80% among pregnant and postpartum mothers since the onset of the pandemic (Ahlers-Schmidt et al., 2020). These mental health risks occur not just in the postpartum period, but have also been found among pregnant women who have displayed less vigor, more anxiety, depression, and hostility than seen at pre-pandemic levels (Smorti et al., 2022). Although strong partner support has previously served as a buffer against negative mental health outcomes in pregnant women during pre-pandemic times, this protective factor does not appear as effective for women in the midst of the pandemic.

Increases in Family Violence

One of the disastrous effects of the pandemic's need for virtual confinement within the home was the increase in family violence that accompanied the escalating pressures on parents. Greater time spent at home posed a risk to some women and children when home was not necessarily a safe space. National surveys in the USA indicated aggression increased during the first months of the stay-at-home orders (Killgore et al., 2021). Rates of intimate partner violence (IPV) rose significantly during the pandemic (Boserup et al., 2020; Jetelina et al., 2020), and more parents endorsed increased stress and perceptions of feeling unsafe due to emotional and physical abuse (Gadermann et al., 2021). Further, these higher rates of IPV are concerning as they are inevitably accompanied by children witnessing more inter-partner conflict (Ferrara et al., 2021). In the context of the pandemic social restrictions, greater social support still buffered the adverse impact of IPV, consistent with pre-pandemic research (Raj et al., 2020). Use of smartphone apps (like the MyPlan app) designed for safety planning, resources, and mental health supports and services were leveraged during the pandemic as a means to reach and help victims even remotely.

Increased rates of family violence were not limited to IPV. Although official reports for child maltreatment dropped precipitously, unofficial accounts indicated an increase in maltreatment given that the key reporters to protective services who oversee children (educational, social service, medical, and mental health professionals; U.S. Department of Health and Human Services, 2021) suddenly lost access to children (Bullinger et al., 2021; Jonson-Reid et al., 2020; Rapoport et al., 2020). Increased family time at home resulted in greater need for parental monitoring and discipline, including more opportunities for parent-child conflict, including physical and psychological aggression (Connell & Strambler, 2021; Lawson et al., 2020; Sari et al., 2021) even controlling for pre-pandemic levels (Rodriguez et al., 2021). Furthermore, the pandemic wielded significant financial hardship that likely contributed to increased neglect of children's physical needs in terms of food, health, and safety (Bullinger et al., 2021). The economic blow to families from lost or reduced employment coincided for many with the loss of access to free and subsidized school meals (Schanzenbach & Pitts, 2020), contributing to potential neglect (Rodriguez et al., 2021). Indeed, parents' social isolation and economic stress led to greater aggressive and physically and emotionally neglectful parenting behaviors (Lee et al., 2021b).

Child and Adolescent Mental Health

Naturally, children and adolescents experienced similar increases in psychological difficulties with the onset of the pandemic, including affective and anxiety disorders (Tang et al., 2021; Zhou, 2020). Children and adolescents underwent, and are still undergoing, dramatic and negative changes to their lives, including their daily routines, learning environments, continuity of learning (with breaks and moves from in-person to online learning), health care, and missed life events (e.g., graduation ceremonies, vacations, family gatherings). Youth are also largely cut off from their peers and social networks, as well as valuable and enjoyable activities. Many have also faced the loss of loved ones, close friends, or other mentors (e.g., teachers) in their lives due to serious illness related to COVID-19 and in some cases death related to COVID-19 (Rapa et al., 2020). In 2021, the NIH reported that 1.5 million youth lost a primary or secondary caregiver during the pandemic, a number that has increased significantly since. The losses and fears faced by youth have been associated with anxiety and depression and exacerbation of current mental health issues (Singh et al., 2020). What we are calling "secondary effects" are those changes related to a system shift because of COVID-19, such as parents losing a job (e.g., many in the restaurant business were affected by this), lower family income, parents working from home resulting in environmental and relationship changes, and parents caring for other family members with COVID-19 and remaining in quarantine due to disease exposure or a loved one's illness (Mak et al., 2020).

Mental health professionals and organizations immediately recognized the risk that the pandemic posed for children's mental health and worked to advocate for resources devoted to aiding children and parents during this difficult time, including the APA. Collectively, many resources for parents, including coping strategies specific to COVID-19, psychoeducation, and ways to support learning and resiliency were developed. There were several "calls to action," including efforts to leverage lessons learned from prior public health crises and disasters (APA, 2020a, 2020b; Tang et al., 2021; Zhou, 2020). For example, Gruber et al. (2021) issued a call to action in caring for mental health during the pandemic, highlighting children's emotional and mental health as being at risk, and urging the need to care for at-risk youth. The APA also offered critical guidance for families via a COVID guidance hub. The Centers for Disease Control (CDC) developed guidance for parents to assist their youth in coping during COVID-19, which included psychoeducational materials related to COVID-19 stressors and life changes that can engender stress and psychological challenges for children.

Concerning Public Health Disparities

Yet some groups inequitably bore the brunt of the pandemic's impact. Emerging work has indicated that the impacts of the pandemic, similar to other adversities and traumatic events, appear to be more adverse for higher-risk sub-groups. For example, adolescents – particularly girls – acknowledged higher rates of depression and suicidality (Mayne et al., 2021). Manzar et al. (2021) observed that social media reports of suicide risk among adolescents increased significantly during periods of lockdown. Socioeconomically marginalized communities and communities of color were disproportionately confronted with the economic blow coupled with greater morbidity and mortality (Bottan et al., 2020; Fortuna et al., 2020), apart from facing grief from the volume of loss of life among loved ones. The pre-pandemic so-called "digital divide" became acutely problematic as millions struggled to attain and sustain reliable Internet access in a world suddenly expecting everyone to have equal online access. Youth from more economically disadvantaged families had more educational challenges, including a lack of educational resources to complete virtual learning such as reliable and speedy Internet access and electronic devices, as well as greater psychological symptoms (Gruber et al., 2021). Some resources were made available to provide under-resourced families with Internet access, laptops, and iPads for homeschooling, and although helpful, it is clear that these resources were not available to all families in need. Children of color particularly lost contact during the sudden transition to the "remote learning" experiment (Dorn et al., 2020; Francis & Weller, 2022). These youth may also lack access to "telehealth" and other virtual services. During periods of lockdown, children in low-income families often faced more isolation and could be more likely to face neglect, violence, or abuse (Bryant et al., 2020; Masonbrink & Hurley, 2020; Phelps & Sperry, 2020; Singh et al., 2020). Parents in low-income families were also disproportionately impacted by job insecurity and loss, followed by further stress on the family, and this could negatively impact their children (Singh et al., 2020). Rural communities as well experienced obstacles stemming from this digital divide (Esteban-Navarro et al., 2020). Continuing a connection outside the home thus proved challenging for many families, spotlighting the current infrastructure weaknesses that fail to ensure universal broadband access to a digital environment – a clear priority area to address proactively.

Additional groups also encountered unique challenges during the pandemic. Youth who are considered "gender minority" – youth who do not identify with their gender assigned at birth – also represent an at-risk group, as prior work has noted these individuals have higher levels of mental health problems and isolation (Bockting et al., 2013; Mak et al., 2020). This unfortunate reality remained true during the pandemic. Longitudinal research demonstrated that sexual and gender minorities demonstrated increased anxiety and depression symptoms with the onset of the pandemic compared to cisgender youth (Flentje et al., 2020; Perl et al., 2021), as well as poorer coping strategies (Krueger et al., 2021). Further, many transgender youth had poorer emotional status before the pandemic, which increased during the restrictions (Perl et al., 2021). Sexual and gender minority children who had found peer support at school were suddenly faced with home confinement, potentially within families who were substantially less supportive or even openly hostile (DeMulder et al., 2020).

Furthermore, parents of children with disabilities and special needs were particularly stressed responding to their children's behaviors (Siracusano et al., 2021). These parents were taxed in their efforts to adequately meet the needs of their children given prolonged, limited access to respite care and the expectations to oversee their education, often with insufficient support (Dickinson et al., 2021). Foster parents were also suddenly confronted with additional stress (Miller et al., 2020) disconnected from the welfare system supports while trying to provide their foster children with a sense of stability during a patently unstable era. Children in foster care were also identified as vulnerable to child maltreatment during the pandemic given the elevated stress on their caregivers (Wong et al., 2020).

Youth with prior existing mental health challenges were also at greater risk. This issue was worsened as many lost access, or at least in-person access, to needed mental health services. Not all children and adolescents were able or willing to engage in telehealth, which was detrimental to many children. For instance, Lantos et al. (2022) noted that mental health consumers who had lower visit rates during the start of the pandemic were at risk for suicidal ideation and attempts. Adolescents who were psychiatrically hospitalized also were at higher risk for suicidal ideation and cited stresses related to isolation during COVID-19 as being related to depression and suicidal thoughts (Thompson et al., 2021). Reinforcing screening efforts of pediatricians and teachers, and providing education about screening and its importance, may improve abilities to identify at risk adolescents. Additionally, encouraging health professionals at all levels to ask the "difficult" screening questions during telehealth visits can increase chances to identify adolescents experiencing suicidal ideation.

The Task Force Workgroup's Pandemic Response

Early in the pandemic in 2020, the APA formed an interdivisional task force including a workgroup focused on children, youth, and families. Our workgroup was formed during the first taskforce meeting, as the larger taskforce immediately recognized the need to understand and address the effect of the pandemic on children and families. Our group included just a few individuals who met virtually, with additional members joining the workgroup over time and others discontinuing their involvement. Since May 2020, the primary focus of our workgroup has been to collect and distribute COVID-19-related resources aimed at children, caregivers, and families as well as child- and family-serving professionals. We remain particularly concerned about the adverse impact of the pandemic on certain sub-groups who may be more vulnerable- specifically young children, trauma-exposed children, families with limited resources and prior mental health challenges, and under-served families and communities. We recognized that the public health efforts to curb the transmission of COVID-19 are paramount in preventing the spread of the disease, yet these guidelines have had a tremendous negative impact on caregivers and families as discussed. We have worked to gather resources to address these various impacts including the loss of childcare, closures of schools and other child-oriented activities, transitions to virtual or e-learning, and isolation from family members, friends, and childcare providers who help with childcare and ease the burdens of parenthood. We established a regularly updated Google Drive with links to "webinars" (live-streamed or pre-recorded); websites with online resource materials; and public guidance from government agencies, all designed to be relevant for children, adolescents, and families. Such resources were circulated through workgroup members' social networks and professional listservs in an effort to advise those still working with children, youth, and families as well as to reach the public directly. We also established a Facebook page along with other social media outlets to further disseminate resources and news stories pertinent to families.

As the pandemic continued into the 2020–2021 academic year, it became clear that many children were struggling with remote learning, particularly young children and those with attentional challenges and academic delays. Supporting children with schoolwork became an additional conflict issue for many caregivers, struggles which are more pronounced among families from underserved communities. We therefore worked to provide guidance to families about how to allocate special times and spaces for children to work – an important topic posted on our social media accounts. Helping parents decide whether to return their child to school upon reopening or continue at-home learning has been another key topic area. Such decisions are often complicated. For example, for those children losing ground in learning required skills where the school is safe, a return to school may be best. However, vulnerable adults may also live in the home, where a return to school could pose too much risk of exposure to illness. Teens struggling with isolation and depression symptoms may need alternative safe reunions with friends. Some families crafted "bubbles" where several families of similar age children agreed to only interact with each other and avoid interactions outside the bubble to lower the infection risk. Other families set up special "schools" in outdoor spaces during the warm weather. Again, making these decisions was challenging for many families, and we attempted to provide decision trees to assist parents as they contemplate their options.

A prime focus of our workgroup has been to understand what was happening to children who were living in homes, who could be struggling not only academically but psychologically as well. For example, the risk of unreported child abuse and neglect rose given children were experiencing substantially fewer contacts outside the home who might notice their bruises or malnutrition. We interfaced with the COVID Hospital Workers workgroup to distribute a *Psychology Today* blog about this pressing concern, which was selected to receive special attention given its important message to help parents and children deescalate tensions and endure the pandemic. That blog post also provided an additional avenue to disseminate links to resources for families and the professionals working with them. Our workgroup also collaborates with the COVID IPV workgroup to offer roundtables to provide guidance to professionals and the public to help protect children who are often unseen victims of the pandemic. As schools reopen and communities return to the streets, recognizing a child in need of help and how to best to offer that support is important for the general public as well as child.

We also quickly learned that even in instances where both parents shifted to working from home and participated in child care, the heaviest burden fell on mothers. As noted above, by the end of the first year, evidence emerged that women's employment suffered the greatest workforce decline across all sociodemographic groups, especially women with career aspirations. Many employment positions disappeared, and women were among the first to be eliminated, particularly for women of color. For working mothers juggling caring for children while working from home, we are just beginning to understand the toll on the advances women have made in the workplace. When families struggled, mothers reduced their work hours. As the post-pandemic era approaches, the workgroup has incorporated suggestions to help women not lose that workforce progress by connecting with other APA groups such as those in Division 35, The Society for Women.

Parents sought ideas on how to manage a rise in child behavior problems (with resources provided through the Centers for Disease Control and Prevention [CDC]) as well as guidance on how to communicate in developmentally appropriate ways about the pandemic and its repercussions (with task force links to videos from the CDC as well as the Annenberg Learner). We provided links to the National Child Traumatic Stress Network (NCTSN) that had resources for parents and children dealing with trauma. Workgroup members interfaced with other task force workgroups to lead relevant discussions on those groups' webinar series or to craft articles to post as blog entries to widen the reach to an audience seeking guidance about issues facing children and families. Videos directed parents to best practices in remote learning and provided guidance for scheduling children's activities, including suggestions on lesson planning and links to educational content. Special materials and resources were provided for families with children with intellectual and/or developmental disabilities. Foster parents were offered resources developed by Healthy Foster Care America. New updates on the public health crises from the CDC were linked through the workgroup's connections to disseminate guidance on evolving pandemic health risks.

Telemental Health

Connections to online mental health resources for self-help were provided for parents to address their own mental health needs as well as to identify the mental health concerns experienced by their children. Apart from webinars and written materials, one of the notable beneficial outcomes of the pandemic was the escalated transition to telemental health, with an exponential increase in the utilization of telehealth particularly among behavioral health providers (Suran, 2022). Although equity issues from the digital divide remain with regard to ensuring reliable Internet access in order to readily utilize such services, progress was made during the pandemic to enable greater public access to care overall. Many mental health organizations have scaled up to ensure opportunities for telemental health beyond the pandemic (Molfenter et al., 2021). Ensuring privacy within the home setting remains a challenge that mental health professionals need to monitor when delivering services to parents and/or children given that delivery of services in the home could foreseeably limit dialogue. These privacy issues are particularly challenging when addressing family violence concerns. Given the workgroup's ability to communicate directly to mental health professionals, the latter became a conduit for disseminating materials and identifying the evolving concerns of families. It is important that youth with mental health problems were able to access telehealth and support during the pandemic, as without support suicide attempts could escalate. However, during telehealth visits with adolescents, screening opportunities could be missed, and it remains critical for mental health care providers to be aware of the need to assess depression and screen for suicidal ideation during telehealth appointments (Lantos et al., 2022).

Throughout this process, we also have provided COVID-19-related resources to support professionals who are working with children, caregivers, and families affected by the pandemic. Apart from the roundtables and blog posts noted above, we maintain a listing of resources that are referenced in the blog post and on social media Facebook and Twitter accounts. This compendium of resources includes mental health resources parents can utilize to identify concerns in their children and ideas for how to offer support; mental health support resources for parents; downloadable pandemic-related children's books; and relevant webinars for families and/or family-serving professionals. We also provide guidance on how we arrived at our resources and what obstacles we encountered in disseminating them, including how we resolved them.

Challenges and Lessons Learned

Some of our hardships have been to recruit a sufficient workforce for the workgroup. Given that everyone is facing challenges with the pandemic, it has been difficult for our group to have sufficient work capacity to promote our efforts. Another challenge has been to reach the more vulnerable groups we are attempting to target. We also have noted that many families have become inundated with fact sheets, resources, and webinars. What families really need are concrete resources: time, money, and childcare. We are empathic to these needs, but are unable to provide families with these supports. In terms of our lessons learned, we have seen the value in not duplicating efforts and working with other related groups as mentioned. We quickly realized not to spend our limited workgroup capacity time developing new resources, but to work to disseminate the valuable resources that were already in existence. We have also tried to leverage existing groups and platforms to reach larger audiences. We continued to build on these efforts, increasing our reach to children, families, and child-serving professionals to learn about and disseminate the emerging guidelines of professional practice that are consistent with the major professional organizations serving this population.

Among the greatest challenges the workgroup faced was identifying additional avenues to interface with the public in an effort to expand its reach. Using social media platforms was useful but required routine updating from workgroup members who were simultaneously managing their own escalating demands during the pandemic (as were the mental health professionals with whom the workgroup was communicating). Similar to other sectors across the globe, workgroup members turned to videoconferencing to problem solve and identify new strategies to widen its reach. Such videoconferencing represents another advantageous approach that gained in popularity at the outset of the pandemic, also enabling the very webinars the group sought to publicize. Yet finding times to meet as a workgroup was challenging for many of the working parents in the workgroup who were faced with the same juggling responsibilities as the families the group sought to reach – resulting in briefer video meetings. Establishment of rapid-response teams that can meet for short periods to efficiently identify needs during a crisis could be formed pre-crisis, similar to other emergency response systems.

On the one hand, the Internet represented an opportunity to reach more families who were often confined to their homes for protracted periods of time. On the other hand, many families were cut off from the schools, workplaces, and medical settings that they had relied upon to gain additional resources and supports. Setting up more interconnected networks across systems of care could provide more nodes of access for families to connect in times of crisis. When families have multiple points of contact through educational, health, and social service professionals, they have pre-existing contacts that can be more readily tapped during periods of global crises. By interconnecting across systems of care, reaching families may become more efficient so that resources can be more quickly and widely disseminated.

Children in low income families may not have Internet access or computers, effectively "shutting off" their access to educational opportunities (Phelps & Sperry, 2020). If educators could reach out, by dropping off books and homework packets to homes, this had the potential to help these children access educational opportunities during periods of lockdown. Mental health providers can play a vital role in guiding teachers, pediatricians, and nurses to ask about and assess adverse experiences to screen for indicators of trauma may assist in appropriate referrals (Bryant et al., 2020). Ensuring that preventive and crisis services are provided online, free of charge, may be another way that mental health providers can assist children and adolescents residing in low-income families where there is a computer and Internet access. Developing short messages for delivery via cellular telephone is another way to improve "mental health messaging." Moreover, ensuring that educators and health professionals learn strategies to enhance resilience and social support for children also will improve feelings of well-being in children as they face adversity related to COVID-19. Because sexual minority, transgender, and nonconforming youth, and especially those with multiple mental health concerns, are at high risk for suicide and significant emotional stress, they are a risk group to identify for outreach and support during times of crisis (Mak et al., 2020). Providing outreach via online support groups, monitored by a behavioral health specialist, is one idea for ensuring outreach to the vulnerable group to increase their support during times of isolation.

If future crises strike, several predictable issues are critical for professionals to monitor given the world witnessed how intricately societal structures and supports are interwoven and thus vulnerable to collapse. The lessons of the COVID-19 pandemic can inform proactive efforts to diversify and interconnect the infrastructure of supports for children and families so that new global challenges do not repeat the chaos that unfolded at the start of this decade. When the COVID-19 pandemic was initially recognized worldwide in early 2020, parents were suddenly confronted by an unprecedented escalation in their daily demands that the existing infrastructure was ill equipped to support. As discussed, supporting parents and child-serving professionals was a key focus of the APA Children and Families Task Force. We worked to compile and disseminate psychoeducation, resources, and strategies to facilitate resilient outcomes among children and adolescents during the pandemic and we hope that these efforts were helpful. We largely worked to provide resources electronically through social media platforms, specifically Facebook and Twitter. However, we worried about reach.

The pandemic is a significant adversity for many youth. It is important to work to help promote healing among those who are significantly struggling as well as enhance resiliency. It is vital to allow children to feel connected to family and friends and build on their resilience factors to improve social and emotional functioning. Children need to discuss and understand what is happening, in relation to their school functioning, involvement in activities, family relationships, extended family, and key life events (e.g., graduation, holidays) in their lives. Encouraging youth to share feelings, and providing a safe space for expressing worries and concerns for one's health and the family's health, provides a means for supporting youth as they share about how the pandemic frightens and saddens them, and how it has changed their lives (Rapa et al., 2020; Spuij et al., 2015). Providing them with a safe space to explore feelings and what they see in the world helps them express emotions and understand how the pandemic is influencing their life course and that of their family. Helping them integrate this experience will help them develop their life stories around and through the effects of the pandemic on their personal worlds. Rates of mental health problems have increased, some may even say sky-rocketed, as a result of the anxiety and depression associated with experiencing COVID-19's impact of their lives and that of family and close friends. Thus, this is a critical public health concern.

Advocating for children, and bringing their issues to the fore, may improve attention to their mental health and their needs for feeling safe and expressing their fears and concerns during a pandemic, such as COVID-19 (Masonbrink & Hurley, 2020). Youth and their families may benefit from "psychological first aid" to provide support to the child and family (p. 8, Singh et al., 2020). Instrumental support, consisting of food and funds for rent and gas and utilities may "lift" spirits of parents, and children, and have a positive effect in slowly improving family conditions and lifting burdens for the child and family. The NCTSN offers a wealth of information and guidance for identifying and helping children cope with trauma.

Lessons Learned in Providing Telehealth Mental Health Services

As discussed, during the lockdown and its aftermath, mental health services have been delivered online. Telemental health, in many ways, has been a new frontier in delivery of all types of health services, and has great potential for the delivery of mental health services (Cain et al., 2016; see Hilty et al., 2017 for a review of competencies). We are still learning how to most efficiently and effectively provide online psychological services, and we describe some of the "lessons learned" from our group.

The APA offered important "tips" for successful telehealth with children. For instance, it is important to initially explain how the telehealth session will work in a developmentally appropriate manner. Therapists may also allow the child to share items from home and drawing with the child during sessions may help build rapport and engage the child (Martinez et al., 2021). The relaxed nature of being at home can also make it difficult to maintain the therapeutic atmosphere. Children may be difficult to engage in teletherapy, as they can become distracted by other sites on the Internet (e.g., games, surfing the web) or, if the session is "in their room," by toys and fun things to do. If they are in a room where they can hear family and pets, noise and other interactions can distract them. It may be appropriate to consider shorter sessions, or inviting parents to sessions to work as a team to help the child focus and discuss critical issues during the therapy session. Privacy can be an issue, as if rooms are "open" or others can walk in they can hear conversations and this can endanger the confidential nature of sessions. Practical recommendations include reducing noise at the clinician's site, avoiding (if possible) taking notes during sessions, and ensuring that the clinician knows of emergency contacts a client can access, if the client is in another state (Martinez et al., 2021). In telemental health sessions, therapists should also screen parental emotional functioning, being ready to speak with parents privately and refer them for mental health services as necessary. Similarly, therapists should be attuned to signs of abuse of neglect of children and make appropriate contacts with protective services, when children are at risk.

In the future, translating short-term, evidence-based therapies for delivery as teletherapies, with careful consideration for reaching youth in low-income families to ensure they can access care, will improve abilities to provide mental health services via the web and through existing technologies to youth during crises (Singh et al., 2020). Mental health professionals have opportunities to be leaders in helping the world recover from the negative impact of the pandemic. We can educate teachers, parents, and health care providers about the importance of allowing children and adolescents to express feelings, teach anxiety-coping strategies (e.g., relaxation, meditation, breathing), feel safe, achieve a sense of security, and promote resilient functioning, increasing social support and stressing child strengths that facilitate positive child functioning (e.g., having a mentor, involvement in sports, strong, positive peer relationships, practicing relaxation techniques, having hobbies, being involved in extracurricular activities, involvement, and personal interests) (Alvord & Grados, 2005; Richards et al., 2016). We hope that our efforts to aid children and families during the COVID-19 pandemic have been of some benefit as well as that, in the event of future disasters, our struggles and lessons learned can be leveraged to better support the psychological functioning of children, parents, and families.

References

Alvord, M. K., & Grados, J. J. (2005). Enhancing resilience in children: A proactive approach. *Professional Psychology: Research and Practice, 36*(3), 238 –245. https://doi.org/10.1037/0735-7028.36.3.238

American Psychological Association (APA) (2020a). *COVID-19*. Retrieved from https://www.apa.org/topics/covid-19

American Psychological Association (APA). (2020b). *COVID-19 telehealth and children*. Retrieved from https://www.apa.org/topics/covid-19/telehealth-children.

Adams, E. L., Smith, D., Caccavale, L. J., & Bean, M. K. (2021). Parents are stressed! Patterns of parent stress across COVID-19. *Frontiers in Psychiatry, 12*, 300. https://doi.org/10.3389/fpsyt.2021.626456

Ahlers-Schmidt, C., Hervey, A., Neil, T., Kuhlmann, S., & Kuhlmann, Z. (2020). Concerns of women regarding pregnancy and childbirth during the COVID-19 pandemic. *Patient Education and Counseling, 103*(12), 2578–2582. https://doi.org/10.1016/j.pec.2020.09.031

Allotey, J., Stallings, E., Bonet, M., Yap, M., Chatterjee, S., Kew, T., et al. (2020). Clinical manifestations, risk factors, and maternal and perinatal outcomes of coronavirus disease 2019 in pregnancy: Living systematic review and meta-analysis. *British Medical Journal, 370*, m3320. https://doi.org/10.1136/bmj.m3320

Atyeo, C., Pullen, K. M., Bordt, E. A., Fischinger, S., Burke, J., Michell, A., Slein, M. D., Loos, C., Shook, L. L., Boatin, A. A., Yockey, L. J., Pepin, D., Meinsohn, M. C., Nguyen, N., Chauvin, M., Roberts, D., Goldfarb, I. T., Matute, J. D., James, K. E., Yonker, L. M., et al. (2021). Compromised SARS-CoV-2-specific placental antibody transfer. *Cell, 184*(3), 628–642.e10. https://doi.org/10.1016/j.cell.2020.12.027

Avena, N. M., Simkus, J., Lewandowski, A., Gold, M. S., & Potenza, M. N. (2021). Substance use disorders and behavioral addictions during the COVID-19 pandemic and COVID-19-related restrictions. *Frontiers in Psychiatry, 12*, 7. https://doi.org/10.3389/fpsyt.2021.653674

Bockting, W. O., Miner, M. H., Swinburne Romine, R. E., Hamilton, A., & Coleman, E. (2013). Stigma, mental health, and resilience in an online sample of the US transgender population. *American Journal of Public Health, 103*(5), 943–951. https://doi.org/10.2105/AJPH.2013.301241

Boserup, B., McKenney, M., & Elkbuli, A. (2020). Alarming trends in US domestic violence during the COVID-19 pandemic. *American Journal of Emergency Medicine, 38*, 2753–2755. https://doi.org/10.1016/j.ajem.2020.04.077

Bottan, N., Hoffmann, B., & Vera-Cossio, D. (2020). The unequal impact of the coronavirus pandemic: Evidence from seventeen developing countries. *PLoS One, 15*, e0239797. https://doi.org/10.1371/journal.pone.0239797

Bryant, D. J., Oo, M., & Damian, A. J. (2020). The rise of adverse childhood experiences during the COVID-19 pandemic. *Psychological Trauma: Theory, Research, Practice, and Policy, 12*(S1), S193–S194. https://doi.org/10.1037/tra0000711

Bullinger, L. R., Raissian, K. M., Feely, M., & Schneider, W. J. (2021). The neglected ones: Time at home during COVID-19 and child maltreatment. *Children and Youth Services Review, 131*, 12. https://doi.org/10.1016/j.childyouth.2021.106287

Cain, S., Nelson, E.-L., & Myers, K. (2016). Telemental health. In M. K. Dulcan (Ed.), *Dulcan's textbook of child and adolescent psychiatry* (pp. 669–688). American Psychiatric Publishing, Inc.. https://doi.org/10.1176/appi.books.9781615370306.md33

Calvano, C., Engelke, L., Di Bella, J., Kindermann, J., Rennenberg, B., & Winter, S. M. (2021). Families in the COVID-19 pandemic: Parental stress, parent mental health and the occurrence of adverse childhood experiences: Results of a representative survey in Germany. *European Child & Adolescent Psychiatry*. Advance Online Publication. https://doi.org/10.1007/s00787-021-01739-0

Cameron, E., Joyce, K., Delaquis, C., Reynolds, K., Protudjer, J., & Roos, L. E. (2020). Maternal psychological distress & mental health services use during the COVID-19 pandemic. *Journal of Affective Disorders, 276*, 765–774. https://doi.org/10.1016/j.jad.2020.07.081

Coates, R., Ayers, S., & de Visser, R. (2014). Women's experiences of postnatal distress: A qualitative study. *BMC Pregnancy and Childbirth, 14*(1), 359. https://doi.org/10.1186/1471-2393-14-359

Connell, C. M., & Strambler, M. J. (2021). Experiences with COVID-19 stressors and parents' use of neglectful, harsh, and positive parenting practices in the northeastern United States. *Child Maltreatment, 26*, 255–266. https://doi.org/10.1177/10775595211006465

Conto, C. A., Akseer, S., Dreesen, T., Kamei, A., Mizunoya, S., & Rigole, A. (2020). *COVID-19: Effects of school closures on foundational skills and promising practices for monitoring and mitigating learning loss*. UNICEF Office of Research. Retrieved from www.unicef-irc.org/publications/pdf/COVID-19_Effects_of_School_Closures_on_Foundational_Skills_and_Promising_Practices_for_Monitoring_and_Mitigating_Learning_Loss.pdf

Correll, S. J., Benard, S., & Paik, I. (2007). Getting a job: Is there a motherhood penalty? *American Journal of Sociology, 112*, 1297–1339. https://doi.org/10.1086/511799

DeMulder, J., Kraus-Perrotta, C., & Zaidi, H. (2020). Sexual and gender minority adolescents must be prioritised during the global COVID-19 public health response. *Sexual and Reproductive Health Matters, 28*, 1804717. https://doi.org/10.1080/26410397.2020.180471

Dickinson, H., Smith, C., Yates, S., & Tani, M. (2021). The importance of social supports in education: Survey findings from students with disability and their families during covid-19. *Disability & Society*. https://doi.org/10.1080/09687599.2021.1994371

Donohue, J. M., & Miller, E. (2020). COVID-19 and school closures. *JAMA, 324*, 845–847. https://doi.org/10.1001/jama.2020.13092

Dorn, E., Hancock, B., Sarakatsannis, J., & Viruleg, E. (2020). *COVID-19 and learning loss—disparities grow and students need help*. Retrieved from https://www.mckinsey.com/industries/public-and-social-sector/our-insights/covid-19-and-learning-loss-disparities-grow-and-students-need-help?cid=eml-web.

Edlow, A. G., Li, J. Z., Collier, A. Y., et al. (2020). Assessment of maternal and neonatal SARS-CoV-2 viral load, transplacental antibody transfer, and placental pathology in pregnancies during the COVID-19 pandemic. *JAMA Network Open., 3*(12), e2030455. https://doi.org/10.1001/jamanetworkopen.2020.30455

Engzelli, P., Frey, A., & Verhagen, M. D. (2021). Learning loss due to school closures during the COVID-19 pandemic. *PNAS, 118*, e2022376118. https://doi.org/10.1073/pnas.2022376118

Esteban-Navarro, M., Garcia-Madurga, M., Morte-Nadal, T., & Nogales-Bocio, A. (2020). The rural Digital Divide in the face of the COVID-19 pandemic in Europe: Recommendations from a scoping review. *Informatics, 7*, 54. https://doi.org/10.3390/informatics7040054

Ferrara, P., Franceschini, G., Corsello, G., Mestrovic, J., Giardino, I., Vural, M., et al. (2021). Children witnessing domestic and family violence: A widespread occurrence during the Coronavirus disease 2019 (COVID-19) pandemic. *Journal of Pediatrics, 235*, 305–306. https://doi.org/10.1016/j.jpeds.2021.04.071

Flentje, A., Obedin-Maliver, J., Lubensky, M. E., Dastur, Z., Neilands, T., & Lunn, M. R. (2020). Depression and anxiety changes among sexual and gender minority people coinciding with onset of COVID-19 pandemic. *Journal of General Internal Medicine, 35*, 2788–2790. https://doi.org/10.1007/s11606-020-05970-4

Fortuna, L. R., Tolou-Shams, M., Robles-Ramamurthy, B., & Porche, M. V. (2020). Inequity and the disproportionate impact of COVID-19 on communities of color in the United States: The need for a trauma-informed social justice response. *Psychological Trauma: Theory, Research, Practice, and Policy, 12*, 443–445. https://doi.org/10.1037/tra0000889

Francis, D. V., & Weller, C. E. (2022). Economic inequality, the Digital Divide, and remote learning during COVID-19. *Review of Black Political Economy, 49*, 41–60. https://doi.org/10.1177/00346446211017797

Francom, G. M., Lee, S. J., & Pinkney, H. (2021). Technologies, challenges and needs of K-12 teachers in the transition to distance learning during the COVID-19 pandemic. *TechTrends, 54*, 589–601. https://doi.org/10.1007/s11528-021-00625-5

Fernandes, D. V., Canavarro, M. C., & Moreira, H. (2021a). Postpartum during COVID-19 pandemic: Portuguese mothers' mental health, mindful parenting, and mother–infant bonding. *Journal of Clinical Psychology, 77*, 1997–2010.

Fernandes, D. V., Canavarro, M. C., & Moreira, H. (2021b). The role of mothers' self-compassion on mother–infant bonding during the COVID-19 pandemic: A longitudinal study exploring the mediating role of mindful parenting and parenting stress in the postpartum period. *Infant Mental Health Journal, 42*, 621–635.

Flaherman, V. J., Afshar, Y., Boscardin, W. J., Keller, R. L., Mardy, A. H., Prahl, M. K., Phillips, C. T., Asiodu, I. V., Berghella, V., Chambers, B. D., Crear-Perry, J., Jamieson, D. J., Jacoby, V. L., & Gaw, S. L. (2021). Infant outcomes following maternal infection with severe acute respiratory syndrome Coronavirus 2 (SARS-CoV-2): First report from the Pregnancy Coronavirus Outcomes Registry (PRIORITY) study. *Clinical Infectious Diseases, 73*(9), 1, e2810–1, e2813. https://doi.org/10.1093/cid/ciaa1411

Flannery, D. D., Gouma, S., Dhudasia, M. B., et al. (2021). Assessment of maternal and neonatal cord blood SARS-CoV-2 antibodies and placental transfer ratios. *JAMA Pediatrics, 175*(6), 594–600. https://doi.org/10.1001/jamapediatrics.2021.0038

Gadermann, A. C., Thomson, K. C., Richardson, C. G., Gagne, M., McAuliff, C., Hirani, S., & Jenkins, E. (2021). Examining the impacts of the COVID-19 pandemic on family mental health in Canada: Findings from a national cross-sectional study. *BMJ Open, 11*, e0432871. https://doi.org/10.1136/bmjopen-2020-042871

Gassman-Pines, A., & Gennetian, L. A. (2020). COVID-19 job and income loss jeopardize child well-being: Income support policies can help. *Society for Research in Child Development*, https://www.srcd.org/sites/default/files/resources/FINAL_SRCDCEB-JobLoss.pdf

Gruber, J., Prinstein, M. J., Clark, L. A., Rottenberg, J., Abramowitz, J. S., Albano, A. M., Aldao, A., Borelli, J. L., Chung, T., Davila, J., Forbes, E. E., Gee, D. G., Hall, G., Hallion, L. S., Hinshaw, S. P., Hofmann, S. G., Hollon, S. D., Joormann, J., Kazdin, A. E., Klein, D. N., … Weinstock, L. M. (2021). Mental health and clinical psychological science in the time of COVID-19: Challenges, opportunities, and a call to action. *American Psychologist, 76*(3), 409–426. https://doi.org/10.1037/amp0000707

Hammerstein, S., Konig, C., Dreisorner, T., & Frey, A. (2021). Effects of COVID-19-related school closures on student achievement: A systematic review. *Frontiers in Psychology, 12*, 746289. https://doi.org/10.3389/fpsyg.2021.746289

Hawrilenko, M., Kroshus, E., Tandon, P., & Christaki, D. (2021). The association between school closures and child mental health during COVID-19. *JAMA Network Open, 4*, e2124092. https://doi.org/10.1001/jamanetworkopen.2021.24092

Hilty, D. M., Maheu, M. M., Drude, K. P., Hertlein, K. M., Wall, K., Long, R. P., & Luoma, T. L. (2017). Telebehavioral health, telemental health, e-Therapy and e-Health competencies: the need for an interprofessional framework. *Journal of Technology in Behavioral Science, 2*(3), 171–189. https://doi.org/10.1007/s41347-017-0036-0

International Labor Organization (2021). ILO Monitor: COVID-19 and the world of work, Seventh edition. Retrieved from https://www.ilo.org/wcmsp5/groups/public/---dgreports/---dcomm/documents/briefingnote/wcms_767028.pdf

Jetelina, K. K., Knell, G., & Molsberry, R. J. (2020). Changes in intimate partner violence during the early stages of the COVID-19 pandemic in the USA. *Injury Prevention, 27*. https://doi.org/10.1136/injuryprev-2020-043831

Jonson-Reid, M., Drake, B., Cobetto, C., & Ocampo, M. G. (2020, April 14). *Child abuse prevention month in the context of Covid-19*. Washington University Center for Innovation in Child Maltreatment Policy, Research and Training.

Kashen, J., Glynn, S. J., & Novello, A. (2020). *How COVID-19 sent women's workforce progress backward*. Center for American Progress. Retrieved from https://www.americanprogress.org/article/covid-19-sent-womens-workforce-progress-backward/.

Killgore, W. D. S., Cloonan, S. A., Taylor, E. C., Anlap, I., & Dailey, N. S. (2021). Increasing aggression during the COVID-19 lockdowns. *Journal of Affective Disorders Reports, 5*, 100163. https://doi.org/10.1016/j.jadr.2021.100163

Kmec, J. A. (2011). Are motherhood penalties and fatherhood bonuses warranted? Comparing pro-work behaviors and conditions of mothers, fathers, and non-parents. *Social Science Research, 40*(2), 444–459. https://doi.org/10.1016/j.ssresearch.2010.11.006

Kochnar, R. (2020, June 11). *Unemployment rose higher in three months of Covid-19 than it did in two years of the Great Recession*. https://www.pewresearch.org/facttank/2020/06/11/unemployment-rose-higher-in-three-months-of-covid-19-than-it-did-in-two-years-of-the-great-recession/

Krueger, E. A., Barrington-Trimis, J., Unger, J. B., & Leventhal, A. M. (2021). Sexual and gender minority young adult coping disparities during the COVID-19 pandemic. *Journal of Adolescent Health, 69*, 746–753. https://doi.org/10.1016/j.jadohealth.2021.07.021

Lambert, L. (2020, May 28). Over 40 million Americans have filed for unemployment during the pandemic-real jobless rate over 23.9%. *Fortune*. https://fortune.com/2020/05/28/us-unemployment-rate-numbers-claims-this-weektotal-job-losses-may-28-2020-benefits-claims-job-losses/

Landivar, L. C., Ruppanner, L., Scarborough, W. J., & Collins, C. (2020). Early signs indicate that COVID-19 is exacerbating gender inequality in the labor force. *Socius, 6*, 1–3. https://doi.org/10.1177/2378023120947997

Lantos, J. D., Yeh, H. W., Raza, F., Connelly, M., Goggin, K., & Sullivant, S. A. (2022). Suicide risk in adolescents during the CoViD-19 pandemic. *Pediatrics, 149*(2), 7 pages. Article e2021053486. https://doi.org/10.1542/peds.2021-053486

Lawson, M., Piel, M. H., & Simon, M. (2020). Child maltreatment during the COVID-19 pandemic: Consequences of parental job loss on psychological and physical abuse towards children. *Child Abuse & Neglect, 110*, 104709. https://doi.org/10.1016/j.chiabu.2020.104709

Lee, S. J., Ward, K. P., Chang, O. D., & Downing, K. D. (2021a). Parenting activities and the transition to home-based education during the COVID-19 pandemic. *Children and Youth Services Review, 122*. 105585. https://doi.org/10.1016/j.childyouth.2020.105585

Lee, S. J., Ward, K. P., Lee, J. Y., & Rodriguez, C. M. (2021b). Parental social isolation and child maltreatment risk during a pandemic. *Journal of Family Violence*. Online First: https://doi.org/10.1007/s10896-020-00244-3

Leonhardt, M. (2022, Feb 9). 16,000 childcare providers shut down in the pandemic. It's a really big deal. *Fortune*. https://fortune.com/2022/02/09/child-care-providers-shut-down-pandemic/

Lin, Y. N., Liu, Z. R., Li, S. Q., Li, C. X., Zhang, L., Li, N., Sun, X. W., Li, H. P., Zhou, J. P., & Li, Q. Y. (2021). Burden of sleep disturbance during COVID-19 pandemic: A systematic review. *Nature and Science of Sleep, 13*, 933–966. https://doi.org/10.2147/NSS.S312037

Linardon, J., Messer, M., Rodgers, R. F., & Fuller-Tyszkiewicz, M. (2022). A systematic scoping review of research on COVID-19 impacts on eating disorders: A critical appraisal of the evidence and recommendations for the field. *International Journal of Eating Disorders, 55*, 3–38. https://doi.org/10.1002/eat.23640

Livingston, G., & Parker, K. (2019). *8 facts about American dads*. Pew Research Center. Retrieved from https://www.pewresearch.org/fact-tank/2019/06/12/fathers-day-facts/

Mak, J., Shires, D. A., Zhang, Q., Prieto, L. R., Ahmedani, B. K., Kattari, L., Becerra-Culqui, T. A., Bradlyn, A., Flanders, W. D., Getahun, D., Giammattei, S. V., Hunkeler, E. M., Lash, T. L., Nash, R., Quinn, V. P., Robinson, B., Roblin, D., Silverberg, M. J., Slovis, J., Tangpricha, V., … Goodman, M. (2020). Suicide Attempts Among a Cohort of Transgender and Gender Diverse People. *American Journal of Preventive Medicine, 59*(4), 570–577. https://doi.org/10.1016/j.amepre.2020.03.026

Manzar, M. D., Albougami, A., Usman, N., & Mamun, M. A. (2021). Suicide among adolescents and youths during the COVID-19 pandemic lockdowns: A press media reports-based exploratory study. *Journal of child and adolescent psychiatric nursing, 34*(2), 139–146.

Martinez, R. G., Seager, I., van Dyk, J. L., Kroll, N. D., & Bursch, B. (2021). Recommendations for building telemental health relationships with youth: A systematic review and resource for clinicians. Evidence-Based Practice in Child and Adolescent Mental Health, Ahead of Print, Article: 1970050, 14 pages. https://doi.org/uc.idm.oclc.org/10.1080/23794925.2021.1970050

Masonbrink, A. R., & Hurley, E. (2020). Advocating for children during the COVID-19 school closures. *Pediatrics, 146*(3). e20201440. https://doi.org/10.1542/peds.2020-1440

Mayne, S. L., Hannan, C., Davis, M., Young, J. F., Kelly, M. K., Powell, M., Dalembert, G., McPeak, K. E., Jenssen, B. P., & Fiks, A. G. (2021). COVID-19 and adolescent depression and suicide risk screening outcomes. *Pediatrics, 148*(3), e2021051507, 11 pages. https://doi.org/10.1542/peds.2021-051507

Miller, C. C. (2020). Nearly half of men say they do most of the home schooling; 3 percent of women agree. *The New York Times*. Retrieved from https://www.nytimes.com/2020/05/06/upshot/pandemic-chores-homeschooling-gender.html

Miller, J. J., Cooley, M. E., & Mihalec-Adkins, B. (2020). Examining the impact of covid-19 on parental stress: A study of foster parents. *Child & Adolescent Social Work Journal, 39*, 147–156. https://doi.org/10.1007/s10560-020-00725-w

Molfenter, T., Heitkamp, T., Murphy, A. A., Tapscott, S., Behlman, S., & Cody, O. J. (2021). Use of telehealth in mental health (mh) services during and after covid-19. *Community Mental Health Journal, 57*, 1244–1251. https://doi.org/10.1007/s10597-021-00861-2

Nearchou, F., Flinn, C., Niland, R., Subramaniam, S. S., & Hennessy, E. (2020). Exploring the impact of COVID-19 on mental health outcomes in children and adolescents: A systematic review. *International Journal of Environmental Research and Public Health, 17*, 8479. https://doi.org/10.3390/ijerph17228479

Patrick, S. W., Henkhaus, L. E., Zickafoose, J. S., Lovell, K., Halvorson, A., Loch, S., Mia. L., & Davis, M. M. (2020). Well-being of parents and children during the COVID-19 pandemic: A national survey. *Pediatrics, 146*, https://doi.org/10.1542/peds.2020-016824

Perl, L., Oren, A., Klein, Z., & Shechner, T. (2021). Effects of the COVID19 Pandemic on Transgender and Gender Non-Conforming Adolescents' Mental Health. *Psychiatry Research, 302*, 114042, 4 pages. https://doi.org/10.1016/j.psychres.2021.114042

Perry, N. B., Donzella, B., Troy, M. F., & Barnes, A. J. (2022). Mother and child hair cortisol during the COVID-19 pandemic: Associations among physiological stress, pandemic-related behaviors, and child emotional-behavioral health. *Psychoneuroendocrinology, 137*, 105656. https://doi.org/10.1016/j.psyneuen.2021.105656

Petts, R. J., Carlson, D. L., & Pepin, J. R. (2021). A gendered pandemic: Childcare, homeschooling, and parents' employment during COVID-19. *Gender, Work and Organization, 28*(S2), 515–534.

Phelps, C., & Sperry, L. L. (2020). Children and the COVID-19 pandemic. *Psychological Trauma: Theory, Research, Practice, and Policy, 12*(S1), S73–S75. https://doi.org/10.1037/tra0000861

Ponti, L., & Smorti, M. (2019). Mediating role of labor on the relationship between prenatal psychopathologic symptoms and symptoms of postpartum depression in women who give birth vaginally. *Journal of Obstetric, Gynecologic, and Neonatal Nursing, 48*, 627–634. https://doi.org/10.1016/j.jogn.2019.09.003

Raj, A., Johns, N. E., Barker, K. M., & Silverman, J. G. (2020). Time from COVID-19 shutdown, gender-based violence exposure, and mental health outcomes among a state representative sample of California residents. *eClinicalMedicine, 26*, 100520. https://doi.org/10.1016/j.eclinm.2020.100520

Rapa, E., Dalton, L., & Stein, A. (2020). Talking to children about illness and death of a loved one during the COVID-19 pandemic. *The Lancet Child & Adolescent Health, 4*(8), 560–562. https://doi.org/10.1016/S2352-4642(20)30174-7

Rapoport, E., Reisert, H., Schoeman, E., & Adesman, A. (2020). Reporting of child maltreatment during the SARS-CoV-2 pandemic in New York City from March to May 2020. *Child Abuse & Neglect, 116*, 104719. https://doi.org/10.1016/j.chiabu.2020.104719

Richards, M., Lewis, G., Cornelli Sanderson, R., Deane, K., & Quimby, D. (2016). Introduction to special issue: Resilience-based approaches to trauma intervention for children and adolescents. *Journal of Child & Adolescent Trauma, 9*(1), 1–4. https://doi.org/10.1007/s40653-016-0081-4

Rodriguez, C. M., Lee, S. J., Ward, K. P., & Pu, D. F. (2021). The perfect storm: Hidden risk of child maltreatment during the COVID-19 pandemic. *Child Maltreatment, 26*, 139–151. https://doi.org/10.1177/1077559520982066

Sari, N. P., van IJzendoorn, M. H., Jansen, P., Bakermans-Kranenburg, M., & Riem, M. M. E. (2021). Higher levels of harsh parenting during the COVID-19 lockdown in the Netherlands. *Child Maltreatment, 27*, 156–162. https://doi.org/10.1177/10775595211024748

Scarpellini, F., Segre, G., Cartabia, M., Zanetti, M., Camp, R., Clavenna, A., & Bonati, M. (2021). Distance learning in Italian primary and middle school children during the COVID-19 pandemic: A national survey. *BMC Public Health, 21*, 1035. https://doi.org/10.1186/s12889-021-11026-x

Schanzenbach, D. W., & Pitts, A. (2020). *Estimates of food insecurity during the COVID-19 crisis: Results from the COVID Impact Survey, Week 1 (April 20–26, 2020).* Institute for Policy Research Rapid Research Report. https://www.ipr.northwestern.edu/news/2020/food-insecurity-triples-for-families-during-covid.htm

Schmidt, S. J., Barblan, L. P., Lory, I., & Landolt, M. A. (2021). Age-related effects of the COVID-19 pandemic on mental health of children and adolescents. *European Journal of Psychotraumatology, 12*, 17. https://doi.org/10.1080/20008198.2021.1901407

Singh, S., Roy, D., Sinha, K., Parveen, S., Sharma, G., & Joshi, G. (2020). Impact of COVID-19 and lockdown on mental health of children and adolescents: A narrative review with recommendations. *Psychiatry Research, 293*, 113429. https://doi.org/10.1016/j.psychres.2020.113429

Siracusano, M., Riccioni, A., Gialloreti, L. E., Segatori, E., Arturi, L., Vasta, M., Porfirio, M. C., Terribili, M., Galasso, C., & Mazzone, L. (2021). Parental Stress and Disability in Offspring: A

Snapshot during the COVID-19 Pandemic. *Brain Sciences, 11*, 1040. https://doi.org/10.3390/brainsci11081040
Smith, J. (2021). From "nobody's clapping for us" to "bad moms": COVID-19 and the circle of childcare in Canada. *Gender, Work and Organization, 29*, 353–367.
Smorti, M., Ponti, L., & Tani, F. (2019). Maternal depressive symptomatology during pregnancy is a risk factor affecting newborn's health: A longitudinal study. *Journal of Reproductive and Infant Psychology, 39*, 492–497. https://doi.org/10.1080/02646838.2019.1581919
Smorti, M., Ponti, L., Ionio, C., Gallese, M., Andreol, A., & Bonassi, L. (2022). Becoming a mother during the COVID-19 national lockdown in Italy: Issues linked to the wellbeing of pregnant women. *International Journal of Psychology, 57*(1), 146–152. https://doi.org/10.1002/ijop.12806
Spitzer, M. W. H., Gutsfeld, R., Wirzberger, M., & Moeller, K. (2021). Evaluating students' engagement with an online learning environment before and after COVID-19 related school closures: A survival analysis approach. *Trends in Neuroscience and Education, 25*, 100168. https://doi.org/10.1016/j.tine.2021.100168
Spuij, M., Dekovic, M., & Boelen, P. A. (2015). An open trial of 'Grief-Help': A cognitive–behavioural treatment for prolonged grief in children and adolescents. *Clinical Psychology & Psychotherapy, 22*(2), 185–192. https://doi.org/10.1002/cpp.1877
Subbaraman, N. (2022). How does COVID affect mother and baby? *Nature, 591*, 193–195.
Suran, M. (2022). Increased use of medicare telehealth during the pandemic. *JAMA, 327*, 313. https://doi.org/10.1001/jama.2021.23332
Tang, S., Xiang, M., Cheung, T., & Xiang, Y. T. (2021). Mental health and its correlates among children and adolescents during COVID-19 school closure: The importance of parent-child discussion. *Journal of Affective Disorders, 279*, 353–360. https://doi.org/10.1016/j.jad.2020.10.016
Thompson, E. C., Thomas, S. A., Burke, T. A., Nesi, J., MacPherson, H. A., Bettis, A. H., Kudinova, A. Y., Affleck, K., Hunt, J., & Wolff, J. C. (2021). Suicidal thoughts and behaviors in psychiatrically hospitalized adolescents pre-and post-COVID-19: A historical chart review and examination of contextual correlates. *Journal of Affective Disorders Reports, 4*, Article 100100, 4 pages. https://doi.org/10.1016/j.jadr.2021.100100
Thorell, L. B., Skoglund, C., del al Pena, A. G., Baeyens, D., Fuermaier, A. B. M., Groom, M. J.,… Christiansen, H. (2021). Parental experiences of homeschooling during the COVID-19 pandemic: Differences between seven European countries and between children with and without mental health conditions. *European Child & Adolescent Psychiatry, 31*, 649–661. https://doi.org/10.1007/s00787-020-01706-1
Twenge J. M. & Joiner T. E. (2021). U.S. Census Bureau-assessed prevalence of anxiety and depressive symptoms in 2019 and during the 2020 COVID-19 pandemic. *Depression & Anxiety, 37*, 954–956. https://doi.org/10.1002/da.23077
United States Department of Health and Human Services. (2021). *Child Maltreatment 2020.* Retrieved from https://www.acf.hhs.gov/sites/default/files/documents/cb/cm2020.pdf
U.S. Bureau of Labor Statistics. (2020). *A-10. Unemployment rates by age, sex, and marital status, seasonally adjusted.* Retrieved from https://www.bls.gov/web/empsit/cpseea10.htm
Verdery, A. M., Smith-Greenaway, E., Margoli, R., & Daw, J. (2020). Tracking the reach of COVID-19 kin loss with a bereavement multiplier applied to the United States. *PNAS, 117*, 17695–17701. https://doi.org/10.1073/pnas.2007476117
Vieira, L. G., Camargo, E. L., Schneider, G., Silva, G. P., Thomazini, M., Possani, M. A., Matioli, M. R., & Ibiapina, A. R. (2020). Repercussions of the COVID-19 pandemic on the mental health of pregnant and puerperal women: A systematic review. *medRxiv*. https://doi.org/10.1101/2020.08.17.20176560
Wamser-Nanney, R., Nguyen-Feng, V., Lotzin, A., & Zhou, X. (2021). Parenting amidst COVID-19: Pandemic-related stressors, inequities, and treatment utilization and perceptions. *Couple and Family Psychology: Research and Practice*. Advance online publication. https://doi.org/10.1037/cfp0000189

Wong, C. A., Ming, D., Maslow, G., & Gifford, E. J. (2020). Mitigating the impacts of the COVID-19 pandemic response on at-risk children. *Pediatrics, 146*, e20200973. https://doi.org/10.1542/peds.2020-0973

Zambrano, L. D., Ellington, S., Strid, P., et al. (2020). Update: Characteristics of symptomatic women of reproductive age with laboratory-confirmed SARS-CoV-2 infection by pregnancy status — United States, January 22–October 3, 2020. *Morbidity and Mortality Weekly Report, 69*, 1641–1647. https://doi.org/10.15585/mmwr.mm6944e3externalicon

Zhou, X. (2020). Managing psychological distress in children and adolescents following the COVID-19 epidemic: A cooperative approach. *Psychological Trauma: Theory, Research, Practice, and Policy, 12*(S1), S76–S78. https://doi.org/10.1037/tra0000754

Rachel Wamser-Nanney PhD is an Associate Professor in the Psychological Sciences Department at the University of Missouri- St. Louis.

Christina M. Rodriguez PhD is a clinical child psychologist, Professor of Psychology at Old Dominion University, and Director of Clinical Training of the Virginia Consortium Program in Clinical Psychology.

Lauren Mizock PhD is core faculty in the Clinical Psychology PhD Program at Fielding Graduate University and in private practice in San Francisco.

Laura Nabors PhD, ABPP is a professor in the School of Human Services in the College of Education, Criminal Justice, and Human Services at the University of Cincinnati.

Chapter 5
Vibrant Older Adults

Irit Felsen, Jenni Frumer, Marilyn P. Safir, Tracey Farber, and Mary Beth Quaranta Morrissey

Our chapter highlights the unique experiences during the pandemic of vibrant older adults. This group comprises individuals older than 60 years old who had been actively involved in multiple social, cultural, and professional activities and interest groups until the outbreak of the COVID-19 pandemic and the social distancing restrictions associated with it. While awareness of the vulnerability of this group to the coronavirus, especially the risk to frail older adults, was amplified in public discourse and by the media in the early months of 2020, their unique needs and challenges have not been sufficiently addressed. This omission was partly due to the lack of differentiation in public and professional discourse to reflect the tremendous diversity within the older adult population. Our mission therefore, became to advance professional awareness and knowledge about the psychological experiences of this group during the COVID-19 pandemic. In addition, we felt it important to address ageism, including internalized subjective ageism, among our own professional colleagues. To that effect, we began hosting online conversations with older

I. Felsen (✉)
Department of Psychology, Columbia University, New York, NY, USA
e-mail: Ivf2101@columbia.edu

J. Frumer
MorseLife Health System, NOW for Holocaust Survivors, Palm Beach, FL, USA
e-mail: jfrumer@jennifrumer.com

M. P. Safir
School of Psychological Sciences, University of Haifa, Haifa, Israel

T. Farber
Student Success Center, Tel-Aviv University, Tel-Aviv, Israel

M. B. Quaranta Morrissey
Wurzweiler School of Social Work, Yeshiva University, New York, NY, USA
e-mail: Mary.morrissey@yu.edu

C. R. Figley et al. (eds.), *Pandemic Providers*,
https://doi.org/10.1007/978-3-031-27580-7_5

psychologists who shared their professional expertise and their personal viewpoint about their experiences during COVID.

Consistent with the work of group members, the OAWG explored the impact of the trauma of the Holocaust and its related intergenerational transmission on the experiences of Holocaust survivors and their offspring during the pandemic. A previous meta-analysis of 71 studies already demonstrated that many community-dwelling Holocaust survivors continue to suffer from elevated post-traumatic symptoms for many decades (Barel et al., 2010). Empirical studies also demonstrated heightened preoccupation and elevated stress reactions among offspring of survivors with regard to life-threatening challenges (Baider et al., 2008; Solomon et al., 1988) and to potential threats of annihilation (Shrira, 2015). This specific preoccupation reflects part of a more general preoccupation with surrounding threats (Shrira, 2015), a sensitivity that manifests as a "hostile world scenario" (Shmotkin, 2005). Such findings suggest that survivors, now in their 80s and older, and the "second generation" (2G), now in their 60s and early 70s, might be a group of older adults who are particularly vulnerable to the impact of the pandemic.

This chapter opens with the story of the origin of the OAWG, which has shaped its mission. It follows with the personal, lived experiences of a vibrant octogenarian group member who was widowed shortly before the onset of the pandemic. The insights shared from "within" this unique perspective of an older researcher-practitioner, and her peers' lived experiences, illuminated phenomenological, lived aspects that otherwise would have remained elusive and unarticulated. The importance of the actual voice of the older individuals in the discourse *about* the older population cannot be over-emphasized.

The subsequent parts of the chapter then offer a review of various interventions by group members during the pandemic, including individual clinical work with Holocaust survivors conducted through home-visits during COVID-19 in Johannesburg, South Africa, the challenges encountered by a multi-level health system offering social services to Holocaust survivors in Florida, USA, and observations from online psychosocial interventions conducted during 2020–2021 with over 3500 Holocaust survivors and their offspring from the USA, Canada, Israel, Hungary, and other countries.

Some of the products of the OAGW include an empirical study, papers published in peer-reviewed journals, and book chapters (Shrira & Baumel-Schwartz) currently in publication, a series of 20 webinar lectures online (Felsen, 2020–2021, https://www.youtube.com/playlist?list=PL98TejO6Vy3qoYCkt71NEKjfHw431dvet), and additional articles and online presentations in trauma-related publications and in the media (Shrira & Felsen, 2021; Felsen, 2021a, b) addressing the vulnerabilities and resiliencies of these unique segments within the older adults population and educating other professionals about the long-reach impact of trauma in responses to the novel challenges of the recent couple of years. Our findings expand previous research in Holocaust families, which paved the way and offered a framework for the study of the effects of historical trauma in other populations. Insights gleaned from our work during the COVID-19 pandemic continue to contribute to this body of knowledge and can be relevant to other trauma-exposed populations. Finally, an additional product of the OAWG has been the collection of articles, webinars, and other resources from the media that are related to older adults and the COVID-19 pandemic. This repository serves as a historical documentation for the pandemic as it has been reflected in the media. The collected items have specifically privileged newspaper articles and other materials that would be harder to reconstruct in the future, in comparison to peer-reviewed professional publications.

Drawing on our interventions and collective experiences of group members, the chapter outlines novel ways to address the psychosocial needs of vibrant older adults during future times when social distancing might be required, as well as to expand the options available during "normative" times. The chapter concludes with lessons from a public health perspective articulated by a group member who has done extensive work in the intersection of mental health, law, and public health policy. Put together, the chapter offers future actionable suggestions that were gleaned from the experiences of OAWG during the COVID-19 crisis.

The Origin Story and Emergent Mission Statement of the Older Adults Work Group

The origin story of the Older Adults Work Group is a living illustration of some of the silver linings of the COVID-19 pandemic, which forced forth awareness to multiple inequities and inconvenient socio-cultural realities that have been neglected far too long, ageism being one of them (Ayalon et al. 2021).

2020 was not a good year to turn 60, but that is when I did. Very shortly before that, my husband and I, freshly empty nesters, moved from the suburbs to the city. Having raised our children in a large house with multiple levels, we had to part with the accumulation of 25 years of "stuff," in order to fit into our new spacious, yet smaller city apartment. We ran up and down three flights of stairs, carrying loads and loads of books and boxed items to be delivered to the local charities, putting long days of grueling physical labor into preparing our house to be sold. As we were doing all that, we felt no different than our 30-year-old selves. But then COVID-19 hit, and all of a sudden, I was one of the "60 years and older," who were at greater risk for complications and death from the coronavirus (Centers for Disease Control and Prevention (CDC), 2020). I, who snickered at the slower pace and lower stamina of my twenty-something-year-old daughters who were helping us during the move but not keeping up with their parents' pace, suddenly became the "older adult" who had to be "protected" by extra precautions. In New York City, where we moved in, the ambulances were endlessly driving by, and 1000 people were dying of COVID daily. A very high proportion of these deaths were of those 60 and older. The threat of death was very real, and almost everyone knew someone who lost a loved one to the pandemic. At 7:00 pm, as shifts in hospitals changed across town, people banged pots and pans in the windows to express their gratitude and admiration for health heroes and essential workers, who were risking their lives daily in medical facilities but also in grocery stores.

The call by Prof. Charles Figley and Division 56 to gather as a COVID-19 Task Force seemed a very appropriate idea for trauma psychologists, in those early weeks of acute and yes, unprecedented trauma. As we gathered via Zoom, then a relatively novel form of social communing, we were about seventy psychologists on the call. Most of us were trauma division members, but it was decided that members of other divisions, as well as other mental health professionals, would be welcome to join us. Having come together we all valued the opportunity to share our confusion and distress at the morbidly surrealistic transformation of the world as we had known it. The first couple of meetings were focused on the formation of a distinct mission and a name for our group. The Interdivisional COVID-19 Task Force, as it was decided, was divided into smaller groups, each of which was to be dedicating its time and focus to the needs of a particular population considered especially vulnerable to the effects of the pandemic. During two consecutive weekly meetings, the work groups were formed, and the mission of the Task Force was articulated as the collection and collation of relevant materials to be made available to professionals and others focused on the needs of each of the interest groups. At the end of this process, some eleven work groups were formed, each chaired by the person who suggested the group. As Figley was concluding the successful completion of this phase, I pointed out that no group was suggested to address the most publicized "vulnerable population," those older than 60, whose ranks I had just joined. This was a glaring, in fact, shocking omission, given the zeitgeist and the prominence of the issue in the media and in the public discourse. It was even more shocking since, as I looked at the Zoom screen, most participants were older than I was. *We* were the "older adults" who were that most vulnerable group! *We* were members of the cohorts whose elevated risk was highlighted by public figures, by the media, and by health campaigns encouraging the public to use social distancing and wear masks to protect each other and in particular, to protect *us*, their parents and grandparents.

COVID-19 was a "time machine" that suddenly transported me into a life phase I had not yet grown into and was not ready for. It forced an unnaturally abrupt shift in my subjective perceptions of my age, and of my aging. Many of my colleagues in the Task Force, who were discussing the needs of vulnerable "others," were a decade or much older than I was. While focusing on the various vulnerable sub-populations, and forming our Work Groups, we were blatantly denying our own vulnerability. Helping others might often be the best way to turn vulnerability to resilience. However, in this case, identifying only as the "helpers" reflected also defensive efforts, not only about the risk associated with COVID-19, but also the dichotomy between "us," the professionals, and "them," and our refusal to count ourselves among the "older" ones. Almost too dramatic to be true, the origin story of our group was a shrill wake-up call about ageism among psychologists, in fact, among aging psychologists. The focus of our group has emerged from this formative moment, which crystallized our wish to highlight the needs of older adults *like ourselves* – actively engaged older adults who have expertise and experience, who can still contribute tremendously in their professional capacities and to society at large.

The "graying of the population" in America and in the Western World is rapidly changing the social landscape. These global demographic changes require appropriate changes in policies and re-framing of attitudes about the later years. The full decade of life that has been added to the average life expectancy of American adults since 1950 has added a new life phase to the modern life cycle. Whereas people used to live only a few years after retirement, set at 65 and 67, old age now spans 30 or more years that include a tremendous diversity in terms of individual levels of objective and subjective aging. With improved healthcare and general life conditions, many older adults in the USA are enjoying several decades of reasonably good health and functioning. These years allow people the opportunity to continue to be socially and culturally active, to remain involved in their professional and occupational circles, and to contribute to their families and to society in multiple ways. Many of us on the Task Force were past what would have been retirement age in previous years; and some were indeed retired. Yet here we were: some of us still working full time or part time, and others retired, yet joining with colleagues in a professional capacity, contributing expertise, making new connections, and developing new projects to respond to novel challenges.

Our Work Group is a reflection of the lived experience of being an Older Adult in these times of "New Aging." One of the social phenomena evoked by COVID-19 pandemic was that it called attention to older adults, attention that some felt was negative, painting all older adults as frail and lonely. However, the spotlight might have nonetheless led to the recognition of another social important inequity, ageism. In the context of the Task Force, the origin story of our Work Group highlighted the need to do away with the dichotomy between "us" and "them" regarding older adults. Older Adults are us. Our group asks, therefore, how has the pandemic affected us, not "them." We write this chapter from this perspective, integrating our personal lived experiences and our professional perspectives during this unusual time.

Furthermore, this chapter describes work conducted by our members during the COVID-19 pandemic, with particularly vulnerable sub-groups within the population of interest to us. As trauma experts, several of us have been focused in our clinical and research work on aging Holocaust survivors and their now-aging adult children. We continued to intervene with these populations during the pandemic. The work which will be reviewed demonstrates the effects of extreme trauma in previous life phases on the experiences of aging trauma survivors during the pandemic, as well as the effects of both intergenerational transmission of trauma and resilience in the responses of the second generation during these challenging times. Research on Holocaust survivors and their families has provided frameworks for the study of historical trauma and intergenerational trauma in multiple other populations (Danieli, 1988; Duran et al., 1998; Yellow Horse Brave Heart et al., 2011; Cross, 1998). Our work with this population during the COVID-19 pandemic, as will be described in the sections that follow, continues to show the relevance of massive trauma for survivors and their descendants in coping with various aspects of the pandemic and with the socio-political and cultural upheaval that accompanied it.

The observations, which will be described below, suggest both unique vulnerabilities and resilient coping that are associated with a legacy of trauma which can inform research and clinical work with other trauma-exposed groups. Continuing to deepen the understanding of historical trauma and intergenerational transmission and its persistent effects later in life is particularly relevant in these times of global crisis. Over the next years, mental health professionals will encounter high numbers of individuals with trauma histories, due to the fact that we are currently witnessing the highest numbers of refugees and displaced populations since after the end of WWII, and due to the global death-toll and economic crises caused by the pandemic.

This chapter will describe the work our group members have done during the COVID-19 pandemic and will conclude with the future-oriented public health perspective and Dr. Morrisey's work to educate healthcare and legal professionals, and recommendations for advancing the well-being of older adults. Dr. Frumer, who is the Director of NOW for Holocaust Survivors Initiative at Morse Life Health System, will share some of her experiences and challenges faced directing multilevel services for aging Holocaust survivors during the pandemic. My own focus in clinical work and research has been on the intergenerational transmission of effects related to the Holocaust in the now-aging children of survivors. Dr. Frumer and I will share our observations from multiple online gatherings of survivors and of children of Holocaust survivors, some were offered by Frumer and me, under the auspices of the Morse Life Health System, and others offered by me for various social networks and organizations of "second generations." These gatherings, attended by over 3500 participants, have rendered poignant observations about the effects of intergenerational transmission of trauma on the experiences of adult children of Holocaust survivors during COVID-19. Findings from an empirical study based on a sample drawn from these webinars will be described. We will articulate our conclusions, regarding the important psychosocial function of online gatherings for groups that share the same particular background of trauma or intergenerational, historical trauma, or another collective challenge. We propose that such virtual shared-background groups function as a uniquely useful novel resource for older adults during the pandemic and beyond.

Dr. Safir initially volunteered to join our group and then had second thoughts about whether she "belonged," since her academic pursuits had nothing to do with aging. I was fortunate to be able to convince her that her unique perspective, combining her professional skills with her lived experiences and her "insider's view" about concerns of her peers during this time, were invaluable to us. Indeed, Safir will share some of her poignant insights, experiences, and anecdotes that could only be told "from the inside," reflecting the way she and her peers and friends experienced the pandemic in Israel.

Inspired by my colleagues and by many friends, patients, and esteemed older adults in my personal and professional life, I suggested the term "vibrant older adults" to emphasize the focus of our group on this particular segment of the population of older adults that does not receive sufficient attention and is often undifferentiated from physically or cognitively frail older adults. Our focus on this segment of the older adult population does not in any way diminish the importance of work to be done in relation to the latter group, but it was a decision based on the limited resources of our group.

The "lumping together" of people who have very diverse needs is a manifestation of ageism and one of the areas in which profound changes must take place. Differentiated attention and efforts to identify the unique needs of various groups within the wider population of older adults is necessary to protect the well-being of all older adults, with sensitivity to diversity, equity, and inclusion. While not focusing specifically on COVID-19 anymore, our interest in the needs of vibrant older adults and our emphasis on advocacy for this sub-population within our professional groups and beyond has been a direct outcome of the pandemic and of this Task Force.

The Older Adults Work Group: Who Are We?

Among the older adult authors of this chapter are several who fall themselves within the definition of "older adults," namely, those 60 years and older, a demarcation that has become so much more accentuated in public and the personal awareness since the beginning of the COVID-19 pandemic. We, personally, represent the group of people we study and advocate for, i.e., active, vibrant older adults.

Dr. Frumer, PhD, LCSW, MEd came out of retirement as the CEO of a large human service organization and launched herself into an intensively demanding new career. She is the VP of Strategic Initiatives and the Director of the NOW for Holocaust Survivors Initiative at MorseLife Health System. She established Jenni Frumer & Associates, LLC; a consultant for leadership development and organizational management. She is also a consultant for the Global Leaders Initiative (GLI). She is an officer on the board of the International Center for the Multigenerational Legacies of Trauma (ICMGLT) and maintains a private practice, specializing in intergenerational trauma. Additionally, Frumer is adjunct faculty teaching classes in social work, business, and qualitative research.

Dr. Safir, PhD, is a vibrant octogenarian professor emerita at the University of Haifa, who, in addition to her academic career and clinical work as a leading sex therapy expert, has had an illustrious record of achievements as a social and feminist activist, both during her early years in the USA and later in Israel. She is a Professor (emerita) of Clinical and Social Psychology at the University of Haifa, Israel. Safir has been a social activist since her college days at Syracuse. She was active in the Civil Rights Movement and worked with Warren Hagstrum and Sol Olinski doing community organization in the 15th ward, serving as Ward Chair for the Democratic Party. She participated in The Meredith March from Tennessee through Mississippi 1966. She was the Founder and Past Director of Women's Studies Program at the University of Haifa, the Academic Director of the Post-Graduate Program in Sex Therapy at the University of Haifa, and the Director of the CBT VR Laboratory at the University of Haifa. In addition, Safir was a pioneer of Israel's new Women's Movement, which began in Haifa in 1970, a founder of the second President of The Israeli Association of Cognitive Behavior Therapy and also a founder of the Israeli Association for Sex Therapy, where she served on the Board of Directors. She is also a founding member of the Executive Committee and first President of the *Israel Association for Feminist and Gender Studies* (1998–2002), a Founding Director and President of the Board of *Nisan –Young Women's Leadership Program* (1995–2001), and a founder of the *Israel Women's Network* (1984) where she served three terms on the Executive Board. Currently, Safir is on the Board of the University of Haifa's Faculty Union representing the retired faculty who number slightly more than 300 individuals, between the ages of 68 and 90 plus, and she has coordinated the activities of this organization and the services it provided to its members throughout the COVID-19 pandemic. Dr. Safir was still leading a clinical lab at the University when the pandemic happened.

Mary Beth Quaranta Morrissey, PhD, MPH, JD, is a gerontological social work researcher and healthcare attorney concentrating in health and public health law and policy. Her phenomenological research on suffering and resilience among older adults has given voice to older persons and informs her law and policy practice. In her New York State, national and international roles, she is leading efforts to expand the next generation of public health strategies for palliative care in the progressive realization of older adults' right to health, including elimination of all forms of systemic racism and discrimination. Morrissey is also working with the State Society on Aging of New York, the American Public Health Association, and the International Network for Elder Abuse Prevention to strengthen the rights of older people, including older immigrants and persons with dementia, and work toward the achievement of a UN Convention on the Rights of Older Persons.

Tracey Farber, PhD, a clinical psychologist, has just made tremendous life-changing moves, immigrating from her native South Africa to Israel, starting a private practice, and working as a psychotherapist at the University of Tel Aviv Psychological Service. In Johannesburg Farber specialized in working with traumatized clients, and she continues to supervise and train psychotherapists in Johannesburg over Zoom. Farber recently published in the *Journal of Trauma and Loss – International Perspectives on Stress and Coping* (2021), and has an academic book based on her PhD research currently in publication. Her research is on catastrophic grief, trauma, and resilience in aging child Holocaust survivors. She developed a model of resilience based on her research and has presented her model to mental health workers, employees, students, parents, and teachers both in Johannesburg and Tel Aviv.

Irit Felsen, PhD, is currently in full-time private practice and also teaches as an adjunct professor at Columbia University and Yeshiva University. Felsen is the co-chair of the Trauma Work Group in the NGO on Mental Health in Consultative Relationship to the UN. Her research and clinical work focus on the long-term effect of the Holocaust and other massive traumatic events and the intergenerational transmission of effects related to trauma in survivor families. Her work was published in peer-reviewed journals and book chapters focusing on the long-term effects of the Holocaust on survivors, and the effects of intergenerational trauma. Recently, she has been writing about the effects of COVID-19 on survivors and offspring of survivors.

Making, Unmaking, and Remaking a "Vibrant Elder"

Marilyn P. Safir

Israel began its COVID lockdown in March 2020. I had retired from teaching in 2006, but continued my research at the university, attended international meetings, and continued my involvement in social activism. I was widowed after 50 years of marriage about 10 months before the lockdown and had reset my life as a newly single, independent individual. I returned from a 5-week trip through the USA, visiting family and friends, and resumed my involvement with academic and social activities and activism. Suddenly, being active and independent was forbidden. I found myself spending more and more time following news of the new epidemic, and a mounting concern, as I, at age 82, was in the age group of those most endangered and likely to die of COVID. Up to this point of time, I had not paid much attention to my "advanced" age, except for anger at the exorbitant cost of travel insurance. The government informed us we should stay home, and that we could not walk more than 100 meters from our homes. We were restricted to certain times for grocery shopping, and non-essential places were closed. I began receiving phone calls from the Haifa Municipality Social Services, as 80 and over was now an endangered population. These very intrusive, annoying callers (probably volunteers) – rather than asking if I need anything or if I wanted help, assumed that volunteers should be sent to take care of me. Suddenly I became aware that I was being viewed as really "older," and perhaps as a result, incompetent!

As an avid reader, involved with various academic research projects, I was already spending my time at home on my computer. As a member of the American Psychological Association, I began following more closely various materials coming through the Internet. I am a Founding Fellow of Division 56 (Trauma Division), and I received an email from Charles Figley, a member of this division, calling for a Zoom Meeting to discuss what we, who professionally deal with trauma, might do in these traumatic times. Figley proposed a task force to deal with the anxieties and trauma surrounding the coronavirus epidemic. I enthusiastically joined the meeting and the discussion. During this discussion, I was struck by Irit Felsen's interruption, calling the group's attention to the fact that no one had mentioned active Elders who live independently and insisting that a specific Work Group ought to focus on this population. I immediately jumped in and said, as a member of this "independent older adults" group – that this specific task force was necessary, and I volunteered to join. I also joined another task force, led by Lenore Walker, in an area that I do research in and promote as a social activist. This group was established to find ways for women to deal with interpersonal violence that would obviously become even more significant in lockdown situations.

The next day, I began to have second thoughts about joining a research group on the elderly. As an elder, Felsen's focus group was very important to me – but I had never done research in this area. I wrote to Felsen raising my concerns that my knowledge of "Elders" is personal – not related to research. Dr. Felsen supported my involvement in the group as I could bring the perspective of an Elder. I have been an active member of this WG and my knowledge has greatly expanded from the personal.

I am going to share my personal story of the impact of this period. I have previously mentioned my annoyance and even anger at receiving phone calls from individuals who assumed that being over 80, I was no longer able to take care of myself. I was angry with the restrictions placed on movement in general. My response was to take my dog out for walks four to five times a day (rather than the usual twice daily). My anger was probably also connected to the mourning of the death of my husband and the major life changes that were related to his illness. He had been diagnosed with a non-aggressive bladder cancer in 2015 and received outpatient treatment. We had been living in an area of private homes in a three-story house that we built in 1972, with a lovely ¼ acre garden. We had been discussing renovations and considered putting in an elevator, as Efraim's arthritic knees had become painful. We changed course with the diagnosis of cancer. We decided that we would sell the house, remove all the pressures related to maintaining it, and move into an apartment. I had taken charge of supervising the building of our house. Now I took charge of its sale, of finding a new home, and dealing with its renovations. Efi was still working and managing his two businesses. We settled into our new apartment. Shortly thereafter, on one of Efi's examinations of the bladder cancer, we learned the cancer had changed course to an aggressive form. He underwent, over a 4-month period, a series 12 chemotherapy treatments, which was very successful. However, his surgeon suggested that he undergo surgery to remove the bladder. I have since learned that in the USA this surgery for men over 75 (Efi was 79) is deemed unnecessary. He went in for surgery with a 1-week hospitalization in February. Because of various complications, he was hospitalized through June, went through eight surgeries, moved in and out of the ICU, until he finally died in mid-June 2019. I was at the hospital daily, from about 9 am until 6 pm. There is a shortage of nursing staff, and it was clear to me that my eyes were necessary to make sure that Efi received the care he needed, when he needed it. To no avail. Needless to say, this was a very traumatic period. One of the things we had to deal while Efi was hospitalized, was to move power of attorney for Efi to me, because some treatment decisions were made when Efi was not in a condition to make a decision. We were able to do this after the first 3 weeks he was hospitalized. I had previously decided – years before – that I wanted to have in my file "*Do Not Resuscitate*." I did not want to be maintained artificially on machines. I wrote letters to my son and daughter, to Efi, and to a good friend of this decision. I discovered following Efi's death that this was not adequate. Having gone through these traumatic 5 months brought my concern about future medical care and mortality to the forefront. I discussed this with my family doctor, and we sat for over an hour filling out a form regarding various potential medical interventions. I indicated what I was willing to undergo, and what treatment I refused. I chose two individuals who have Power of Attorney to determine that my wishes will be followed. This is on file with the Ministry of Health. So, this has been a very significant period dealing with mortality. A major result from this traumatic period is that I have stopped cooking. This was not a conscious decision. As before

Efi's death we often had friends over for dinner, this change has impacted my social life.

During the 10 months of this mourning period, predating COVID-19, I had not realized I had become less social in general. In addition, I have had to deal with some major health problems on my own. However, being part of the Task Force been very significant, both personally and professionally. I made new friends through these groups, I have been intellectually stimulated, and in writing this short memoire I can see that these involvements have helped me overcome the trauma of Efi's illness and hospitalization, the mourning process, and the anxieties of the COVID epidemic. Being a member of the two work groups helped bring me back to being interested and involved – moving toward becoming a vibrant elder again.

Home Visits for Holocaust Survivors During COVID-19: Revisiting Trauma and Resilience

Tracey Farber

This is a description of the therapeutic interventions home visits that were undertaken during the lockdown from March 2020 to September 2020 during the beginning of COVID-19 at Jewish Community Services in Johannesburg, South Africa. As a clinical psychologist, my research for the PhD degree focused on the long-term effects of trauma and features of resilience in children and adolescents who were interned in concentration camps during the Holocaust. Based on the results of my research, I initiated the psychosocial services for Holocaust survivors – the first of its kind – at Jewish Community services in South Africa. Until then, the small survivor community had no dedicated psychological services. In that period of time, I supervised social workers who provided home visits and services to survivors. I also saw survivors and second-generation survivors in my general private practice in Johannesburg, where I specialized in working with traumatized clients. As the COVID-19 lockdown began, I was grateful to have permission and to get a license from the Jewish community services to visit isolated "at risk" survivors in their homes. David, Ann, and Yankel were visited in their homes, while Sara was seen on video over the Internet (to protect their confidentiality these are not their real names). During the home visits I maintained social distance and wore a mask at all times. The home visits continued for a period of 6 months until I emigrated to Israel.

YANKEL

Yankel was referred as he was very depressed and requested to see a therapist. I visited Yankel at his flat in Johannesburg. He spoke about his ongoing grief regarding his adult daughter who had died 2 years previously. Yankel struggled to come to terms with this loss. In addition, he felt that his faith in G-D had been shaken, and he was afraid that his unresolved grief was a burden for his wife to carry. The death of his daughter also triggered his previous grief for the family he had lost and also the loss of faith he had endured after he survived the Holocaust. He reported that it was a relief for him to be able to discuss these thoughts and feelings freely, as they were difficult to discuss with his family, and he felt overwhelmed by grief. He spoke of his anger regarding the loss of his daughter and the "senseless grief" that he had felt after losing his extended family during the Holocaust.

Yankel was seen for three sessions at his home. Before the scheduled 4th session, he called to tell me not to come as he was struggling to breathe. Sadly, he was rushed to ICU and died later that week as a result of the COVID 19 virus.

I attended Yankel's funeral in person – it was a very small funeral as it was during the pandemic. It was a very sad event; his wife could be heard sobbing inconsolably as she was deeply shocked and grief stricken. I had an opportunity to reflect on our short time together in therapy, and I understood that it was an opportunity for Yankel to express his grief, anger, despair, and his lack of faith before he died. He expressed that he felt relieved to have had the opportunity to discuss these difficult emotional experiences.

SARA

Sara is a survivor from Poland who lived at a facility for aging adults and as such she was under a strict lockdown. For this reason, I was not able to visit her and so I saw her for online video sessions on a weekly basis. The trauma of being in lockdown triggered Sara's experience of being imprisoned during the Holocaust in a concentration camp. This was exacerbated by her isolation in her unit, which meant that during this time, she had no face-to-face human contact. As a result, she was at times frustrated, angry, and hopeless. She repeated many times to me "I thought I had been through my time in 'geheinem' (hell), and now I found myself in 'gheinem-again." This psychologically difficult situation was worsened by her uncomfortable health issues that caused her pain and discomfort.

Online therapy provided her with the opportunity to articulate her sense of despair and outrage. She also spoke about how trapped she felt, and how she missed her family members. The isolation and her experience of "imprisonment" seemed to trigger her memories of her Holocaust experience where she was interned in a concentration camp – in other words she felt like she was living in "hell for the second time in her life." She revisited the loss of her father and spoke of the other family members that she had lost during the Holocaust, and she told me that she struggled to "block these feelings out "as she was alone all day with no distraction. Although she felt helpless, sad, and angry, Sara expressed her gratitude for the opportunity to discuss her difficult feelings. This seemed to lessen her extreme sense of isolation that was both real and also a trigger for her memories of suffering as a child survivor during the Holocaust. Sara was finally able to be reunited with her family after the lockdowns.

ANN

Ann is a survivor from France who was seen for home visits during the period from March to September 2020. I initially visited her at her son's house and thereafter at her apartment on a weekly basis. Ann was frustrated and angry that she had not moved into a retirement village. She verbalized her anger and her distress about this over and over. A major source of pain and sorrow was her experience of being rejected by many of her friends. This experience triggered her early experience of being rejected by her biological mother when she was a child.

Ann said that her experience of not belonging had been with her all her life. She said that at two and a half years old her family sent her away into hiding as the Germans invaded France. Ann said that between the ages of two and a half until four and a half years old, she has fragmented memories. She was moved around and she was hidden in different places and she had no constant attachment figure. Finally, at four and a half she met a Catholic widow and a mother of three children. She remembered this lady Camille telling the people she was with – that she had three children to feed and could not foster/hide Ann. Years later when Ann was an adult – Camille told Ann that when she saw her sad little face, she could not say "no." Ann remembered Camille extending her hand and saying "Vien avec moi" (French for "come with me"). Ann reported that she had felt wanted and deeply loved in Camille's home. She got on well with her other "siblings" and Camille was very loving. Camille reported years later to Ann that she used to cry out in her sleep and her language was very poor. At seven and a half, her Jewish parents who had survived the Holocaust came to fetch her. She was heartbroken to leave Camille and her family. She said that she kept in touch with Camille and visited her in France twice over the course of her adult life and stayed in touch with her "siblings" until their deaths. She said that her biological mother was harsh and rejecting and she missed her Catholic family all her life.

Ann's story shows how her early attachments were disrupted at the critical age of two and a half – a time when young toddlers start to explore the world and gain some sensory-motor independence. For the age of two and a half until four and a half years old she was moved around with no consistent adult figures that she rememberd. This is particularly traumatic for a child as she was deprived of adult figures on whom she could depend. Her world was destabilized causing her normal development of attachments to be disrupted. Her disrupted attachment history as a young child is likely to have resulted in a disorganized/anxious attachment, which is reflected in her report that she felt an inner sense of emptiness and loneliness, and in her frequent complaints about feeling hurt and let down by others. Ann expressed her distress during the COVID-19 lockdown where she felt isolated and again, she felt that there was no one to look after her. She felt that she didn't belong, and was left to looking after herself when she felt lonely and vulnerable. She said that the pain of her friends rejection of her made her feel abandoned, angry, and alone. In her despair she said that she wished that COVID-19 would take her and kill her – then there would no longer be suffering. I was a witness to her deep despair and I listened to her stories about Camille, and her memory and experience of being loved and feeling that she belonged. When she remembered Camille and her late husband, she could momentarily view herself from a perspective of being loved. At such moments she felt less alone. Although she could engage with the memory of the good objects in her internal world and remember what it felt like to be loved, these experiences did not mitigate against her sense of feeling rejected, but perhaps provided some moments of reprieve.

In her final session with me she cried as she said goodbye. She said it helped her to know that "someone cared." At the time of my departure, she moved to a facility for aging Jews and she was less socially isolated.

DAVID

I have known David for many years. I visited him in his apartment on a weekly basis from March 2020 to September 2020 during lockdown. David lives in an apartment in Johannesburg where his maid Karen takes care of him, and she and her children are his "family." He said that in general he coped well with the isolation of COVID-19, as he was an "introvert" and not very keen on being around people. It was clear that his resilient world view enabled him to cope with this new challenge.

David spoke a lot about the death of his father and his own sense of survivor guilt as his father had died as a "Musselman" – emaciated and starving. By contrast, David managed to survive. When he spoke about his 16 family members who died at Auschwitz, he said that he would never understand why he lived and they died. He spoke of his late wife and his marriage. He spoke about his regrets, namely, that he felt that he did not offer his wife enough support. He also spoke of his great love for her. As I listened, it felt as if he was organizing his memories and reviewing his life as aging people do – in the stage of integrity versus despair (Erikson, 1964). David spoke in-depth about his experience of being in the concentration camps. Although I had heard most of these stories before, they were nuanced with his current sense of feeling helpless and trapped, possibly triggered by the difficulties and restrictions of COVID-19. He said that he felt that being imprisoned as a young teenager had left him feeling "emasculated," and that this feeling had never left him. He had tried taking up shooting to overcome his sense of helplessness, and had become an expert shooter, to some extent, helping him to overcome his sense of being helpless.

It seemed that he used the psychotherapy as a final opportunity to speak about the deep traumas that he experiences of being emasculated as an adolescent in the concentration camps. This wound seemed to have stayed with him from his adolescence until his senior years. It was also an opportunity for him to speak about his regrets in his marriage, and he exposed his vulnerability in a very poignant way.

David would often say that he was an atheist as a result of the suffering in the Holocaust. During the period of this therapy, he made reference to his atheist position a few times. It was interesting that in our final session he said that he had been reading a book about Jewish history and he was now starting to think that perhaps there is a G-D. He continued to tell me, that when he marveled at all the miracles that happened in the history of the Jewish people – that only the existence of a G-D could explain them. From this perspective, it seemed that he also used the therapeutic process to explore his ambivalent spiritual feelings regarding his faith in the Creator. It is possible that the therapeutic space, at this late stage, offers survivors the opportunity to explore issues of faith that many of them have struggled with over the course of their life trajectories.

In his final session David said that he would miss me; it was a sad goodbye. He continues to be visited by his social worker from Jewish Community Services.

Concluding comments Child Holocaust survivors faced multiple traumas and losses. Some were interned in concentration camps, others hidden by gentiles, some suffered abusive treatment by their rescuers, while others developed deep loving connections with the rescuers and these were ruptured again upon reunification with a survivor parent whom they sometimes did not recognize. The multiple traumas suffered by young child survivors involved in most cases a sudden and violent separation form parents and other caretaker figures, and without social support for enduring the crises they were going through. Mourning was not possible, as the children needed to be "good," hide any distress, and avoid overtaxing their caretakers. Some children maintained the hope of reuniting with parents, further preventing them from mourning their loss. The nature of the losses suffered by child survivors during the Holocaust was catastrophic in terms of its massive scale, duration, lack of preparation, and lack of support, and later with knowledge of the gruesomeness of the way loved ones perished. As such, we used the term "catastrophic grief" (Farber, 2019; Farber et al., 2022) to describe the grief of child Holocaust survivors. Under such conditions, there is greater risk of developing complicated prolonged traumatic grief and severe depression (Herman, 1992; Rozalski et al., 2017). Kluger (2002) maintains that without the closure of mourning rituals, the survivor is "condemned to go on mourning".

Complicated grief is characterized by intense yearning for the deceased, feeling a lack of meaning after the loss, an inability to trust others, and impairment in daily functioning (Horowitz et al., 1993). Loss and traumatic bereavement are core themes in understanding the experiences of Holocaust survivors (Witztum & Malkinson, 2009). Several authors suggest that life-long mourning in survivors is a form of maintaining attachment and connection with loved ones murdered in the Holocaust (Klein & Holder, 2012; Witztum & Malkinson, 2009) Witztum and Malkinson (2009) highlight the need to understand that Holocaust survivors experienced both severe trauma *and* devastating loss, which is so overwhelming that, as Danieli asks (1988), "How can one ever mourn this" (p. 230)? I proposed the term "catastrophic grief" to capture the degree to which awareness of loss leaves aging child survivors with a sense of having suffered permanent ruptures in self-formation and a life-long experience of distress that is beyond consolation. I also posit that the grief observed in many ageing child survivors appeared unlike that related to the negative cognitions and mood associated with posttraumatic stress disorder (PTSD) (DSM-5, APA, 2013), nor was it appropriately captured by the conditions of complex bereavement (DSM-5, APA, 2013) or complicated grief (Horowitz et al., 1993). The survivors described in this chapter, like other survivors described in another study (Farber et al., 2022), were not all clinically depressed, and many were highly functional and manifested a robust ability to compartmentalize their ongoing grief despite its intensity (Farber et al., 2018). Survivors also frequently expressed "survivor guilt" and anger. As is often the case in situations of trauma in which survivors feel impotent to intervene and/or appreciate that they could equally have perished, catastrophic grief may be accompanied by survivor guilt. The term "survivor guilt," first coined by Niederland (1964) and observed by others (Hass, 1995), should be clearly distinguished from guilt associated with perceived or actual moral transgressions (Krell, 1984). "Survivor guilt" pertains to the cognitive and emotional experience of those who are fortunate enough to have survived while so many others, and so many loved ones, did not.

Anger is another feature that seemed to persist in the experience of some of the child survivors. In genocides such as the Holocaust, there is an appreciation that harm was deliberately inflicted by perpetrators and bystanders who were purposefully cruel and murderous. The added recognition of such inhumanity fuels intense anger and rage, particularly about the deaths of family members. It has been proposed that in traumatic bereavement, anger may represent a reaction to abandonment and unresolved mourning for loss experienced (Auerhahn & Laub, 1984; Lifton, 1967).

We have proposed the conceptualization of a "Trauma Trilogy" (Farber et al., 2018, 2022) as a way of understanding how catastrophic grief, survivor guilt, and anger are often entwined in aging child survivors. Such enduring trauma-related affects might constitute a vulnerability in aging child survivors when facing novel challenges, such as the pandemic, with the disruption to life and the isolation it has caused.

During COVID-19 it was apparent from my experience that for Holocaust survivors, traumas were re-triggered, yet also resilience skills were evident in their coping with periods of isolation and lockdowns. I am most grateful to have had this opportunity to visit the survivors in lockdown and offer supportive psychotherapy, as it gave me an opportunity to witness both their traumas and their remarkable resilience. During the time that I did the home visits, I started to think about the importance of offering psychotherapy to aging survivors as well as to aging trauma survivors in general, as it offers an important "last chance" to re-organize the traumas within their internal world, to prepare for the next stage. Even though stories may be repeated, the aging clients have feelings and experiences that need to be witnessed. Dori Laub (Felman & Laub, 1992), Holocaust survivor and psychoanalyst, underscored the importance of the role of the caring listener in witnessing the trauma and suffering of Holocaust survivors. It seems that even in old age, perhaps even more so than in earlier life phases, this need to be witnessed continues, and offers an important function of containment and working-through. In addition, the therapist listens and helps the individuals to make sense and meaning of both their traumatic experiences and also their resilience-building, nourishing life experiences. This type of work can potentially help aging survivors to have an opportunity to be witnessed one last time, in an attempt to reach some integration of both traumatic and life affirming experiences. Finally, having a therapeutic space offers the aging person an opportunity to potentially clarify spiritual issues which may be relevant at this final life stage.

Psychoeducational Interactive Online Webinar for Aging Children of Holocaust Survivors: Sharing Current Experiences in the Safety Provided by a Shared Legacy

Irit Felsen

During 2020–2021, I was approached by multiple social networks and organizations catering to adult children of Holocaust survivors, the "second generation" or "2G," among them, MorseLife Health System and Dr. Frumer, requesting me to provide a combination of a psychoeducational lecture and a facilitated interactive gathering to discuss the current experiences of the participants in response to the pandemic and to the national and global socio-political turmoil that characterized this particular year in the USA. Most offspring of Holocaust survivors are now entering their own aging, and so were also part of the population identified as being at elevated risk for complications from the coronavirus. During 2020–2021, over 3500 individuals from the USA, Canada, Israel, Hungary, and additional parts of the world participated in these interactive virtual meetings.

The following sections describes some of the main themes that were expressed during the interactive discussions, as well as findings from an empirical study that utilized a convenience sample of participants from these webinars. These observations are thus based on a self-selected sample and do not reflect the experience of the larger population of 2G. However, the mere number of participants who attended the meetings suggests that our observations reflect the experiences of a significant group within the larger population of 2G.

Empirical Findings

An empirical study (Shrira & Felsen, 2021), conducted between the months of June and August 2020, utilized a convenience sample drawn from the participants in online webinars for children of Holocaust survivors who responded to questionnaires online and rated posttraumatic stress disorder (PTSD) symptoms for their parents and for themselves. Additionally, COVID-19-related worries, feelings of loneliness, and the level of social support during the pandemic were also assessed. The respondents were divided into four groups: 2G with two parents with probable PTSD, with one such parent, with no such parent, and comparisons whose parents did not undergo the Holocaust.

The results demonstrated that 2G with two parents with PTSD reported the highest levels of PTSD symptoms. Controlling for respondents' own PTSD, 2G with two parents with PTSD reported higher levels of psychological distress relative to comparisons. Moreover, those who perceive one or both parents as having (probable) PTSD reported higher loneliness relative to 2G without parental PTSD or comparisons, despite the fact that there were no differences among these groups in the actual level of social support they reported. This subjective difficulty in benefiting from perceived available social support during difficult times, resulting in elevated feelings of loneliness, might represent an "invisible" vulnerability in 2G. Experiences of loneliness in the intergenerational relationships while growing up have been retrospectively described by adult children of Holocaust survivors. The relational experience of such "failed intersubjectivity" in some families of Holocaust survivors (Wiseman, 2008) thus might sensitize 2G to more intense subjective feelings of loneliness during challenging times and in response to social distancing. Parental PTSD thus appeared to be a risk factor associated with increased vulnerability of 2G to psychological distress and subjective loneliness. The critical influence of parental PTSD is consistent with other findings (Lambert et al., 2014; Leen-Feldner et al., 2013), and supports the perspective that prior exposure to traumatic or stressful events, in this case, exposure to historical trauma (SAMHSA, 2014), sensitizes individuals to novel threats (Hyer et al., 1995; Solomon, 1993).

There were no differences among the groups in our study in COVID-19-related worries. This finding might reflect that fact that the participants were mostly retired and enjoyed a relatively good financial situation, which protected them from both direct exposure to the virus and from the financial worries related to loss of income. The findings from our study suggested that the distress experienced by 2G with parental PTSD, which was reflected in higher levels of anxiety and depressive symptoms, was more general, possibly related to the cascade of socio-political crises that occurred since the pandemic began, rather than to the health risk or other concerns directly associated with COVID-19. Such concerns, articulated by participants in the interactive gatherings, are described below.

Qualitative Observations from Interactive Gatherings of 2G

An overarching sense of hypervigilance and anxiety connected with Holocaust-related associations was expressed by participants in the interactive gatherings of children of Holocaust survivors, alongside a recognition of the hardiness and an inherent preparedness for disaster that was also attributed by them to their parents' legacy of endurance and resilience during the Holocaust and in the lives they built afterwards. Common themes shared by participants (Felsen, 2021a, b) revealed associations to the Holocaust evoked by shortages in the initial months of the pandemic, as well as the rise in sales of guns and ammunition, which triggered intense anxieties about the eruption of potential violence by fellow citizens. The televised police killing of George Floyd and mass demonstrations that followed intensified anxieties about both violence perpetrated by the police and worries about mob behavior. Images of shattered glass in the streets were described as particularly triggering reminders of the infamous Kristallnacht, "Night of Shattered Glass," which took place between November 9 and 10, 1938, in which Nazis vandalized Jewish synagogues, businesses, and homes, and killed about 100 Jewish people.

The participants described a heightened hypervigilance, which has always characterized them and has enabled them to sense the dangers of COVID-19 ahead of others. They described having been prepared for disaster, in fact, having anticipated disaster, from as early an age as they can remember. They felt that they, as 2G, were better equipped to handle the difficulties of the situation, in comparison to non-Holocaust-related peers and relatives, and that this emotional preparedness and better coping were due to the perspective they have as children of Holocaust survivors and to adaptive strategies learned from the parents. Such co-existent vulnerabilities and resiliencies are consistent with the literature about families of Holocaust survivors (Shmotkin et al., 2011). However, in contrast to the adaptive value of such coping strategies during challenging times, such as the COVID-19 pandemic, 2G also commented about the cost of their chronic hypervigilance to their own well-being and to the atmosphere of their family relationships during normative, calm times.

Many participants gave words to the observation from the empirical study about a subjective feeling of loneliness. This theme is particularly relevant as it reflected a particular vulnerability among these older adults. Exacerbated subjective experiences of loneliness and isolation can be of particular concern regarding the mental health burden of the pandemic (Moreno et al., 2020) and other, potential future similar situation.

Social distancing disrupted many relationships and activities, and a vulnerability to more intense subjective sense of loneliness can put 2G (and other groups who experience intergenerational transmission of trauma) at a heightened risk in the face of such challenges.

Some 2G feared their reactions to events that triggered strong feelings related to the Holocaust would be judged as extreme by their non-Holocaust-related friends and relatives. In contrast, other 2G felt that the difficulties expressed by non-Holocaust-related others are exaggerated, and so they feared that people would be offended if they shared that as children of survivors, their perspective is less extreme, based on a comparison with what survivor parents endured during the Holocaust. Regardless of individual differences, there was an overwhelming sense of comfort expressed by participants about being able to share their feelings with others who are also children of Holocaust survivors, because of the prominence of the Holocaust and its relevance to their personal experiences. Despite differences in the individual responses to the events, there was a feeling that the shared intergenerational experiences conferred meanings which others cannot comprehend.

The Impact of the Pandemic on Community-Dwelling and Residential Care: Perspectives from the *NOW for Holocaust Survivors Initiative* in Palm Beach County (Jenni Frumer, PhD, LCSW, MSEd)

It is suggested that Holocaust survivors demonstrated unique psychological reactions to the COVID-19 pandemic (Cohn-Schwartz et al., 2020). Their early life history, advanced age, and general health-related conditions may have retraumatized them during the pandemic. Yet, others demonstrated resilience during a difficult and uncertain time.

I have worked with Holocaust survivors and their families for almost 4 decades, first in human services setting and more recently, for the past 3 years, ironically to coincide with the pandemic, for MorseLife Health System in Palm Beach, Florida. MorseLife is a leader in the care of older adults, and home to the NOW for Holocaust Survivors Initiative, a philanthropic-funded program to support Holocaust survivors and their families. The following chapter briefly describes some of the observable and stated experiences of Holocaust survivors and their offspring, the 2Gs or children of Holocaust survivors during the pandemic.

Initially, the news of the coronavirus and the toll it was taking on older adults was alarming but did not feel threatening. Once the large healthcare campus, which boasts independent and assisted living, memory residential care, affordable housing, short-term care, and a rehabilitation center serving over 800 older adults went into lockdown, did the magnitude of the impact become almost unbearable. MorseLife also serves over 2800 older adults who reside in the community, a few hundred of them, are Holocaust survivors.

The absence of a daily routine was one of the first indications of both physical and emotional struggle for so many. This was followed by an extreme sense of vulnerability and fear of engaging physically with others for fear of being infected. Many survivors either chose to or were forced to cancel the daily or weekly services they received from the formal caregivers from home health agencies that they so deeply depended on. Services generally ranged from transportation to doctor appointments (which had also shut down), grocery shopping, assistance with housekeeping (laundry and light housekeeping), assistance with bathing and dressing, meal preparation, and medication administration.

For some survivors, it felt like they were back in hiding (from the Nazis and their collaborators), fearful of being "exposed." Others expressed experiences of incarceration, not being allowed to venture out of their apartment, room, or house. Food was delivered, but it was placed on the doorstep and many continued to feel obsessed, worrying if they would have enough until the next delivery. The preoccupation with food and whether it would last can be considered a trigger from earlier trauma exposure when almost all survivors were deprived of nutrition. So many survivors admitted that they had the need to hoard food and did not eat all the meals that were delivered to their apartment or room on campus just in case the meals stopped being delivered. Many living in the community called relentlessly, to confirm the date and time of food delivery. Since it was difficult to pinpoint the time of delivery exactly, it led to greater anxiety for so many survivors. Personnel themselves felt the impact of a great sense of helplessness and perceived they in some significant ways were contributing to the distress of so many survivors.

We all remember there were no more smiles, as everyone wore facial masks, and on the healthcare and residential housing campus, personnel also wore gloves and sometimes shields. The only visible interaction with another human was their eyes and voice.

While all the survivors I interacted with were careful not to compare the pandemic to the Holocaust, a common theme in our conversations centered around how the current situation and the need to stay-at-home triggered earlier memories of conditions that often resulted in traumatic reactions. Memories were activated and the general confinement triggered fear. On a theoretical level, we continue to gain a greater understanding of how certain situations or environments may trigger memories of the past – the pandemic was doing an exceptionally good job of being a trigger for so many survivors and their children. Children of survivors, for maybe the first time, not only imagined but viscerally experienced a threat to self and life. For them, this threat against their own and their parents' lives was prolonged moments of deeper understanding and compassion for what their survivor parents may have experienced during the Holocaust. Not being able to freely engage physically with family members resonated with the 2Gs. Conversations with the children of survivors had a distinct refrain. While in no way comparable to the events of the Holocaust, when Jews were hunted down and murdered; when it was a crime to be born Jewish, there are threads that resonated at a deep emotional level when older adults feel like a target when life changes so drastically almost overnight, their eyes were opened in a different way. I observed a greater outpouring of love, devotion, and a rekindling of commitment to honoring their survivor parents and their stories.

The observable effects of prolonged isolation were visible at a psychosocial level, and in some cases, also cognitively. Survivors tearfully expressed a sense of "losing their minds" and because they were forced to stay away from loved ones, felt they would "die alone…after all the trauma and loss [they went through] during the Holocaust." It was the uncertainty of the circumstances that was hardest to bear.

While not all survivors were able to quickly adapt to or access technology, however, those who used technology to communicate, or took advantage of engaging in educational programs, expressed some relief in being able to connect with others. Interestingly, even while learning new skills, it did not necessarily decrease their worry, depression, or anxiety.

Resilience

Among the turmoil and distinct threat during the pandemic, as the literature suggests, early-life trauma can both sensitize and buffer Holocaust survivors from new adversities (Shrira et al., 2010; Bachner et al., 2018). Many survivors see themselves as examples of survival and resilience. One 94 survivor stated "… at least even though I am confined, and I hate the feeling of being stuck, like in-hiding, I know I can open my front door and stick my head out, without it being shot at by a German soldier." Another survivor commented on the lack of availability of toilet paper during this time and stated "… I did not see toilet paper for years [during the Holocaust] so this is nothing to panic about… it isn't the end of the world." Her statement, accompanied by a smile, and flippant hand gesture was not intended to be submissive. She further expressed a deep sense of resilience in her words and behaviors every time I interacted with her. For her, the pandemic was temporary and she claimed the past had prepared her well.

Loneliness and Social Isolation

Social isolation has been defined as social disconnectedness; the physical separation from others and the perceived isolation, resulting in feelings of loneliness and lack of support (Cornwell & Waite, 2009). The survivors I engaged with suffered from physical and emotional social isolation, resulting for the most part in severe feelings of loneliness. As a result of the pandemic, families were not able to visit. Too often, even the staff did not "visit" and were required to pass meals and medications through cracks in the doors of apartments and rooms in residential care. Loneliness, defined as a perceived state of social and emotional isolation, has been associated with cognitive and functional decline (Donovan et al., 2016). In my interaction with survivors and their families, I was continually struck by how palpable and observable it was to see how survivors struggled with acute psychological stress, symptoms of depression, bereavement, and other experiences of social disconnection. These types of reactions to quarantine and forced social isolation – feeling like a prisoner – tended to amplify difficulties in overall physical, emotional, and cognitive functioning of so many survivors.

One of the first studies assessing the psychiatric correlates of loneliness among older adults during the COVID-19 found that the association between loneliness and psychiatric symptoms was significant and robust only among participants with older subjective ages (Shrira et al., 2020). Among those with young subjective ages, there were no adverse correlates of loneliness. These findings highlight the moderating effects of subjective age regarding the effects of stress, and the importance of further research into the factors that are associated with, or support, younger subjective age. Understanding better the relationship between subjective age, loneliness and psychiatric symptoms will help identify who are older adults at risk, especially when opportunities for social contact are greatly reduced.

Lessons Learned

While presumptuous to suggest we have the answers, I think it is worth mentioning some of the obvious and not-so-obvious lessons we take with us from the pandemic and especially from the survivors served by MorseLife. I keep learning about the effects of the pandemic on Holocaust survivors and their families. Interventions to reduce the threat of infection among the survivors served to continue to be front and center during this endemic stage of the pandemic. I continue to learn about how a global pandemic has translated into more local understandings of how much social isolation resonates with survivors and their families. Professionally, I have a keen awareness of these issues. We have learned considerations and how to put greater effort into mitigating social isolation and loneliness for all older adults. Post-pandemic, there is more support and recognition of the importance of intervention to reduce social isolation and loneliness. We continue to learn how resilient survivors can be. We have learned how much more compassionate caregivers have become, especially those who have identified more with survivors' experiences at the hands of the Nazis. Ultimately, there is collective, greater sensitivity to and recognition of the ill effects of relational deprivation on older adults. For so many survivors, their families are the living testimonies to winning the war and defying Hitler's plan for the total annihilation of the Jewish people. Surviving the COVID-19 pandemic was both a curse, a significant disruption and a real threat to lives, and also a blessing in that many survivors and their families found a deeper connection.

Older Adult Trauma and Resilience: A Public Health Priority

Mary Beth Quaranta Morrissey

My experience in the Older Adults Working Group has been rewarding. I first learned of the Working Group from colleagues in the wider APA Interdivisional COVID Task Force. I was immediately engaged at my first meeting when I learned the group leaders and interlocutors would be studying trauma among older adults during the pandemic. I had been working on public health policy issues related to the pandemic in the role of chair of the New York State Bar Association's (NYSBA) first COVID Task Force under the aegis of the Health Law Section, and later serving as member of NYSBA's Task Force on Nursing Homes and Long-Term Care (2021). Both these Reports were adopted by NYSBA's House of Delegates (2020, 2021) and have highlighted the trauma experienced by older adults in the pandemic environment.

I eventually connected with Irit Felsen, Jenni Frumer, and other members of the group at one of their first meetings. Dr. Frumer shared that she was beginning her research exploring intergenerational trauma among Holocaust refugees. I was reminded that I had never left behind my own personal story as a child growing up next door to a woman by the name of Beatrice Peltzman whose family had been killed in the Holocaust. As children, my brother Kevin and I – along with Beatrice's three sons – heard Beatrice recite many times her story of escaping the Nazis, climbing out a window to the roof of her residence. Beatrice's parents and brother, who was a famous pianist in Europe, were killed by the Nazis. I carried the story of Beatrice's and her family's lived experience of intergenerational trauma well beyond my early youth to the present day and have understood its meanings and historical significance.

Beatrice's story also provided a context of meaning for understanding the trauma of older adults who experienced terrible suffering during the pandemic. Now at a point later in my career and equipped with formal knowledge in gerontology, gerontological social work research, and health and public health policy, I recognized the suffering of older adults in its many forms – abandonment, social isolation, limited or no access to family or friends, physical suffering that accompanied COVID for those older adults who had been unlucky enough to contract the virus, and perhaps most dramatically the trauma and smell of death; the death of loved ones and friends and the impact upon whole communities. And these traumatic experiences and losses had been compounded by not being able to grieve and mourn in keeping with social and cultural customs and traditions.

The question that emerged early on in the work of the group was whether the lived experience of older adults in the new pandemic environment was a public health crisis of its very own embedded in the larger contexts of the declared COVID public health emergency and global health crisis. And if so, how could we better understand the legal, social, and economic determinants of the older adult public health crisis and its layers of complexity? The work done by the New York State Bar had made clear that during the public health emergency in New York we were operating under crisis conditions. The normal operations of the health and public health systems in New York had been disrupted. Resources were in scarce supply, and that scarcity extended to staffing shortages and supplies of PPE, for example. New York's most prominent bioethicists had been writing prolifically about these issues and calling attention to the potential for ageism and discrimination in decisions about resource allocation. Advocates in the disabilities community joined in the outcry about violations of the human rights of older people and people with disabilities. In institutional settings, such as nursing homes, the intersectionality of age, race, disability, and vulnerability was perhaps most pronounced. There is a robust body of evidence that nursing home residents were disproportionately impacted by the pandemic. Older people in correctional facilities also received little attention in the media, and were certainly denied access to vaccines and other public health protections until much later in the course of the pandemic.

Little is also known at this point in time about the experience of Holocaust refugees during the pandemic, most of whom are now advanced in age. What does their experience look like and who will tell their story? The leaders and members of the Older Adults Work Group are committed to that project and support the ongoing work of the Group's scholars who are moving this research forward, drawing on diverse methods of inquiry.

As a matter of public policy, the COVID Older Adults Work Group will continue to advocate for recognition of older adult trauma as a public health concern. Disseminating older adult trauma research will better inform public health policymaking and funding for adequate services and supports for older adults, including supporting resilience.

Conclusions Irit Felsen,PhD

By 2050, the US older adult population will have doubled from earlier in this century to 83.7 million people and reports have shown that the workforce is woefully underprepared to meet the mental health needs of this population (Hinrichsen et al., 2018). Advances in medicine and improved life and work conditions have created a new and growing sub-group within this population of older adults: those who are relatively well, who want, need, and are able to continue to contribute to families and to society.

This chapter aims to call attention to the needs of this relatively new and relatively neglected segment among older adults, those whom we termed "vibrant older adults," whose unique needs and challenges are invisible not only in the social discourse but even among psychologists. As our experience has shown, this omission reflects not only a knowledge gap, as other studies have found, but also ageism and subjective discomfort among psychologists about being perceived by others, and perceiving ourselves, as older adults.

Furthermore, this chapter describes work conducted by our members during the COVID-19 pandemic, with particularly vulnerable sub-groups within the population of vibrant older adults. As trauma experts, several of us have been focused in our clinical work and in research on aging Holocaust survivors and their now-aging adult children. We continued to intervene with these populations during the pandemic. The work reviewed here demonstrates the effects of extreme trauma in previous life phases on the experiences of aging trauma survivors during the pandemic, as well as the effects of intergenerational transmission of both trauma and resilience (Shmotkin et al., 2011) in the responses of the 'second generation' during these challenging times. Research on Holocaust survivors and their families has provided frameworks for the study of historical trauma and intergenerational trauma in multiple other populations (Duran et al., 1998; Yellow Horse Brave Heart et al., 2011; Cross, 1998). Our work with this population during the COVID-19 pandemic, as described in the different sections of the chapter, continues to show the relevance of massive trauma for survivors and their descendants in coping with various aspects of the pandemic and with the socio-political and cultural upheaval that accompanied it. The observations reflect both unique vulnerabilities and resilient coping that are associated with a legacy of trauma. Our observations can inform research and clinical work with other trauma-exposed groups. Continuing to deepen the understanding of historical trauma and intergenerational transmission and its persistent effects later in life is particularly relevant in these times of global crisis. Over the next years, mental health professionals will encounter high numbers of individuals with trauma histories, due to the fact that we are currently witnessing the highest numbers of refugees and displaced populations since after the end of WWII, and due to the global death-toll and economic crises caused by the pandemic. It is our hope that the lessons learned from the experiences of survivors of the Holocaust and their offspring during the global COVID-19 pandemic and the unique socio-political upheaval during 2020–2021 will enhance the understanding and the preparedness of the mental health professionals dealing with future potential challenges.

References

American Psychiatric Association. (2013). *Diagnostic and statistical manual of mental disorders* (5th ed.). American Psychiatric Association.

Auerhahn, N. C., & Laub, D. (1984). Annihilation and restoration: Post traumatic memory as pathway and obstacle to recovery. *International Review of Psychoanalysis, 11*, 327–344.

Ayalon, L., Chasteen, A., Daiehl, M., Levy, B. R., Neupert, S. D., Rothermund, K., Tesch-Römer, C., & Wahl, H.-W. (2021). Aging in times of the COVID-19 pandemic: Avoiding ageism and fostering intergenerational solidarity. *The Journals of Gerontology: Series B, 76*(2), e49–e52. https://doi.org/10.1093/geronb/gbaa051

Bachner, Y. G., Carmel, S., & O'Rourke, N. (2018). The paradox of well-being and Holocaust survivors. *Journal of the American Psychiatric Nurses Association, 24*, 45–52. https://doi.org/10.1177/1078390317705450

Baider, L., Goldzweig, G., Ever-Hadani, P., & Peretz, T. (2008). Breast cancer and psychological distress: Mothers' and daughters' traumatic experiences. *Supportive Care in Cancer, 16*(4), 407–414. https://doi.org/10.1007/s00520-007-0320-1

Barel, E., Van IJzendoorn, M. H., Sagi-Schwartz, A., & Bakermans-Kranenburg, M. J. (2010). Surviving the Holocaust: A meta-analysis of the long-term sequelae of a genocide. *Psychological Bulletin, 136*(5), 677–698.

Centers for Disease Control and Prevention (CDC). (2020). *Coronavirus disease 2019 (COVID-19) older adults.*

Cohn-Schwartz, E., Sagi, D., O'Rourke, N., & Bachner, Y. G. (2020). The coronavirus pandemic and Holocaust survivors in Israel. *Psychological Trauma: Theory, Research, Practice, and Policy, 12*(5), 502–504. https://doi.org/10.1037/tra0000771

Cornwell, E. Y., & Waite, L. J. (2009). Measuring social isolation among older adults using multiple indicators from the NSHAP study. *Journal of Gerontology Psychological Sciences and Social Sciences, 64B*, 38–46.

Cross, W. E. (1998). Black psychological functioning and the legacy of slavery: Myths and realities. In Y. Danieli (Ed.), *The handbook of multigenerational legacies of trauma* (pp. 387–403). Plenum Press.

Danieli, Y. (1988). Confronting the unimaginable: Psychotherapists 'reactions to victims of the Nazi Holocaust'. In J. P. Wilson, Z. Harel, & B. Kahana (Eds.), *Human adaptation to extreme stress* (pp. 219–238). Plenum Press.

Danieli, Y. (Ed.). (1998). *The handbook of multigenerational legacies of trauma*. Plenum Press.

Donovan, N. J., Wu, Q., Rentz, D. M., Sperling, R. A., Marshall, G. A., & Glymour, M. M. (2016). Loneliness, depression, and cognitive function in older U.S. adults. *International Journal Geriatric Psychiatry*, 564–573.

Duran, E., Duran, B., Yellow Horse Brave Heart, M., & Yellow Horse-Davis, S. (1998). Healing the American Indian soul wound. In Y. Danieli (Ed.), *The handbook of multigenerational legacies of trauma* (pp. 341–355).

Erikson, E. H. (1964). *Childhood and society* (2nd ed.). W. W. Norton.

Farber, T. R. (2019). *Integrity versus despair: The experiences of traumatised child Holocaust survivors* (Unpublished doctoral dissertation). University of the Witwatersrand, Johannesburg.

Farber, T., Eagle, G., & Smith, C. (2018). Catastrophic grief and associated defences in elderly child Holocaust survivors. *Psycho-Analytic Psychotherapy in South Africa, 26*(2), 49–83.

Farber, T., Smith, C., & Eagle, G. (2022). The trauma trilogy of catastrophic grief, survivor guilt and anger in aging child Holocaust survivors. *Journal of Loss and Trauma, 27*(2), 99–119.

Felman, S., & Laub, D. (1992). *Testimony: Crises of witnessing in literature, psychoanalysis, and history*. Taylor & Francis.

Felsen, I. (2020–2021). *Next generations lecture series*. https://www.youtube.com/playlist?list=PL98TejO6Vy3qoYCkt71NEKjfHw431dvet

Felsen, I. (2021a). "Web-based, second-best togetherness": Psychosocial group intervention with children of Holocaust survivors during COVID-19. *American Journal of Orthopsychiatry, 91*(2), 171–180.

Felsen, I. (2021b). "The canary in the mine": Re-traumatization and resilience in offspring of Holocaust survivors during the Covid-19 pandemic. *Trauma Psychology, Division 56 Trauma News Letter,* Fall 2020, *15*(3).

Hass, A. (1995). Survivor guilt in Holocaust survivors and their children. *A Global Perspective on Working with Holocaust Survivors and the Second Generation, 35*, 163–183.

Herman, J. L. (1992). *Trauma and recovery: From domestic abuse to political terror*. Pandora Publishers.

Hinrichsen, G. A., Emery-Tiburcio, E. E., Gooblar, J., & Molinari, V. A. (2018). Building foundational knowledge competencies in professional geropsychology: Council of Professional

Geropsychology Training Programs (CoPGTP) recommendations. *Clinical Psychology: Science and Practice, 25*(2), e12236. https://doi.org/10.1111/cpsp.12236

Horowitz, M. J., Bonanno, G. A., & Holen, A. (1993). Pathological grief: Diagnosis and explanation. *Psychosomatic Medicine, 55*(3), 260–273. https://doi.org/10.1097/00006842-199305000-00004

Hyer, L., Summers, M. N., Braswell, L., & Boyd, S. (1995). Posttraumatic stress disorder: Silent problem among older combat veterans. *Psychotherapy: Theory, Research, and Practice, 32*, 348–364. https://doi.org/10.1037/0033-3204.32.2.348

Klein, H., & Holder, A. (2012). *Survival and trials of revival: Psychodynamic studies of Holocaust survivors and their families in Israel and the diaspora*. Academic Studies Press. https://doi.org/10.1515/9781618111074

Kluger, R. (2002). *Still alive: A Holocaust girlhood remembered*. Feminist Press at the City University of New York.

Krell, R. (1984). Holocaust survivors and their children: Comments on psychiatric consequences and psychiatric terminology. *Comprehensive Psychiatry, 25*(5), 521–528.

Lambert, J. E., Holzer, J., & Hasbun, A. (2014). Association between parents' PTSD severity and childrens' psychological distress: A metaanalysis. *Journal of Traumatic Stress, 27*(1), 9–17. https://doi.org/10.1002/jts.21891

Leen-Feldner, E., Feldner, M. T., Knapp, A., Bunaciu, L., Blumenthal, H., & Amstadter, A. (2013). Offspring psychological and biological correlates of parental posttraumatic stress: Review of the literature and research agenda. *Clinical Psychology Review, 33*(2013), 1106–1133. https://doi.org/10.1016/j.cpr.2013.09.001

Lifton, R. J. (1967). *Death in life: Survivors of Hiroshima*. Random House.

Moreno, C., Wykes, T., Galderisi, S., Nordentoft, M., Crossley, N., Jones, N., Cannon, M., Correll, C. U., Byrne, L., Carr, S., Chen, E. Y. H., Gorwood, P., Johnson, S., Kärkkäinen, H., Krystal, J. H., Lee, J., Lieberman, J., López-Jaramillo, C., Männikkö, M., & Arango, C. (2020). How mental health care should change as a consequence of the COVID-19 pandemic. *Lancet Psychiatry*. https://doi.org/10.1016/S2215-0366(20)30307-2

Niederland, W. G. (1964). Psychiatric disorders among persecution victims: A contribution to the understanding of concentration camp pathology and its after-effects. *The Journal of Nervous and Mental Disease, 139*(5), 458–474. https://doi.org/10.1097/00005053-196411000-00006

New York State Bar Association. New York State Bar Association COVID-19 Resolutions. (2020). Retrieved June 17, 2021, from https://nysba.org.app/uploads/2020/02/Final-NYSBA-COVID-19-Resolutions_11-7-20-with-single3link.pdf

New York State Bar Association. New York State Bar Association Health Law Section COVID-19 Report. (2020). Retrieved June 17, 2021 from https://nysba.org/app/uploads/2020/09/Health-Law-Section-COVID-19-Report-September-20-2020.pdf

New York State Bar Association. (2021). New York State Bar Association Nursing Homes and Long Term Care Report. NYSBA.

Rozalski, V., Holland, J. M., & Neimeyer, R. A. (2017). Circumstances of death and complicated grief: Indirect associations through meaning made of loss. *Journal of Loss and Trauma, 22*(1), 11. https://doi.org/10.1080/15325024.2016.1161426

SAMSHA. (2014). *Trauma informed care in behavioral health services*. https://store.samhsa.gov/product/TIP-57-Trauma-Informed-Care-in-Behavioral-Health-Services/SMA14-4816

Shmotkin, D. (2005). Happiness in face of adversity: Reformulating the dynamic and modular bases of subjective well-being. *Review of General Psychology, 9*(4), 291–325. https://doi.org/10.1037/1089-2680.9.4.291

Shmotkin, D., Shrira, A., Goldberg, S., & Palgi, Y. (2011). Resilience and vulnerability among aging Holocaust survivors and their families: An intergenerational overview. *Journal of Intergenerational Relationships, 9*(1), 7–21. https://doi.org/10.1080/15350770.2011.544202

Shrira, A. (2015). Transmitting the sum of all fears: Iranian nuclear threat salience among offspring of Holocaust survivors. *Psychological Trauma: Theory, Research, Practice, and Policy, 7*(4), 364–371. https://doi.org/10.1037/tra0000029

Shrira, A., & Baumel-Schwartz, J. (Eds.). *The handbook of second generation* (Taylor and Francis, in publication).

Shrira, A., & Felsen, I. (2021). Parental PTSD and psychological reactions during the COVID-19 pandemic among offspring of Holocaust survivors. *Psychological Trauma: Theory, Research, Practice, and Policy.* Advance online publication. https://doi.org/10.1037/tra0001014

Shrira, A., Hoffman, Y., Bodner, E., 7 Palgi, Y. (2020). COVID-19-Related Lonliness and Psychiaatric Symptoms Among Older Adults: The Buffering Role of Subjective Age. *The American Journal of Geriatric Psychiatry, 28*(11), 1200–1204.

Shrira, A., Palgi, Y., Ben-Ezra, M., & Shmotkin, D. (2010). Do Holocaust survivors show increased vulnerability or resilience to post-Holocaust cumulative adversity? *Journal of Traumatic Stress, 23*(3), 367–375. https://doi-org.ezproxy.cul.columbia.edu/10.1002/jts.20524

Solomon, Z. (1993). *Combat stress reaction: The enduring toll of war*. Plenum Press.

Solomon, Z., Kotler, M., & Mikulincer M. (1988). *American Journal of Psychiatry, 145*(7), 865–868.

Wiseman, H. (2008). On failed intersubjectivity: Recollections of loneliness experiences in offspring of Holocaust survivors. *American Journal of Orthopsychiatry, 78*(3), 350–358.

Witztum, E., & Malkinson, R. (2009). Examining traumatic grief and loss among Holocaust survivors. *Journal of Loss and Trauma, 14*(2), 129–143. https://doi.org/10.1080/15325020902724511

Yellow Horse Brave Hearth, Chase, J., Elkins, J., & Altschul, D. B. (2011). Historical trauma among Indigenous Peoples of the Americas: concepts, research, and clinical considerations. *Journal of Psychoactive Drugs, 43*(4), 282–290. https://doi.org/10.1080/02791072.2011.628913

Chapter 6
The Hospital, Health and Addiction Workers, Patients and Families

Maureen O'Reilly-Landry, Patricia O'Gorman, and Robert M. Gordon

Introduction

Origin

Maureen O'Reilly-Landry

Our group was present from the very beginning of the Task Force when in March 2020, Dr. Maureen O'Reilly-Landry reached out to APA colleagues to inquire about joining the APA COVID Task Force she assumed already existed. As a medical psychologist and psychoanalyst whose professional work focused on medically induced psychological stress and trauma, she was acutely aware of the potential for significant emotional fallout from this unfolding worldwide health crisis. But it was a personal situation that provided the true motivation to get involved: with both a husband and son working as physicians in a New York City hospital, the first epicenter of the COVID-19 crisis, she wanted a meaningful way to use her own skills to join their valiant mission to address the potential devastation of the novel coronavirus. She was also very worried about them.

In her capacity as Co-Chair of the Psychoanalysis and Healthcare Committee of APA's Division of Psychoanalysis (39), she emailed colleagues to find out who chaired the COVID-19 Task Force. Drs. Judie Alpert and Kathleen Kendall-Tackett responded immediately, though neither they nor anyone they spoke to could find

M. O'Reilly-Landry
Columbia University, Psychiatry Department, New York, NY, USA

P. O'Gorman
Saranac Lake, New York, NY, USA; https://www.patriciaogorman.com

R. M. Gordon (✉)
New York University Grossman School of Medicine, New York, NY, USA
e-mail: Gordon@nyulangone.org

C. R. Figley et al. (eds.), *Pandemic Providers*,
https://doi.org/10.1007/978-3-031-27580-7_6

such a group. Members of the Trauma Division, however, thought it was an excellent idea. Dr. Carolyn Allard, then President of the Trauma Division, put out a call and within days, a COVID-19 task force was created. Dr. Charles Figley, who would head the group, suggested it be interdivisional, and so it is, with Division 39 as one of the founding members.

Maureen now saw her purpose: to create a work group within the Task Force that would address the adverse psychological sequelae for those working in hospitals treating patients with COVID-19. A few weeks later, Susan McDaniel, a leader in Health Psychology (Division 38), and Past President of APA, responded to Maureen's original email stating, "I can't believe I missed this, but I did in the COVID-deluge. Would my help still be useful?" Absolutely, Maureen responded. Susan, too, thought it an excellent idea, and joined our group.

Our group's strength derives from having arisen from the bottom up, rather than as a directive from leadership. As such, it is driven by the collective experience, training, and passions of our individual members. Individuals with collective expertise in acute and chronic trauma, medical and health psychology, PTSD, addictions, grief, compassion fatigue and vicarious trauma, cultural, racial, and socioeconomic disparities, moral injury, crisis intervention, psychological first aid, psychoanalysis, existentialism, somatic therapies, psychological resilience, post-traumatic growth, stress reduction, and policy and legal issues, all joined together in an effort to mitigate the adverse psychological sequelae in COVID hospitals. Shortly after its inception, Patricia O'Gorman, trauma and addiction specialist from rural New York State, joined the group and Maureen asked her to serve with her as co-chair. The number of patients dying from the opioid epidemic was already up by 13% from 2019, without accounting for those also dying from the rapid increase in alcohol consumption as a direct result of the pandemic. The realization that we were addressing an epidemic within a pandemic gave us all pause. With Patricia's expertise, the scope of our group broadened even further to include outpatient and addiction settings.

Along the way, we encountered some unanticipated issues: What can we call ourselves when we interface with medical organizations and the public? Is it permissible to use the imprimatur of APA at all, given we had not been appointed by the leadership? Was it the case that we were in the APA, yet not of the APA? Where is the boundary between merely providing resources and engaging in consultation? Facilitated by group members Dr. Lu Steinberg, a member of the APA Council, and attorney Dr. Mary Beth Morrissey, these issues became part of discussions with APA legal counsel.

Mission

Maureen O'Reilly Landry

Nowhere is American was the potential for pandemic-related trauma greater than for those in Emergency Rooms and Intensive Care Units in hospitals treating COVID-19 patients. In addition to the personal fear of contagion from a virus about which so little was understood and against whose deadly effects there was often inadequate protective gear, medical clinicians also bore witness to overwhelming numbers of sick bodies that far exceeded the hospital's capacity to treat. Difficult decisions needed to be made about who warranted immediate attention and who must of necessity be ignored. In places that were hardest hit, dead bodies piled up, while some that were still living languished unattended. Efforts to contain the spread of the virus meant that once admitted to the hospital, families and loved ones must be left behind, an emotionally devastating situation for all.

The Hospital, Health and Addiction Workers, Patients and Families Work Group arose originally out of concern for the psychological well-being of medical "first responders" working in hospitals treating patients infected with COVID-19: physicians, nurses, respiratory therapists, and all medical clinicians. Of particular concern were those working in Emergency Rooms and Intensive Care Units, where acute psychological trauma was expected to be greatest.

We quickly realized that all "essential workers" performing valuable and necessary jobs in highly infected hospital environments and where encounters with death and dead bodies were common occurrences, would be at great risk for emotional stress and psychological trauma. We understood that we needed to include all people working in COVID hospitals: non-medical clinicians, spiritual counselors, and non-clinician essential workers such as janitors, food preparers, and support staff.

We are unusual in our desire to address the unique needs of the often-overlooked non-clinical staff ("unsung heroes") such as housekeeping, who put themselves and their families at risk, but who receive little attention for their sacrifice. We appreciated that lower social status, economic insecurity, crowded home conditions, membership in racial/ethnic minority groups, compounded by relative invisibility and lack of recognition for their sacrifices might all serve to increase vulnerability to emotional distress and trauma.

Soon thereafter, hospitalized COVID-19 patients and their families also fell under our umbrella of concern. We recognized the double trauma of being seriously ill while also in enforced isolation from loved ones, and the simultaneous suffering of family members not permitted to give comfort to their gravely ill loved ones. For the treating clinicians, bearing witness to their patient's emotional suffering amplifies the emotional stress already placed on them. This circle of psychological distress and trauma is then taken home, affecting the families of those working in these settings.

We recognize the enormous grief and trauma, as well as the spiritual and existential issues that have arisen during the pandemic. Our focus is on reducing distress, developing resiliency, and facilitating post-traumatic growth by addressing traumatic stress, moral injury, compassion fatigue, depression, suicide, and other negative psychological sequelae during this worldwide health crisis.

Our group's overarching goal has been to reduce and, when possible, prevent COVID-related psychological trauma, and facilitate resiliency and even post-traumatic growth for those who work or are cared for in medical or addiction centers. Many hospitals and organizations were developing their own programs and resources, so our first goal became to collect, organize, and disseminate

COVID-specific clinical, educational, and training resources, including articles, videos, podcasts, webinars, and tip sheets. Eventually, we began to create and disseminate our own resources described in the subsequent sections of the chapter.

In the summer of 2020, a psychiatrist from South Korea sought us out to tell us about public policy interventions she and her colleagues had developed in her country, and we assisted in the dissemination of their writings in this country. Our group has an international component that includes members representing Qatar, Spain, India, Israel, Iceland, Honduras, and Cuba.

At one of our earlier meetings, a health psychologist advised that dissemination would be our greatest challenge, to which we responded with the creation of a website https://resilienceandcovid.us/, a Psychology Today blog: Psychological Trauma, Coping and Resilience, and a speaker series for psychologists and medical professionals, which will be described in the *Clinical Interventions* and *Speaker Series* sections of the chapter. Our first goal then became to collect, organize, and disseminate these COVID-19-specific clinical, educational, and training resources. We then began to create our own resources by drawing on the collective wisdom of our talented group of trauma-informed experts.

What Kept Us Going?

Maureen O'Reilly-Landry

With many initial fits and starts, our group took quite a while to figure itself out. Looking back on the early phase of the group's evolution, it is hard to comprehend how we made it this far and accomplished what we did. But the answer essentially boils down to this: this group is comprised of the most amazing group of human beings I have ever had the privilege to know. As the group evolved and membership stabilized, I came to appreciate the extraordinary level of accomplishment, expertise, wisdom, and dedication of this group of trauma-informed psychologists and mental health experts. But at the beginning, this had not been so clear to me.

Initial meetings felt daunting as the group's rapidly growing membership looked to me for instruction on what to do. While filled with ideas about what was needed, I lacked knowledge about how to make these things happen, or anyone with whom to share the burden of figuring it out. Eventually, and not a moment too soon, Patricia O'Gorman joined the group. In a conversation outside the weekly meeting, I recognized her as someone I connected with on many levels, both personal and professional, and as a kindred spirit with whom I both could and wanted to work. She accepted my offer to co-chair the group with me, and things began looking up from there.

We worked well together, both of us valuing a collaborative style of discussion and decision-making and a desire to hear from the group members. While I tended to the behind-the-scenes issues that kept the group activities going, Patricia went out of her way to support and encourage group members in their own work. The group is extremely hard working, but like so many psychologists, we tend not to practice the type of self-care we know to be important, particularly when working with trauma. A pivotal moment occurred in the group when, feeling fatigued and overwhelmed, Patricia and I considered reducing the frequency of our meetings and discussed this with the group. At the suggestion of Judy Roth, a valued group member working in the trenches with medical students during the peak of the pandemic, we chose instead to invite individual members to speak about their own work, with emphasis on the challenges and struggles they were encountering. From these sometimes quite emotional meetings emerged a sense of group cohesion and openness, and the group became for many of us a source of support, connection, and energy that has persisted.

As soon as we launched our blog, "Psychological Trauma, Coping and Resilience: COVID-19 and pandemics," I put together a 4-part series to address the trauma taking place in Intensive Care Units of hospitals treating COVID-19 patients. Since little had been written at that time specifically about COVID ICUs, it was necessary to draw on what we already knew prior to the pandemic, though we fully understood this would not address the trauma of the isolation of the patient and separation from families and loved ones. I began this series of my own pre-pandemic experiences of having a son in the ICU, in order to describe the potentially traumatic impact on family members ("When Trauma Hits Home," December 1, 2002, and "The Psychological Trauma of Having a Loved One in the ICU," December 3, 2020b). Next in the series are two blogs by invited guest author Dr. Ethan Lester, a psychologist at Massachusetts General Hospital, describing a program created prior to COVID-19 that had been helping ICU families to cope with ICU stress and trauma ("Making an Emotional Recovery Together in the COVID-19 ICU," December 4, 2020a; and "Managing Emotional Distress in the Hospital and ICU," December 8, 2020b). Finally, couple and family expert and member of our group, Dr. Irina Wren, directly addressed the issues faced by family members specifically in the COVID ICU ("What Can I Do if My Family Member is in the COVID ICU?" December 16, 2020). Because so very many issues became so much worse during the pandemic, COVID-19 brought to light many serious that had previously existed below the radar. We recognized that the plight of family members and staff in the ICU is one of these issues and devoted an installment in our Speaker Series to the topic, "Psychological Trauma in the ICU: The Healing Power of Relationships" (Maureen O'Reilly-Landry, Ph.D. & Denise Carballea, MS, a graduate student in our working group). A subgroup of attendees from this talk joined us in forming a subgroup to address mental health problems of families and staff in ICUs.

That human beings are essentially meaning-making creatures was made evident to me during the early weeks of the pandemic as we all struggled to make sense of what was happening to use and to the world. As I listened to people coming to see me in my private office and then later on video, I heard people reacting to nearly identical situations in completely different, sometimes, even opposite ways, and these differences did not correspond to life circumstances, such as membership in a vulnerable group, level of exposure to the virus, etc. For example, I wondered what could account, for when some medical professionals in infected COVID-19 hospitals experienced fear and dread as they traveled the subway to work, while others felt a sense of emptiness or even guilt on their days off. I came to realize it was in the personal meaning of the situation, which I described in my blog, "Discover Your Personal Meaning in the COVID-19 Experience" (O'Reilly-Landry, March 9, 2021c). There, I posed some questions the answers to which might be helpful in discerning one's own meaning: "What do I most fear?" This may tell you where your values lie. "What do I most fear losing?" This will tell you what you hold most dear. Perhaps we could emerge from this crisis knowing as much about ourselves as about the virus that has given us this opportunity to self-reflect.

Dr. Patricia O'Gorman

It felt like COVID-19 dropped a steel shutter over my life, but as an addiction and trauma psychologist consulting in rural addiction and mental health treatment and recovery system in northern New York State, a mostly improvised area covering 4000 square miles, I knew I could not stop.

In my world where I focus on addiction and trauma, working with veterans with PTSD and addiction, and teenagers as young as twelve with such serious addiction and mental health concerns that they require inpatient care, I already knew an addiction epidemic was raging. I felt a cold pit in my stomach as I considered what COVID-19 would do to intensify this. Unfortunately, I wasn't proven wrong which I documented in a recent post O'Gorman, P Morgan, C Addiction + Covid = A Toxic Cocktail where we explored: Alcohol use disorders are the third-leading preventable cause of death; opioid overdose is the leading cause of accidental death for those under age 44; and breakthrough COVID-infections are more commons among those with SUD's.

Having been raised that "if you are not part of the solution, you are part of the problem," I knew I had to do something: turning to the APA, I explored what efforts I could join. There I found a work group of first responders, the only group vaguely health related, developed by Dr. Maureen O'Reilly Landry, a psychologist whose energy and commitment to patient care, had spurred the APA to begin to systematically address COVID-19.

After attending a few meetings, Maureen asked me to co-chair our workgroup, an honor and responsibility that we have shared since then. We considered what to call ourselves, as our scope was broader than she had initially considered, addiction was now included in our name. Together we explored what was needed, how to address the new stressors psychologists were feeling in working now virtually, most for the first time, and still needing to address the needs of patients, their families, and the healthcare and addiction staff who care for them. We also began to address the one voice that was, and still is, missing in the COVID-19 debate, that of psychologists. We felt that surely, we the profession that focused on behavior, conflicts, and how to heal from them by developing resilience could be of value.

We began to meet weekly in this journey into healthcare, addiction, and COVID-19 creating a collective of sorts, where all had a voice, and an opportunity to write a post for our Psychology Today blog: Psychological Trauma, Coping and Resilience. As someone who has written books on resilience, I was thrilled with our approach. My first blog post in our joint effort was aptly titled O'Gorman, P. On the Covid-19 Battlefield: Providing Psychological Guidance, Hope and Resilience.

Working intensively together, some weeks daily, it was hard to believe I had never met Maureen in person. That is until recently, 2 years after we began working when she joined me in marching in the first St. Patrick's Day Parade in New York City in 2 years, together holding the banner for a new organization to the parade, the "Sober St. Patrick's Day Foundation," an organization on whose Board where I serve. Linking addiction to COVID-19 on St. Patrick's Day, I addressed in O'Gorman, P. On St. Patrick's Day, Be Truly Radical—Celebrate Sobriety: Why During an Addiction Epidemic Within A Pandemic, Choosing Sobriety is Smart.

Our working group has evolved during the past 2 years into an interested, supportive, worldwide community for each other, and for those we served. Currently, we are supporting a colleague on a strike in Spain, another who is setting up a mental health clinic in Qatar, another from Iceland opening up a holistic clinic in Arizona, and a colleague who has moved to Israel. We have spanned the globe with both caring, learning from each other, and using this to help others. We are each connecting with like-minded psychologists, broadening and enriching the scope of our work, and strengthening the impact of our clinical experience in trauma, resilience, and coping to help heal our world.

The Culture of the Work Group

Dr. Janet Plotkin-Bornstein

In March 2020, New York City experienced unimaginable terror and uncertainty, and rapidly became the epicenter of the unfolding global pandemic. As a clinical psychologist and psychoanalyst working in private practice, I had to suddenly pivot from working within the "sacred space" of my physical office in Manhattan, to the disembodied world of "telehealth," of virtual sessions with my patients. In most times of national crisis, we are able to find comfort and support through the psychological and physical presence of others. However, in this unprecedented emergent situation, being physically present with others was deemed to be potentially life threatening. Rather than being a haven of comfort, we all became potential sources of contagion. I grappled with the very nature of emotional intimacy within this new virtual world.

Then, early in the Spring of 2020, I was invited to join Dr. Maureen O'Reilly-Landry, founder of our group, on her most inspired mission to offer the world of healthcare workers, patients, and their families, resources to help them cope with the psychological trauma that was rapidly engulfing our entire world.

Over the course of the past 2 years, our beloved group, with our two co-leaders, Drs. O'Reilly-Landry and Patricia O'Gorman, developed into an exquisitely emotionally intimate group of international and national colleagues. The group taught me, in very palpable ways, that emotional intimacy could be created even from within virtual spaces that encompass diverse geographical, cultural, and theoretical differences.

As I strove to create and nurture emotionally safe, intimate, and meaningful spaces with my patients in this new virtual world, so too, my personal life became deeply impacted by all of my cherished colleagues in our work group. Our weekly Friday meetings became a source of vitality, a renewed sense of hope and purpose, which I was, in turn, able to carry into my clinical work with my patients. The nature of emotional intimacy within this new pandemic world of deep uncertainty and vulnerability continually evolves.

During these 2 years, I have passionately searched the media and Internet for new and relevant information, articles, and stories for our group's website, particularly with my longstanding interests in grief and mourning, and moral suffering, injury, and courage. Patricia lovingly named me "resource detective" of our group. My drive to find and share resources was borne out of my heartfelt desire to make connections with others and ideas, which could help nurture and sustain them through their fear and isolation.

Our group has become a stunningly beautiful chorus filled with the music of soothing connection and deep nourishment, wherein each of our unique voices is honored with an enduring clarity. Our evolving group has created a musical composition in which the whole is infinitely greater than the sum of its parts. The foundation of this composition has been the safe and protective space of our group to allow us to grieve, bear witness to our stories of hardship and love, laugh together, and, most importantly, to create, hold onto, and cherish an enlivening and humane sense of purpose, possibility, vision, and hope. This, most heartfully, captures the true beauty and essence of what it means to be human within our community of dearly beloved and cherished humans.

Objectives of the Chapter

The chapter is organized around the achievements of the group. The initial section involves dissemination of clinical interventions through our *Psychology Today Blogs* and seminar series. The links for the blogs described in this chapter are in the reference section. The following part of the paper consists of personal vignettes of the group members describing their perspective of dealing with trauma during COVID-19 and the various international and national leadership roles that have taken on during this period, and the impact of the pandemic on a national level and public policy implications particularly on underserved populations. The chapter concludes with graduate school students' experiences during this challenging time and lessons learned and future directions.

Achievements of the Group

There have been five major achievements of our working group: (1) highlighting and thinking through some of the most important psychological issues arising in medical and addiction settings during the pandemic, and making suggestions and recommendations for how to address them at the individual, professional, and policy levels; (2) disseminating information on effective and flexible clinical interventions during COVID-19; (3) describing a comprehensive description of trauma; (4) taking on global and international leadership roles during the pandemic; and (5) making recommendations for public policy during COVID-19. The personal reflections in this chapter describe multiple perspectives on trauma and the various leadership and public advocacy roles the group members have undertaken during these challenging times.

Clinical Interventions During COVID-19

Dr. Ann F. Wimpfheimer

The COVID-19 pandemic brought a tremendous increase in depression and related mental health issues. In my clinical practice, I saw a significant increase in patients coming for treatment with depression, anxiety, and relationship difficulties. Couples and families sought help as they experienced much stress, isolation, the trauma of loss, and faced fears and feelings of loneliness and disconnection. My awareness of mind-body connections, the impact of trauma, and the power of resilience and social connections grew as a member of our APA Task Force. Various presentations focused on deepening our mind/body, sensory and somatic approaches, and our role as psychologists acting in the wider societal/political sphere. Additionally, being part of this ongoing group was personally meaningful and sustaining. Social connections and relationships are critical for patients and professionals alike, especially at this difficult, prolonged, and uncertain time of the pandemic when everyone is dealing with so much cumulative trauma and unprocessed grief.

Exploring Racial Inequalities

Together we explored, probed, and discussed how COVID was changing lives. As we became more mindful of how COVID was putting our healthcare disparities under a spotlight. Patricia O'Gorman was able to have a guest post written by a colleague in Child Welfare where I had consulted The Collective Trauma in the Black Community in 2020. Here Drs. Gardner and Kohomban recommended:

- First, there need to be courageous conversations at the local, state, and national levels about the historical and systemic disparity and discrimination afflicted on certain communities, even if it is difficult to admit and certainly difficult for some to hear.
- Second, elevate the voices of credible and trusted messengers in all areas and in all professions.
- Lastly, it will require financial resources that make the statement that this nation is finally willing to tackle once and for all the original sin of racism, which has resulted in and continues to result in profound pain and trauma for so many despite unimaginable advances as a society.

Supporting Those Experiencing Racial Tension and Threats

We began to realize how we could actively support each other in our work and in our personal lives including focusing on racial inequalities, from supporting colleagues in India when COVID-19 spiked, to those in our groups confronted with personal challenges. This was particularly important for Patricia O'Gorman as when the Asian hate incidents spiked, it terrified her, as her family is largely Asian. She shared that "the comfort I received from the group was strengthening, making it a safe place for my pain and to understand how to move forward."

Grief

We created an opportunity to not only learn together but also to support group members in both professional areas and personal areas. We realized that grief was more intense during COVID-19, not just for others, but also for ourselves, making doing clinical work more of a challenge. This I wrote about O'Gorman, P. Three Ways to Grieve When Your Grief Has No Place To Go: Making Space for Personal Loss and Collective Grief While Helping Your Patients:

- Reaffirm a new way of honoring your lost loved one.
- Share your pain.
- Spread joy where you can.

Vaccine Hesitancy

O'Gorman also explored why there was growing vaccine hesitancy, which was chronicled in O'Gorman, P Vaccine Hesitancy: Understanding The Power of NO:

- It is important to understand the reasons why specific groups are not being vaccinated.
- It is not helpful to lump the unvaccinated into political groups that obscure their individual motivation.

- Feelings of powerlessness may be driving decision-making.
- Our messaging needs to stop frightening people, and instead provide positive reasons for why and how individuals can be vaccinated.

Developing Family Compassion Across Different Beliefs

As COVID-19 raged over the holidays and families were splitting, we encouraged compassion O'Gorman, P Compassion: The Needed Ingredient for Holiday Gatherings encouraging family members to consider:

- Family gatherings this holiday season require clear expectations in terms of safety.
- The desire to be with family, vaccinated or not, cannot override the need to stay safe.

Adam R. Klyczek

Reduce COVID Trauma with Psychological First Aid (March 6, 2021)

Psychological First Aid (PFA) is recognized as an effective initial disaster response designed to assess immediate concerns, promote stabilization, and to connect individuals to resources. The approach highlights the importance of safety, calming, connectedness, self-efficacy, and hope (Hobfoll et al., 2007). PFA can and should be employed more broadly in first responders at scenes, emergency rooms, and intensive care units during the pandemic to reduce the development of PTSD and adjustment disorder.

Dr. Denise Bossarte

The following three blogs were written by Dr. Bossarte based on how her personal history was impacted by COVID-19 and various coping strategies she incorporates into her clinical work:

COVID-19 Overwhelm: Self-Care for Abuse Survivors: Cultivating Self-Care Can Ease the Burden of Anxiety Triggered by Unsafe Times (February 5, 2021a)

As a survivor of childhood sexual abuse, the COVID-19 pandemic triggered memories of my experiences as a child that the world was a dangerous place and that I had little control over protecting myself (Bossarte, 2022).

To counter this, I discovered several self-care practices that helped me deal with my fear and anxiety in the immediate moment: deep breathing, self-massage, and visualizing being with people who care for me. I also developed a toolkit of personal self-care practices to help me regularly move out of fear and feeling frozen to a place of calm and ease.

COVID Overwhelm: Photography Self-Care for Abuse Survivors: Tapping into Your Innate Creativity to Ease Your Sense of Disconnection (March 17, 2021b)

One of the supportive practices I have discovered in my healing journey is photography. Even with the COVID-19 pandemic, I have been able to engage in this healing and resilience practice in a way that helps me feel safe and supported.

Multiple studies have shown that being out in nature is very healing. Photography enables me to get outside, into nature and the world. It also gets me outside of my normal criticizing and self-doubting mind. For a time, I can let go of any storyline and open myself up to the beauty and wonder of the ordinary world with the benefit of having beautiful images to enjoy and share later!

COVID-19 Overwhelm: Yoga as Self-Care for Abuse Survivors: Stress Reduction Through Bodywork (April 20, 2021c)

My yoga practice has been a pivotal part of my healing journey from childhood sexual abuse and has sustained me during the COVID-19 pandemic. Yoga allows me to be in a different place where I am the one deciding what is going to happen with my body, and how I am going to treat my body.

You can build your resilience for managing COVID-19 overwhelm through yoga. What type of yoga you practice is not important. Gifting yourself with self-care by getting on the mat on a regular basis is the key.

Dr. Kirk J. Schneider

What Existentialists Can Teach Us About COVID-19 (March 12, 2020)

Existential thinkers including Frankl, Becker, Kierkegaard, May, and Camus have stressed the importance of freedom to choose our attitude toward crises that are beyond our control, to define rather than being defined by our circumstances, to draw upon our imagination, intuition, and spirituality, to connect with loved ones, and to devote oneself to projects outside ourselves.

Dr. Robert M. Gordon

There were two major phases in my writing: the initial blogs focused on how existential and humanistic approaches and values can deepen our work during the pandemic, while the second series of articles emphasized some of more complex challenges psychologists were facing in their clinical work. Each blog included a number of practical tips for clinicians and patients and their families to help them cope during the pandemic.

Phase 1

Existential Interventions During the Age of COVID-19 (January 12, 2021)

Unexpected events, including life-threatening illness or dealing with COVID-19, are often catalysts for thinking about meaning in life, values, and priorities for clients and therapists (Hill, 2018).

- Asking open-ended questions including “When do you feel most engaged in life? and “What provides you with passion, pleasure, and meaning” can facilitate this self-reflective process (Hill, 2018).

Why Am I So Tired? Managing Fatigue During the COVID-19 Pandemic (February 13, 2021d)

Compassion fatigue refers to emotional exhaustion from working with a traumatized population and is a form of caregiver burnout (Figley, 2002). Empathy and emotional energy are driving forces in effective clinical work with suffering, but there is a physical and emotional toll.

- Try not to compare yourself to your pre-COVID-19 self.
- Limit exposure to upsetting news and social media.

Self-Compassion and Kindness During COVID-19 (February 26, 2021c)

Self-compassion means, “treating oneself with kindness, care, and concern in the face of negative events” (Terry & Leary, 2011, p. 352). “Modest acts of kindness are more significant than we recognize…you just need to touch one person each day with compassion” (Burger, 2018, p. 176).

- Practice self-compassion: direct kindness, understanding, and acceptance toward yourself.
- Retain important qualities that foster hope within ourselves and to others, including joy, honesty, curiosity, and courage (Buechler, 2004).

Sustaining Hope in Pediatric Care During COVID-19 (March 21, 2021b)

- "Hope is a choice and gift we give to each other" (Burger, 2018, p. 186).
- Focus on what you and your child can do rather than cannot because overcoming a feeling of helplessness can help cultivate hope.
- Ask the child where they find their strength (Remen, 2000).

Phase 2

Navigating Two Worlds: Resiliency During Pandemic Transitions (April 27, 2021)

In the aftermath of chronic stress or adversity, individuals typically undergo a transition period that involves readjusting to a state of relative safety and adapting behaviors accordingly. Psychological flexibility is an important and modifiable predictor of resilience and has been proposed as an explanation for how resilience works (Bonanno, 2021). A flexibility mindset involves optimism about the future, conviction in our ability to cope and adapt, and the willingness to embrace stressors as challenges (Bonanno, 2021).

- Questions including "What have you discovered about yourself through the pandemic?" and "Are you aware of any aspect of COVID-19 that has changed you for the better?" allow one to construct a more flexible and self-compassionate narrative (Gordon et al., 2021a).
- Your decisions during the transition phase should be consistent with your most important values, what kind of person you want to be, and long-term goals (Harris, 2018).

Improving Communication with Your Partner (August 4, 2021)

As we transition into a new phase of the COVID-19 pandemic, we continue to search for answers, direction, and meaning in a different world to provide a sense of safety, predictability, and normalcy. Dealing with these struggles while maintaining a healthy, collaborative partnership can trigger strong emotions.

- Openly discuss any emotions that may follow feelings of uncertainty and vulnerability (e.g., fear, frustration, sense of urgency, anger, irritability).
- Acknowledge the increased likelihood of committing to actions/ideas as a means of avoiding the discomfort of ambiguity (Holmes, 2015).
- What are your feelings of uncertainty, vulnerability, and fear trying to teach you?

The Psychology Behind COVID-19 Vaccine Hesitancy: Ways to Approach Challenging Conversations (September 17, 2021)

Psychological theories on heuristics and cognitive biases can explain vaccination hesitancy. Understanding the motivational factors and "mental traps" behind the hesitation is critical as it may foster productive conversations with those with different perspectives. Those with hesitancy may ask themselves the following questions:

- What side effects are you most concerned about? Where did you get that information?"
- How would you assess the potential risk of the vaccine's side effects compared to contracting COVID-19?

Cultivating Forgiveness During COVID-19 (March 3, 2022)

The pandemic has highlighted political and racial tensions and healthcare disparities and polarized our political discourse. Forgiveness is a potential way to temper polarized thinking. Perspective taking, active listening, and compassion can facilitate a flexibility mindset when communicating with individuals with different viewpoints during COVID-19.

- Consider the context of someone's life to understand his or her individual point of view.
- Tell yourself that not forgiving is a legitimate act in itself and that withholding forgiveness is a decision as hard won as to grant it (Safir, 1999).

Compassionate Leadership During COVID-19 (May 12, 2022)

Effective leaders inspire a shared vision, enable others, and encourage with the heart. Leadership qualities can be cultivated through modeling compassion, leading with your core values, and viewing stressors such as COVID-19 as challenges. Having a growth and flexible mindset provides a path to resilience by motivating us to engage with stressors (Bonanno, 2021).

- Monitor how your words and actions align with your core values.
- Ask yourself if you have an intentional plan for personal growth.

Blog Posts on Child and Family Issues

We invited Dr. Christina M. Rodriguez, who is a member of the Children and Family Task Force, to write about her own research on the increased incidence of child abuse during the pandemic ("Children At Risk For Maltreatment During the

COVID-19 Pandemic," January 22, 2021). We addressed similarly alarming phenomena related to the effect of addiction on children: Invited guest Rosemary Tisch wrote about addiction and child abuse during COVID-19 ("COVID is Not the Only Public Health Problem Facing America," January 1, 2021), and Dr. Patricia O'Gorman discussed "Suicide by Intentional Overdose in Children" (February 2, 2021c).

Though not an official part of our mission, in response to requests from parents for articles that address their needs, we created a blog series on parenting during the pandemic, a 6-part parenting series: "The Brave New World of Parenting in the Pandemic," Dr. Ellen Luborksy, January 3, 2021; "Bring Creativity and Play to Kid's Lives During COVID," Dr. Ellen Luborksy, January 7, 2021a; "Decode the Message in Your Child's Behavior," Dr. Ellen Luborksy, January 19, 2021b; "Turn Play into a Way to Help Children During the Pandemic," Dr. Ellen Luborsky, January 27, 2021; "Sustaining Pediatric Hope in Pediatric Care During COVID-19," Dr. Robert M. Gordon, Taylor Groth, MA, and Sara Schapiro, March 21, 2021b; and "The Return to School: Tips for Parents of Anxious Children," Dr. Allison Winik, June 29, 2021.

Speakers Series

Our comprehensive speaker series has covered some of the most challenging aspects of the pandemic. We invited national experts to speak at our Friday meetings to discuss their work, which was incorporated into our clinical work. In 2021, the post-COVID condition known as Long COVID began to receive extensive news coverage. The condition appeared to baffle the scientists, and we wanted to better understand this later development of the illness from a psychological/trauma perspective. Its disabling aspects could undoubtedly result in high stress or even trauma for the individual suffering from this condition. However, as a group of trauma-informed psychologists, we are also well versed in the research demonstrating that psychological trauma can adversely affect the body. We wondered whether trauma (either pandemic related or that occurred pre-pandemic) might play a role in the etiology of Long COVID.

To explore this further, we invited Alla Landa, Ph.D., a psychology professor and researcher in the Columbia University Department of Psychiatry, to discuss the possibility that her research might shed light on potential psychological mechanisms involved in Long COVID. Dr. Landa's research has attempted to uncover the etiology of psychosomatic distress and to develop new, effective treatments. Her treatment approach integrates modalities of therapy that have been shown to alleviate psychosomatic distress, including multidisciplinary team care for patients with psychosomatic disorders. We were particularly interested in her paper, "Beyond the unexplainable pain: Relational world of patients with somatization syndromes," which appeared in the *Journal of Nervous and Mental Disease* (Landa et al., 2012).

Two crucial, mutually understood caveats were present in our discussion. First, any ideas we might derive from our conversation would be purely speculative and require their own investigation. The second was an appreciation for the dangers of describing physical symptoms as having a psychological component, as the unsophisticated listener often makes the unfortunate mistake of dismissing the symptom as "all in the head," failing to appreciate the complex interplay between the mind and the body. Dr. Landa accepted our invitation, and we invited others outside our group who were interested in the topic. Her talk generated enormous enthusiasm and requests for a return visit.

Another topical pandemic medical issue was the controversy over "vaccine hesitancy." The long-anticipated development of vaccines against COVID-19, hailed as a public health breakthrough, was met with enormous enthusiasm by some, but reluctance, dissent, and objection by others.

Our group had already published several blog pieces on the topic. Still, we wanted to understand the phenomenon at an even deeper level. We invited Bernice Hausman, Ph.D., Chair of Medical Humanities at Penn State College of Medicine and author of *Anti/Vax: Reframing the vaccination controversy*, to speak to us. Published in 2019, her book chronicles her investigations into the phenomenon of vaccine dissent in its pre-pandemic manifestation. We wanted to explore the possibilities for understanding how we might apply her findings to the current COVID vaccine situation. Again, the response was overwhelmingly positive and enthusiastic, prompting requests for her to return.

When Dr. Hausman returned, she invited colleague Heidi Lawrence, Ph.D., from George Mason University and author of *Vaccine Rhetorics* (2020). Dr. Hausman stated that this time she wanted to listen more than she spoke in order to find out what psychologists had to say about the phenomenon. We have been able to sustain and develop our working group by developing subgroups that were open to new members. For example, our most recent installment, "Psychological Trauma in the ICU: The Healing Power of Relationships" inspired the formation of a separate group consisting of both group members and attendees to devise ways to address the psychological needs of families and staff in the ICU (Table 6.1).

Global Perspectives on Trauma

Dr. Judy Roth

My work abroad with people living in crisis zones has deeply informed my clinical work with medical students and young healthcare providers who were deployed to frontline hospitals as the pandemic hit the city. My crisis work drew from the accompaniment framework, explained below, where we strive to bear witness and

Table 6.1 Speaker Series

Speaker(s)	Date	Topic
Dr. Alla Landa	10/29/21	Can What We Already Know About Mind-Body Disorders Help Us Understand Long-COVID?
Dr. Bernice Hausman	11/12/21	Vaccine Dissent and the Post-COVID Landscape
Dr. Ilene Serlin	2/4/22	Embodied Resilience
Drs. Bernice L. Hausman and Heidi Y. Lawrence	2/18/22	Rethinking Vaccine Hesitancy in a Pandemic: A Discussion
Dr. Mary Beth Morrisey	2/25/22	Vaccine Culture, Pandemic Injustice, and Psychosocial Hazards for Workers
Dr. Wendy dean	3/11/22	Choosing Change After COVID-19: Reframing Distress in the Healthcare Workforce
Drs. Patricia L. Gerbarg and Richard P. Brown	5/13/22	Breath-Body-Mind: A New Global Mental Health Model for COVID-19, Ukraine, and Other Mass Disorders
Dr. Maureen-O'Reilly Landry and Denise Carballea, MS	6/10/22	Psychological Trauma in the ICU: The Healing Power of Relationships

advocate while seeking to open professional communities and mutually empower. Psychological accompaniment is about providing support during social calamity and its aftermath. It is not construed as therapeutic per se – but provides a particular stance of being present, standing in solidarity during existential suffering, amplifying what has been disavowed and unacknowledged (Roth, 2016), which might sow the seeds for "reasonable hope" (Weingarten, 2010). Intrinsic to the engagement is the idea of reciprocity – that those living on the precipice have a great deal to teach us instead of the other way around. We/outsiders can try to listen deeply and have the privilege to help hold anguish, collective pain, and terror, while resisting a public ethos that often dismisses or denies the impact of the unfolding catastrophe.

Our task force group offered a "parking place" of sorts to hold the pain, outrage, psychic numbing, existential despair, and feelings of betrayal that I was hearing from my medical students and young physicians. The group recognized that the clinical work others and I were doing during this time was of a different order and thus in some ways sacred. In my situation, my young patients/students were holding more than they had ever had been prepared for –handling excruciating human realities and decisions quickly with minimal information, in a climate where death and heartbreaking endings shadowed everything. The group's acknowledgment of the sacred was deeply meaningful and protective. Their belief that we were worthy witnesses to an unfolding clinical crisis with something essential to convey helped protect against compassion fatigue (Figley, 2002) and opened the possibility of thinking and giving words to emerging clinical phenomena and new psychosocial challenges.

Dr. Evelyn Rappoport, Somatic Trauma Specialist and Psychoanalyst

My colleagues often ask me about my dedication and passion for somatic trauma healing. I respond: The seeds of my passion and interest took root long before I was born; I was born into trauma, to parents who carried extraordinary histories of survival and resilience. My first experience in a bomb shelter in Haifa, Israel, at age four, during the Sinai War in 1956, felt safe and cozy. I have shadow memories of a pajama-like party with candles, surrounded by friends and family members in the protective safety of the shelter. Events like this in my early childhood shaped my commitment to working with traumatized others, with individuals, groups, diverse communities, and first responders in New York, India, Israel, and Ukraine.

We know that trauma does not discriminate among people; it is a mutual opportunity employer who leaves no one behind. I firmly believe that trauma healing should be available to everyone regardless of religion, ethnicity, disability, or financial status. I have dedicated most of my career to this mission, as have many colleagues, mental health workers on the psychological frontlines.

Everyone has experienced trauma, and everyone is compromised and impacted to some degree. Trauma symptoms, whether a consequence of developmental trauma or critical incident, are often embedded in the body and nervous system, creating habitual patterns of constriction, dissociation, and pain. The corporal body, the living container of our interiority, holds and narrates what words fail to convey. When our survival system becomes overwhelmed by the intensity of the situation, it shuts down and becomes frozen and numb in order to not feel the fear, anxiety, and discomfort of living through the trauma.

Bromberg (1994) stated that the mechanism of dissociation is a defense against overwhelming anxiety that would result in fragmentation. It provides an escape where dramatically incompatible emotions or perceptions are needed to be cognitively processed in the same relationship. The traumatic experience that is causing the incompatible perception and emotion is removed from the cognitive processing system and remains in an unformulated and unsymbolized state (Van der Kolk, 1987). When words fail, somatic narrative (the story the body communicates) links the body (soma), mind (psyche), and heart. Supporting clients with kindness and compassion, and providing the safe space to fully live the felt sense of experience in the moment, enable individuals to enter previously warded-off self-states that were disavowed following acute or chronic trauma. Incorporating the neurophysiology of trauma across physical, emotional, and cognitive domains opens the space for traumatized individuals to reconnect to themselves with embodiment in the present moment. Davies and Frawley (1994) and Stern (1996) emphasized that dissociative self-states cannot be put directly into words, but can only be known through the impact on the therapist-client interaction.

My interest and expertise in somatic trauma healing and posttraumatic growth grew from the feeling that psychotherapy and psychoanalysis were limited in treating trauma. After attending a group with a somatic practitioner, I immediately understood that the missing piece is the body and the autonomic nervous system. I often tell my patients, "Your body is so much more than a pillar for your head." A sense of humor always helps!

After learning about the APA Task Force group developed by Drs. Maureen O'Reilly-Landry and Patricia O'Gorman, I immediately joined hoping to creative a bridge with the New York State Psychological Association (NYSPA) Task Force. Belonging to this group of authentic, like-minded individuals has been a surprising gift. Similar to the feelings I experienced in the bomb shelter in Haifa in 1956, *members of this group have organically co-created a safe space in which softness and love can reach into the deepest levels of emotional pain, vulnerability, and uncertainty in others and ourselves during the pandemic*. Together, we are surviving our traumas. We nurture each other as we dedicate ourselves to trauma healing and compassionate care for individuals, couples, families, diverse groups, and communities. Through the process of restoring ruptured connections and enhancing our interconnectivity, each member of our international and diverse group increases the capacity to reimagine a more hopeful future. Although the sequelae of trauma can be disastrous and catastrophic, my lifelong conviction is that the definition of tragedy is when trauma does not yield to inner growth and a change in perspective on one's priorities and what is most meaningful in life.

Tina Balachandran, MSc, Clinical and Aviation Psychologist

After 18 years in the field and over 10 years in the corporate world, I was aware of the systemic gaps that existed in the field of mental health, but the road of how to address them was steeper than expected. My journey into community care started in 2013 with the vision to create a psychologically healthy and safe space for nationals and residents in Qatar to heal, grow, and flourish. While I had a full-time privileged position within the national airline in Qatar, I engaged in pro-bono work with the community running mental health awareness sessions to break the stigma associated with mental health in the workplace and in safety-critical industries. Right before the pandemic, I decided to move into private practice and stepped down from my role in the airline. The pandemic turned out to be a challenge both personally and professionally in numerous ways.

"I am not what happened to me, I am what I choose to become" (Carl Jung) has become a core belief that has helped me through life's challenges, as well as inspired me to do more during the pandemic. As a member of the APA, I was very excited to hear about the APA COVID-19 Task Force and jumped at the opportunity to join the group. Given my work in crisis and disaster response, aviation, and healthcare, I felt the need to reach out to healthcare workers, fellow mental health professionals, and first responders, as I was able to relate to the stress, distress, and traumatic experiences in the field.

Supporting the mental health of physicians, nurses, and care team members is a critical part of the public health response, as there is a need to create and ensure infrastructure, and responses are available to support the mental health and wellbeing of healthcare staff. I created a framework that focused on providing resources, creating connections, and providing supportive interventions to enhance and sustain current effort to ensure both clinical and non-clinical healthcare staff remain psychologically well and have the required psychological support. This perspective was very much aligned with the goals and objectives of the *Hospital, Health and Addiction Workers, Patients and Families Work Group* to provide resources, create nurturing connections, and provide a supportive space.

I was fortunate to be involved in facilitating support groups for psychologists and therapists in India, providing a safe space for them to talk about their personal and professional challenges during the pandemic. These groups were part of the "Clinician Collaborative" initiative with our APA working group "Professional Support for Psychologists." I shared my experiences during our working group and Dr. Evelyn Rappoport, a member of our working group, was able to volunteer her time in facilitating the group interventions. Meanwhile, I continued working on my personal vision toward a social enterprise focused on increasing awareness around mental health, improving access to mental health services, advocating an integrated and holistic systemic approach to healthcare, and promoting a psychologically healthy and safe workplace.

With a culturally diverse population of over 150 nationalities in Qatar, traditional Western therapeutic approaches are not always efficient in catering to the complexities of psychological care within the community. There is a need to bridge the gaps with therapists from diverse backgrounds who can be culturally sensitive, trauma-informed, and open to incorporating evidence-based approaches with the flexibility of cultural adaptations. It took over 6 years and the pandemic to turn this around into an outpatient community center – Flourishing Minds Clinic, based out of Qatar. With a foundation built on safety, trust, choice, collaboration, empowerment, and respect, the focus is to engage individuals, families, communities, and organizations to motivate, inspire, nurture, and sustain healing and growth.

The supportive space of encouragement, validation, and unconditional positive regard from all of the members of the group provided a much-needed supportive space for me to rejuvenate and continue working toward my vision. I am truly grateful for the connections and friendships that the pandemic has brought me through my work with this wonderful group of human beings from across the globe who are passionate about creating a difference in the world.

Dr. Judy Kuriansky

Participating in this working group has been a valuable experience, with appreciation to everyone for the support, friendship, and professional sharing. Here are my personal and professional reflections and activities during COVID-19.

Personal Impact

When Columbia University Teachers College, where I teach, went on Spring Break in March 2020, I was at home, enduring my share of virtual burials of loved ones, and expecting to catch up on work, when I found myself suddenly coughing, gasping for breath, and unable to move off the couch. I had to accept that I got COVID-19. Ashamed to be so vulnerable, I did not tell anyone except my sister – a social worker at a hospital overrun with COVID patients – who agreed I should hold out going to the hospital where people were dying. Instead, I pounded my chest for air (a technique I learned from climbing Mount Kilimanjaro) and for the first time, prayed to G-d not to die because I had more to give the world. Only when I saw on television that UK Prime Minister Boris Johnson was infected, did I finally feel OK about myself.

Months later, I succumbed to the "fear factor" – which I had never done before, having gone twice to West Africa during the height of the Ebola outbreak – to not travel to Africa to help during the COVID outbreak, only to relent later to attend the funeral in Benin of one of my best friends, their Ambassador to the United Nations. Family trumps fear.

Professional Activities

My way to defy panic is to be productive. Thus, I kept busy by the below.

The Tripartite Model

The scientist-practitioner model we all know has now expanded into the tripartite model I teach my graduate students, adding advocacy, focusing on issues of social justice. Herewith, my activities are in the three areas.

Practice For decades, I have provided psychosocial support trainings centered on the theme of resilience, "on the ground" after terrorist attacks, school shootings, and natural disasters worldwide, including in Haiti, Japan, China, and Africa. However, due to travel restrictions, I had to shift online, providing training in coping strategies for a Chinese peer counseling organization, Nepali psychology staff, and others.

Science: Research

Many of the above trainings included an outcome assessment. Also, a major research project involved an intervention in a remote village in the Democratic Republic of the Congo, implemented by the local team, with modules of positive health behaviors (mask-wearing, hand-washing) and psychosocial techniques, which showed significant positive outcomes. Another pilot project addressed post-traumatic growth, with the most predominant "silver linings" reported being quality time with family and pursuing interests such as reading and cooking.

Policy/Advocacy

As my colleagues in NGOs in consultative status at the United Nations, and the United African Congress (UAC) had done during the Ebola epidemic, we "raised the alarm" early about the imminent dangers of COVID-19 in Africa during a live event during World Interfaith Harmony Week. For sustainability, we held a series of 10 events on COVID-19 in Africa on a variety of topics including economics, food, vaccines, gender, and racism. In addition, I collaborated with the Mission of Costa Rica at the UN about developing a working group for the UN Group of Friends of Mental Health and Wellbeing.

Media

Consistent with my media career as a radio advice host, television feature reporter, and print columnist, these activities continued, including responding to requests on an English-speaking Chinese television station and writing my column for *Black Star News*. For example, I advocated for replacing the reference to "social distance" with "physical distance" since social connection is what *helps* people cope during crisis. In addition, given the proliferation of technology, which became more essential during lockdowns and restrictions, I initiated a book about technology for resilient health systems, especially for low-resource settings, for the COVID-19 recovery period and beyond (to be published by Elsevier this Fall).

Going Forward and Lessons Learned

Clearly, COVID recovery will be a long-haul, for me, with some lingering symptoms, for my students, facing unknowns and family separations, and for my work at the UN, given the pandemic's impact on poverty, vulnerable populations, and people's mental health and well-being. Big lessons learned: dismiss petty worries and cherish people, the planet, and preciousness of life. Like the theme of the anthem I co-wrote with my songwriting partner, Russell Daisey – sung throughout Africa now: "Hope is Alive." And like the Haitian saying, "Where there is life, there is hope."

Dr. Patricia Villavicencio Carrillo

I had the following dream one year into the pandemic:

"They Jumped Off Dancing"

The sidewalk and street are full of people standing in silence. I do not hear a sound, not even a whisper. Some are looking at the buildings on the opposite side of the street; another group is looking down as if there was something on the ground. I could see an empty space in the center of the crowd. I do not stop and I keep walking. There is a woman a few steps away from me, walking slowly through the crowd. I sped up my pace; grab her left arm from behind and ask her what has happened. She turns around, not surprised at all, and answers back "There were four and they jumped off dancing….I can clearly see them jumping off the building dancing."

Dreams have always been fascinating to me. They can be the most creative poetry our unconscious minds can reveal to us. A dream can vividly portray the sensual details of a delicious meal, and the kinesthetic sensations you had swimming in the clear ocean at the age of five during a family vacation. On the other hand, they can be the most terrifying and overwhelming experience if you have suffered a traumatic event. Dreams can be interpreted in numerous ways as attempts at problem-solving and conflict resolution, ways of mastering trauma, explorations of unknown possibilities and paths not chosen in life, wish fulfillment, compensation, communication with the therapist, and integration of the self (Lippmann, 2000).

As a trauma therapist in Spain, I know that many trauma victims experience PTSD symptoms for decades if they do not have the opportunity to undergo trauma-based psychotherapy in order to process overwhelming events that haunt their dreams and in their daily lives. Even before COVID-19, teenage suicide was a growing health issue in my clinical practice. There have been long waiting lists for treatment, which has exacerbated their emotional conditions by the time they begin treatment. Research has indicated that the pandemic has increased the numbers of teenager and young adult suicide and self-harm behaviors worldwide.

Reflecting back on my dream, my initial reaction involved worry and fear about the immediate and long-term impact on the pandemic of the psychological functioning of the younger generation, including suicidal behavior. I realized, however, that suicidal patients would not be jumping off a building smiling and dancing. It took time to process and fully understand that the dream conveyed my deep conviction that neither the COVID-19 pandemic or any personal adversity that I have ever faced has ever undermined by unbreakable spirit. This underlying faith and hope is something I have learned from my loving parents and my patients in my clinical practice who have given me the opportunity to be part of their recovery and healing and learn from each other.

Dr. Betsy Gard discussed how her previous international work on natural disasters and traumatic events provided a perspective working with frontline workers during COVID-19.

I became interested in becoming part of the Work Group as I have served the American Red Cross (ARC) on disasters as a Disaster Mental Health Volunteer for over 30 years. During my time, I have worked as a Manager in Disaster Mental Health and provided training and consultation to hundreds of mental health professionals and frontline workers following hurricanes, floods, tornadoes, bombings, shootings, airline crashes including 9/11, and preparation for possible pandemics. The ARC Disaster Mental Health professionals provided support for both clients and those supporting the disaster team including police, firefighters, EMT's, reporters, and medical staff. I gained valuable experience working as a volunteer during the Ebola pandemic and provided psychological support to returning medical personnel.

I was privileged to go on international disaster missions, including trips to Romania, Belarus, Russia, and China. I was part of a team of surgeons, pediatric ICU physicians, and nurses who went to Port-au-Prince to help victims with crush injuries and was the mental health support person for the multiple teams of medical volunteers following the earthquake. I was also a member of the team that worked on coping with cholera when this became problematic in Haiti.

I am an adjunct professor in the Emory School of Medicine Department of Psychiatry and Behavioral Sciences. I come from a long line of family members dedicated to the medical field, including my grandfather, cousins, a niece, and my daughter who is a pediatric emergency room and trauma physician in Atlanta.

As COVID-19 exploded and frontline workers struggled to cope with the physical and emotional impact, I provided "Drop-In" support for the ARC staff and volunteers, as well as psychologists and nurses from Georgia. Most of these were through telehealth platforms including Teams, Zoom, WebEx, and Doxy. The meetings focused on developing flexible and adaptive coping and self-care strategies, gaining awareness of inner strengths and resiliency, and facilitating discussions of the unique challenges and rewards of working during the COVID-19 pandemic. In addition, resources were posted at the Georgia Psychological Association (GPA), and a recorded Webinar on working with families who had experienced loss and disability was available, free-of-charge on the GPA website. In the fall and winter of 2021, a free CE workshop on Psychological First Aid was provided to any psychologist who provided two pro bono services to nurses and psychologists.

Through my multiple international and national experiences dealing with disasters and trauma, I have learned the importance of frontline workers finding the time for structured self-care including attending support sessions. It would be ideal to provide this support embedded in the places and spaces where frontline workers naturally congregate, such as at the water cooler and coffee pots. This was not possible due to the risk to providers during the pandemic. This unprecedented challenge has required the development of a wide and flexible "menu" of options including different times to be able to "drop-in," on-line resources, on-call mental health support services, and pre-recorded, brief resiliency-based tools. Unfortunately, no programmatic studies were done. However, in my observations, the demand for these ad-hoc, drop-in resources by Zoom, Team, and other virtual platforms was high. We had many attendees and many "thank yous" and expressions of gratitude for providing a forum for meeting, sharing, and learning more information on stress management. As the pandemic dragged on, after the first 12–18 months, attendance dropped and participation was decidedly less. It appeared that there was "Zoom fatigue" and people really missed face-to-face contact and support. Virtual meetings are continuing in certain organizations but it will be interesting to determine, if we continue to have waves of COVID what we might see with these alternative options. I think some of the response will be mediated by whether there is a move back to limiting in-person meetings and education. The issues around masking, quarantines, testing, and vaccinations (including boosting for adults younger than 60) often seem political and economically driven, rather than mediated by what is best for public health

Dr. Soffia Palsdottir

I was born and raised in Iceland and moved to Arizona to pursue my clinical career in the area of clinical health psychology and integrated care with patients with life-threatening illness. I joined the working group to collaborate on how to address the psychological and physical toll during COVID-19 on physicians working with patients with cancer. The pandemic had placed additional stressors on the treatment team at the cancer center where I had been working, including patients not having family members present during treatment due to visitor restrictions and often-delaying treatment and having more advanced cases. Brainstorming with the working group provided new perspectives and ideas to deal with the compassion fatigue, distress, depression, and anxiety and disruptions in the usual work environment the oncology physicians were experiencing. My consultation with physicians emphasized the importance of self-care including spending time with loved ones, healthy nutrition, sleep hygiene, exercise, and avoiding excessive alcohol or substance use, and embracing small wins to protect against burnout and compassion fatigue (Palsdottir, 2021). I subsequently become the Chief Clinical Psychologists at the Mental Health Center of America (MHCA), a new multidisciplinary comprehensive program in Phoenix. At MHCA, we are providing clinical services with a diverse range of patients including first responders who have been heavily impacted by COVID-19 such as ICU nurses, ambulance drivers, fire fighters, teenagers struggling with the mental health impact of the pandemic, and several patients with Long COVID-19. We provide an integrative, mind-body approach including the use of neurofeedback, nutritional psychiatry, hyperbaric chambers, and cold and hot therapies, and meditation.

The National Impact of the Pandemic on Public Policy

Dr. Mary Beth Quaranta Morrissey, PhD, JD, MPH

Public Health Policy: Coming Out of the Shadows

The COVID-19 pandemic has had the unintended, but positive consequence of bringing public health and policymaking finally out of the shadows and into our community conversations, disclosing the significance of public health in our human history. The institutionalization of a new pandemic environment has raised our consciousness of health as a *public good* and driven debate about balancing autonomy and civil liberties and threats to the public's health. There is now a heightened awareness that social and economic determinants beyond the control of the individual, including race, age, gender, poverty, education, income, housing and food insecurity, language, and transportation, shape health experience and outcomes for diverse populations and communities, and contribute to structural inequities and healthcare disparities. The disproportionate impacts of the pandemic upon communities of color experiencing marginalization and vulnerability, such as older New Yorkers residing in nursing homes or incarcerated in correctional facilities, are a paradigmatic example of such inequities and serve as a clarion call for social change and policy reform.

The New York State Bar Association (NYSBA) (and NYSBA's Health Law Section) is one example of a professional organization that has invested considerable social capital over the last 2 years in examining the challenges presented by the pandemic and identifying the policy failures of government. For example, it is now known that thorny decisions about allocation of scarce resources during the pandemic often devolved to the provider and occurred at the bedside without the benefit of uniform Crisis Standards of Care (Institute of Medicine, 2012). Crisis standards are triggered when normal healthcare operations have been disrupted as we have witnessed during the pandemic. However, in the absence of such clear standards and guidance, provider systems, physicians, and health professionals in New York and other states were left to make decisions on their own with little oversight or accountability. Not surprisingly, there have been federal civil rights enforcement actions based upon age discrimination in the design and implementation of allocation of scarce resource guidelines during the pandemic.

In light of these failures in public health policymaking, the NYSBA has mapped out a series of policy recommendations that are worthy of serious consideration by New York and other states. One salient recommendation in the NYSBA reports has been the call for expanding palliative care to mitigate suffering as an ethical minimum during pandemics and building therapeutic palliative environments in the progressive realization of the rights to health and mental health. NYSBA has also been in the forefront in developing vaccine mandate recommendations, advocating for community education to increase acceptance of vaccines especially among communities of black and brown people who have experienced histories of exploitation and colonization. Public health will increasingly be the focus of community conversations and social action in the next decades to ensure participatory democracy in pandemic environments.

Policy Recommendations by Dr. Patricia O'Gorman

We also supported each other in our professional lives which I experienced in sharing my heartbreaking work with adolescents who were being sexually abused and trying to kill themselves as a result of being "babysat" by known abusers. Our group encouraged me to write about this and the steps I took to expand risk factors for assessing risk of abuse, important policy considerations for agencies and private practitioners to incorporate O'Gorman, P. Suicide By intentional Overdose in Children: The Missing Variable in Tackling Teen Suicide is the Addiction Epidemic.

Here O'Gorman recommended adding to standard abuse assessments:

- Substance use by the adolescent
- Access to drugs and or alcohol
- Access to any prescription medication, including those prescribed for their parents or themselves
- Access to OTC medications such as Tylenol, and cough syrups containing dextromethorphan
- Isolation
- Enduring emotional, physical, or sexual abuse
- Witnessing domestic violence
- Being isolated with a known abuser
- A known abuser having access to this youth

Dr. Maureen O'Reilly-Landry

Our work group's meetings were generating powerful ideas to help various groups deal with the pandemic. With experts in their respective fields, we discussed the psychological aspects of vaccine hesitancy, Long COVID, the Intensive Care Unit, and various ways to address the effects of psychological stress and trauma on the body. Our recent Speaker Series about Psychological Trauma in the ICU, for example, generated a new separate group to address the psychological needs of families and staff in the ICU. Yet, there has been frustration about the absence of a more far-reaching public platform from which psychologists, particularly those well versed in the research on psychological trauma, can educate, inform, and advise leaders and decision-makers. Even after the CDC reported that adults, young adults, racial and ethnic minorities, essential workers, and unpaid caregivers reported COVID-related increases in mental health and substance abuse problems, little has been done to address such matters.

I therefore wrote to advocate that trauma-informed psychologists to be placed alongside medical doctors at local, state, and federal levels in order to analyze the highly complex social, psychological, cultural, and historical dynamics driving public health behaviors, which would enable leaders to implement more effective strategies to address these vital matters ("American Needs a Psychologist-in-Chief,"

February 4, 2021b, and "To heal from COVID, America must fix its psychological infrastructure," September 8, 2021a).

I suggested that President Biden "Fix [America's] Psychological Infrastructure" by "including psychologists…who understand the effects of psychological trauma on emotions, behavior, relationships, bodies and medical conditions" in order to help the medical scientists understand the biological nature of medical illness and psychological stage. Psychologists can help elucidate mechanisms involved in development of "Long-COVID" by drawing on our rapidly growing body of scientific knowledge about the complex interactions between the biological, psychological and social aspects of medical illness, including the important insight that emotional stress and trauma (inherent in a pandemic) is known to result in biological changes at the cellular level.

Integrating psychologists into the White House COVID-19 Response Team would also provide a visible platform from which to educate the public about grief and traumatic stress in a way that reduces stigma and encourages people to seek help earlier, when problems are more easily treated. Possibilities to integrate an understanding of psychological and sociological phenomena into social decision-making and to educate the American population about important mental health issues remain import, even beyond COVID-19. If our decision-makers were to have a better grasp of important issues at this deeper level, they would be in a much better position to the impact of our country's deep polarization, social class inequities, and racial trauma. Our group is fortunate to have been joined by Dr. Kirk Schneider, who has been advocating for an Office of Psychological Consultants long before the pandemic.

Dr. Kirk J. Schneider has focused on what psychologists can do on a national level to address the psychological crises arising from the pandemic.

I have been deeply moved by my participation with the Hospital, Health and Addiction Workers, Patients and Families Work Group of the COVID-19 Task Force. This is an inspiring group of professionals, dedicated body and soul to our health and well-being of so many suffering individuals today. My experience with our working group has only reinforced my passionate belief that we are starved for deeper and more comprehensive mental health services in our country. I have written about this in an article calling for a federal office of psychological advisors tasked with providing around the clock "best available evidence" to address the psychosocial crises arising from the pandemic and related issues of political polarization, racism, and violence that have only been exacerbated over the last 2 years. I was inspired in part to write this above piece based on our discussions in our working group and allied publications by such members of our group as Maureen O'Reilly-Landry, Patricia O'Gorman, and Robert Gordon. All members of our group have helped to forge a new and more depth-oriented path for the healing and revitalization of our society and world. I cannot overestimate the rigor and dedication our group to this cause.

Political, social, racial, and environmental crises are exploding today, and we need to mobilize our discipline for action. We are in crisis with gender and sexual injustices, and we are in crisis with mental health. In short, America is poised on the precipice, and if our profession fails to grasp this problem, we are in danger of inflaming it. This is the time for psychology to take the lead in repairing and transforming the world. This has been a driving force in my decision to be a candidate for president of the American Psychological Association this year (2022). My platform this year is due in no small part to the support and resonance that I have experienced in discussions with our group. In that spirit, I call for a renewed focus on "emotionally restorative relationships," as the centerpiece of my campaign. By emotionally restorative relationships, I mean relationships where people feel heard and seen and that get at the roots of their problems. I also call for a "National Corps of Psychologists" to facilitate this focus. Specifically, I call for this Corps to provide highly structured, healing dialogues to address the alarming cultural and political divides in our country. I also call for the Corps to provide equitable access to longer-term, emotionally restorative psychotherapy.

This framework moreover would be integrative, comprising, as appropriate, medical, cognitive-behavioral, psychodynamic, and existential dimensions of practice. The Corps would also foster a wide range of services to enhance individual and public well-being. For example, it could expand the availability of first responders to aid police dealing with mental health emergencies, provide consulting services to organizations in impoverished communities, and bolster the time and quality of psychological services in schools, hospitals, prisons, and governmental and diplomatic settings – wherever such services are in greatest need today.

To fund this National Corps of Psychologists, I would use the platform of APA president to call on the support of government, private industry, and others who care about the state of our profession and world. Such funding in turn would generate the pilot studies, grants, and other forms of support that would help to discern the viability and long-term sustainability of given Corps services. The superb resources of our research as well as applied and practice communities will be very much needed in this timely, broad-based effort. In addition, there is a need for a Presidential Task Force to investigate the merit of urging the US Congress to create an Office of Psychological Advisors to the United States to promote innovative national programs, such as the healing dialogues movement and in-depth therapy in underserved communities and to advise Executive and Congressional leaders on this present existential crises we all face.

Doctoral Student's Perspectives

Adam R. Klyczek (Molecular Neuroscience Doctoral Student)

Reflecting upon the past 2 years since the onset of the pandemic, I realized that we all felt our worlds collapse in on us. Our bubbles suddenly became quite small; the world and life as we knew it drastically changed. Life became surreal and no one had a playbook on how to navigate these extraordinary challenges.

We became sheltered and isolated in our homes either by local mandates or by personal choice. I could feel the unease and pain in others, a familiar feel from my medical work in combat and disaster relief. Consequently, I picked up as many hours as I could on the local ambulance squad. My world began to grow again. Daily, I saw new, but again familiar forms of fear and anguish in my fellow humans' eyes. I could feel it deep in my heart. As a result of being a member of the military, neuropsychology, and traumas divisions (19, 40, and 56, respectively), I was driven to write an article with our Task Force regarding these experiences and the need for psychological first aid for first responders in emergencies during the pandemic. I could still feel deep in my heart the suffering being experienced and exacerbated by the pandemic, particularly in my combat peers enduring PTSD, anxiety, and addiction. Thus, my doctoral research in molecular neuroscience gained personal purpose and meaning.

The transition into the world of academic research from rescue was jolting and refreshing. Felling out of my depth in my new role, I was encouraged to be met with respect and genuine curiosity by my new colleagues; the work I had undertaken to this point was not ignored as sophomoric as I had expected it to be, but rather embraced as an interesting and fruitful platform from which to further develop research, ideas, and the ultimate implications of the research. I have had the opportunity to design the majority of my research at McGill University focusing on the molecular underpinnings of stress, PTSD, and TBI. I am grateful to be able to bring my passion and experience to this endeavor. I am hopeful that my research can provide relevant data that can be utilized to help others overcome adversity and suffering. My unique background and experience has provided a broad and compassionate and empathetic perspective that help nourish all phases of the research process.

Rita M. Rivera, M.S.

I was pursuing my doctoral degree in clinical psychology during the COVID-19 pandemic. I am also a psychologist in my home country of Honduras. As such, during the coronavirus pandemic, I was in a unique position, providing services in-person and via telehealth as a psychology trainee in Florida, USA, while also providing pro-bono services via telepsychology to individuals in Honduras.

My participation in the *Hospital, Health and Addiction Workers, Patients and Families Work Group* impacted my view of the role of psychologists on a societal level, particularly through the support and engagement of fellow members. Psychologists, as well as other mental health practitioners, were and continue to be in the frontlines of the pandemic; we are essential healthcare workers that play a crucial role in the well-being of individuals, communities, societies, and overall systems. Through the discussions, meetings, and work developed by the working group, I observed how professionals across the world came together to foster a sense of resilience and posttraumatic growth. This, in turn, inspired and empowered me to continue my professional activities amidst so much uncertainty and distress. As I reflect on the past years, I am confident that the quality of my clinical, research, and academic work was positively and significantly impacted by the support and resources offered and disseminated by this community. Equally importantly, I have also grown and flourished on an individual and personal level, truly believing and sharing.

Denise Carballea, M.S.

As a graduate student training in an Intensive Care Unit (ICU) during the pandemic, I had the opportunity to experience first-hand the emotional and cognitive toll the prolonged crisis had on the treatment team works and families (2022a, b). We depended on stamina, flexibility, and resilience while navigating this unchartered territory. Being part of this work group, attending and being part of the speaker series with Dr. Maureen O'Reilly-Landry on psychological trauma in the ICU: the healing power of relationship, and writing articles on the impact of the pandemic on medical personnel has been a vital part of my growth as an aspiring psychologist.

The following Table 6.2 summarizes the diverse areas addressed by the working group in the areas of dissemination, advocacy and policy recommendations for underserved populations, and leadership roles.

Lessons Learned and Future Directions

COVID-19 has been a sudden, unexpected, and existentially shattering and potentially traumatic experience for many individuals, resulting in questioning their sense of safety and security in the world (Hoffman, 2021). Whether facing illness or loss of loved ones, anxiety about getting sick or infecting others, social isolation, or economic hardship, people have now been facing unprecedented stressors for over 2 years. In order to address these multiple challenges, the various personal reflections presented in this chapter highlight the clinical need for a broad, integrative view of trauma that incorporates somatic perspectives, bearing witness and advocating for others in a compassionate manner, utilizing a flexible mindset, and therapists' processing their emotional reactions and dreams.

The pandemic has also highlighted political and racial tensions and healthcare disparities, which have further polarized our political discourse. Political, social, and racial crises are exploding today, and we need to mobilize for action, advocacy, and compassionate and creative leadership. The diverse roles taken on by the diverse members of our Task Force reflect the importance of taking on the unique challenges of COVID-19 that incorporate psychodynamic, existential-humanistic, mindfulness, and cognitive-behavioral perspectives. The various local, state, national and international leadership roles described in personal vignettes included facilitating support groups, training in coping strategies, conducting research in positive health behavior interventions and posttraumatic growth, and writing about technology for low resource settings.

Table 6.2 Summary of areas addressed by the working group (2020–2022)

Dissemination		
Addictions	Trauma	Vicarious trauma
Vaccine dissent/ hesitancy and rhetoric	Long COVID	Working with patients with cancer
Psychological trauma in COVID-ICU	Rural healthcare during COVID-19	Effective communication with couples
Grief and loss	Parenting skills	Dealing with stress and fatigue
Reducing COVID-19 trauma with psychological first aid	Self-care for abuse survivors	Stress management strategies for healthcare providers
Resiliency and embodied resilience	Compassion and kindness	Understanding children's play and behavior
Children at risk for maltreatment during COVID-19	Pediatric suicide	Collective trauma of the Black community
Existential issues during COVID-19	Compassionate leadership	Cultivating forgiveness
Advocacy/policy recommendations for underserved populations		
Need for a "Psychologist-in-Chief"	Call for expanding palliative care to mitigate suffering as an ethical minimum	Adding questions to standard abuse assessments
Integrating trauma-informed psychologists on the White House COVID Response Team	Urging Congress to create an Office of Psychological Advisors to promote national programs, such as the healing dialogues movement and in-depth therapy in underserved communities	Calling for a federal office of psychological advisors tasked with providing around the clock "best available evidence" to address the psychosocial crises arising from the pandemic
Palliative care		
Leadership roles		
Starting a mental health clinic in Qatar	Facilitating support groups for psychologists in India	Providing training in coping strategies for Chinese counseling organizations
Research on interventions for positive health behaviors in the Congo	Research on interventions for positive health behaviors in the Congo	Starting a mental health clinic in Arizona

Future directions for psychologists include further development and research on an integrated model of trauma and resilience that incorporates somatic perspectives, the concept of accompaniment, existential-humanistic, cognitive-behavioral, and psychodynamic perspectives. Coursework in graduate school and during internship and postdoctoral training on effective leadership and advocacy can further enhance the roles of psychologists when dealing with global crises. An important future direction of our group will include addressing the psychological needs of families and medical staff in Intensive Care Units, gaining further understanding into the need for addiction treatment given the escalation addiction epidemic during COVID-19, and further exploring the mind-body component of Long COVID.

The present chapter is written while COVID-19 is still at large. The battle is far from over, which makes it impossible to fully assess the extent of its emotional and psychic impact at a global and individual level. The therapeutic process is a much-needed space for patients to cope with the pain brought on by a changed world and sense of self due to COVID-19. Therapists may find this new context as an opportunity to explore existential concerns with patients in deeper ways than before. The prolonged and uncertain nature of the pandemic has also provided an opportunity for each member of our international working group to reflect on personal values and priorities, and what is most meaningful and precious in life (Gordon et al., 2021a).

Author Note The Hospital, Health and Addiction Workers, Patients and Families Work Group at the APA Interdivisional Task Force on the Pandemic would like to thank the group members for their contribution to the chapter including Tina Balachandran, Denise Bossarte, Denise Carballea, Betsy Gard, Adam R. Klyczek, Judy Kuriansky, Soffia Palsdottir, Janet Plotkin-Bornstein, Mary Beth Quaranta Morrissey, Evelyn Rappoport, Rita Rivera, Judy Roth, Kirk J. Schneider, Patricia Villavicencio Carrillo, and Ann F. Wimpfheimer.

References

Bossarte, D. (2022). *Thriving after sexual abuse: Break your bondage to the past and live a life you love*. Passion for Life Press. https://thrivingaftersexualabusebook.com/, https://www.amazon.com/Thriving-After-Sexual-Abuse-Bondage-ebook/dp/B0937GR5MR

Bonanno, G. A. (2021). *The end of the trauma: How the new science of resilience is changing how we think about PTSD*. Basic Books.

Burger, A. (2018). *Witness: Lessons from Elie Wiesel's classroom*. Houghton Mifflin Harcourt Publishing.

Buechler, S. (2004). *Clinical values: Emotions that guide psychoanalytic treatment*. Routledge. https://doi.org/10.4324/9780203767221

Bromberg, P. (1994). "Speak! That I may see you": Some reflections on dissociation, reality and psychoanalytic listening. *Psychoanalytic Dialogues, 4*(4), 517–548. https://doi.org/10.1080/10481889409539037

Carballea, D. (2022a). Intensive care unit providers' mental health during the COVID-19 era. *Florida Psychologist*, 12–13. https://cdn.ymaws.com/www.flapsych.com/resource/resmgr/publications/FPA_Spring_2022_FINAL.pdf

Carballea, D. (2022b). Psychological wounds inflicted on ICU workers during the COVID-19 pandemic. *Trauma Psychology News, 17*(1), 28–30.

Davis, J. M., & Frawley, M. (1994). *Treating adult survivors of childhood sexual abuse*. New York Basic Books.

Figley, C. R. (2002). Compassion fatigue: Psychotherapists' chronic lack of self-care. *Journal of Clinical Psychology, 58*(11), 1433–1441. https://doi.org/10.1002/jclp.10090

Gordon, R. M., Dahan, J. F., Wolfson, J. B., Fults, E., Lee, Y. S. C., Smith-Wexler, L., Liberta, T. A., & McGiffin, J. N. (2021a). Existential-humanistic and relational psychotherapy during COVID-19 with patients with preexisting medical conditions. *Journal of Humanistic Psychology, 61*(4), 470–492. https://doi.org/10.1177/0022167820973890

Harris, R. (2018). *The happiness trap: How to stop struggling and start living* (2nd ed.). Shambhala Publications.

Hausman, B. L. (2019). *Anti/vax: Reframing the vaccine controversy*. Cornell University.
Hill, C. E. (2018). *Meaning in life: A therapist's guide*. American Psychological Association. https://doi.org/10.1037/0000083-000
Hobfoll, S. E., Watson, P., Bell, C. C., Bryant, R. A., Brymer, M. J., Friedman, M. J., et al. (2007). Five essential elements of immediate and mid-term mass trauma intervention: Empirical evidence. *Psychiatry: Interpersonal and Biological Processes, 70*(4), 283–315. https://doi.org/10.1521/psyc.2007.70.4.283
Hoffman, L. (2021). Existential-humanistic therapy and disaster response: Lessons from the COVID-19 pandemic. *Journal of Humanistic Psychology, 6*(1), 33–54. https://doi.org/10.1177/0022167820931987
Holmes, J. (2015). *Nonsense: The power of not knowing*. Crown Publishing Group.
Institute of Medicine. (2012). In D. Hanfling et al. (Eds.), *Crisis standards of care: A systems framework for catastrophic disaster response: Volume 1*. https://doi.org/10.17226/13351, https://commed.vcu/IntroPH/2012/crisisManagement_IOM.pdf
Landa, A., Bossis, A. P., & Boylan, L. S. (2012). Beyond the unexplainable pain: Relational world of patients with somatization syndromes. *The Journal of Nervous and Mental Disease, 200*(5), 413.422. https://doi.org/10.1097/NMD.0b013e3182532326
Lawrence, H. Y. (2020). *Vaccine rhetorics*. The Ohio State University Press.
Lippmann, P. (2000). *Nocturnes: On listening to dreams*. The Analytic Press.
O'Reilly-Landry, M. (2021a, Sept 8). *To heal from COVID, America must fix its psychological infrastructure*, Smerconish.com.
Remen, R. N. (2000). *My grandfather's blessings: Stories of strength, refuge, and belonging*. Riverhead Books.
Roth, J. (2016). Dwelling at the thresholds: Witness to historical trauma across concentric fields. In J. L. Alpert & E. R. Goren (Eds.), *Psychoanalysis, trauma, and community: History and contemporary reappraisals* (pp. 43–66). Routledge.
Safir, S. (1999). *Forgiving and not forgiving: Why sometimes it's better not to forgive*. HarperCollins Publishers.
Schneider, K. J. (2021, Oct 27). *Why Biden needs to appoint a psychological advisor*. smerconish.com/exclusive-content/why-biden-needs-to-appoint-a-psychological-advisor/.
Stern, D. B. (1996). Dissociation and constructivism: Commentary on papers by Davies and Harris. *Psychoanalytic Dialogues, 6*(2), 252–266. https://doi.org/10.1080/10481889609539118
Terry, M. L., & Leary, M. R. (2011). Self-compassion, self-regulation, and health. *Self and Identity, 10*(3), 352–362. https://doi.org/10.1080/15298868.2011.558404
Van der Kolk, B. A. (1987). *Psychological trauma*. American Psychiatric Press.
Weingarten, K. (2010). Reasonable hope: Construct, clinical applications, and supports. *Family Process, 49*(1), 5–25.

Psychology Today Blogs

Bossarte, D. (2021a, Feb 5). *COVID-19 overwhelm: Self-care for abuse survivors*. https://www.psychologytoday.com/us/blog/psychological-trauma-coping-and-resilience/202102/covid-19-overwhelm-self-care-abuse-survivors
Bossarte, D. (2021b, March 17). *COVID Overwhelm: Photography self-care for abuse survivors*. https://www.psychologytoday.com/us/blog/psychological-trauma-coping-and-resilience/202103/covid-overwhelm-photography-self-care-abuse
Bossarte, D. (2021c, April 20). *COVID-19 overwhelm: Yoga as self-care for abuse survivors*. https://www.psychologytoday.com/us/blog/psychological-trauma-coping-and-resilience/202104/covid-19-overwhelm-yoga-self-care-abuse

Connor, F. B., & Gordon, R. M. (2022, May 12). *Compassionate leadership during COVID-19.* https://www.psychologytoday.com/us/blog/psychological-trauma-coping-and-resilience/202205/compassionate-leadership-during-covid-19

Garcia, K., & Gordon, R. (2021, Sept 17). *The psychology behind COVID-19 hesitancy.* https://www.psychologytoday.com/us/blog/psychological-trauma-coping-and-resilience/202109/the-psychology-behind-covid-19-vaccine

Gardner, T. F. & Kohomban, J. C. *The collective trauma of the Black Community in 2020.* https//www.psychologytoday.com/us/blog/psychological-trauma-coping-and-resilience/202012/the-collective-trauma-the-black-community-in

Gordon, R. M. (2021, Jan 12). *Existential interventions during the age of COVID.* https://www.psychologytoday.com/intl/blog/psychological-trauma-coping-and-resilience/202101/existential-interventions-during-the-age?amp

Gordon, R. M., & Groth, T. (2022, March 3). *Cultivating forgiveness during COVID-19.* https://www.psychologytoday.com/us/blog/psychological-trauma-coping-and-resilience/202203/cultivating-forgiveness-during-covid-19

Gordon, R. M., Groth, T., & Schapiro, S. (2021b, March 21). *Sustaining hope in pediatric care during COVID-19.* https://www.psychologytoday.com/us/blog/psychological-trauma-coping-and-resilience/202103/sustaining-hope-in-pediatric-care-during

Gordon, R. M., Persaud, U., & Schapiro, S. (2021c, Feb 26). *Self-compassion and kindness during COVID-19.* https://www.psychologytoday.com/us/blog/psychological-trauma-coping-and-resilience/202102/self-compassion-and-kindness-during-covid-19

Gordon, R. M., Wolfson, J., & Talis, E. (2021d, Feb 13). *Why am I so tired?.* https://www.psychologytoday.com/us/blog/psychological-trauma-coping-and-resilience/202102/twhy-am-i-so-tired

Gordon, R. M., & McGiffin, J. N. (2021, April 27). *How to build resilience during the post-pandemic transition.* https://www.psychologytoday.com/us/blog/psychological-trauma-coping-and-resilience/202104/how-build-resilience-during-the-post-pandemic

Klyczek, A. R. (2021, March 6). *Reduce COVID trauma with psychological first aid.* https://www.psychologytoday.com/us/blog/psychological-trauma-coping-and-resilience/202103/reduce-covid-trauma-psychological-first-aid

Lester, E. (2020a, Dec 4). *Making an emotional recovery together in the COVID-19 ICU.* https://www.psychologytoday.com/us/blog/psychological-trauma-coping-and-resilience/202012/making-emotional-recovery-together-in-the

Lester, E. (2020b, Dec 8). *Managing emotional distress in the hospital and ICU.* https://www.psychologytoday.com/us/blog/psychological-trauma-coping-and-resilience/202012/managing-emotional-distress-in-the-hospital

Luborsky, E. (2002, Jan 3). *The brave new world of parenting in the pandemic.* https://www.psychologytoday.com/us/blog/psychological-trauma-coping-and-resilience/202101/the-brave-new-world-parenting-in-the-pandemic

Luborsky, E. (2021a, Jan 7). *Bring creativity & adventure to kid's lives during the pandemic.* https://www.psychologytoday.com/us/blog/psychological-trauma-coping-and-resilience/202101/bring-creativity-and-adventure-kids-lives

Luborsky, E. (2021b, Jan 19). *Decode the message in your child's behavior.* https://www.psychologytoday.com/us/blog/psychological-trauma-coping-and-resilience/202101/decode-the-message-in-your-childs-behavior

Nordeman Sumarriva, G., & Gordon, R. M. (2021, Aug 4). *How to improve communication with your partner.* https://www.psychologytoday.com/us/blog/psychological-trauma-coping-and-resilience/202108/how-improve-communication-your-partner.

O'Gorman, P., & Morgan, C. (2022, May, 16). *Addiction + Covid = A Toxic Cocktail.*

O'Gorman, P. (2020a, Dec 13). *Three ways to grieve when your grief has no place to go: Making space for personal loss and collective grief while helping your patients.*

O'Gorman, P. (2020b, Dec 2). *On the Covid-19 battlefield: Providing psychological guidance, hope and resilience.*

O'Gorman, P. (2021a, Dec 24). *Compassion: The needed ingredient for holiday gatherings.*

O'Gorman, P. (2021b, Sept 29). *Vaccine hesitancy: Understanding the power of NO*

O'Gorman, P. (2021c, Feb 2). *Suicide By intentional overdose in children: The missing variable in tackling teen suicide is the addiction epidemic.*

O'Gorman, P. (2021d, March 15). *On St. Patrick's day, be truly radical—celebrate sobriety: Why during an addiction epidemic within a pandemic, choosing Sobriety is smart.*

O'Reilly-Landry, M. (2020a, Dec 1). *When pandemic trauma hits home.* https://www.psychologytoday.com/us/blog/psychological-trauma-coping-and-resilience/202012/when-pandemic-trauma-hits-home

O'Reilly-Landry, M. (2020b, Dec 3). *The psychological trauma of having a loved one in the ICU.*

O'Reilly-Landry, M. (2021b, Feb 4). *America needs a psychologist in chief.*

O'Reilly-Landry, M. (2021c, March 9). *Discover your personal meaning in the COVID-19 experience.*

Palsdottir, S. (2021, Sept 14). *When working with cancer patients is traumatic: Self-care to better aide patient care.*

Rodriguez, C. M. (2021, Jan 22). *Children at risk for maltreatment during COVID-19*

Schneider, K. H. (2020, May 12). *What existentialists can teach us about COVID-19.* https://www.psychologytoday.com/us/blog/awakening-awe/202005/what-existentialists-can-teach-us-about-COVID-19

Tisch, R. (2021, Jan 1). *COVID is not the only public health problems facing America.* https://www.psychologytoday.com/us/blog/psychological-trauma-coping-andresilience/202101/covid-is-not-the-only-public-health-problem

Winik., A. *The return to school: Tips for parent of anxious children.* https://www.psychologytoday.com/us/blog/psychological-trauma-coping-and-resilience/202106/the-return-school-tips-parents-anxious

Wren, I. (2020, Dec 16). *What can i do if my family member is in the COVID ICU?.* https://www.psychologytoday.com/us/blog/psychological-trauma-coping-and-resilience/202012/what-can-i-do-if-my-family-member-is-in-the

Wren, I. (2021, Jan 28). *Surviving and thriving as a couple in the pandemic.* https://www.psychologytoday.com/us/blog/psychological-trauma-coping-and-resilience/202101/surviving-and-thriving-couple-in-the-pandemic

Chapter 7
Supporting Mental Health Clinicians During the Pandemic

Melissa Wasserman, Julian D. Ford, and Arlene Lu Steinberg

Introduction: Challenges Facing Mental Health Professionals in the COVID-19 Pandemic

Results of surveys of healthcare workers during the COVID-19 pandemic consistently demonstrate adverse effects on their psychological well-being (De Kock et al., 2021) that were progressively worse over the first year of the pandemic (Sasaki et al., 2021). Front-line providers are at risk for insomnia, anxiety, depression, post-traumatic stress, somatization, and suicidality related to threats to their (and their co-workers' and families') lives and health and exposure to the suffering and deaths of patients and their families and of their co-workers (Li et al., 2021). Systematic programs therefore have been initiated to mitigate the adverse mental health effects on front-line healthcare providers with therapeutic, educational, and social support interventions (Rolling et al., 2021). However, the impact of the pandemic on the psychological well-being of mental health professionals has been largely overlooked. A survey of 110 psychotherapists in the United Kingdom early in the pandemic found that pressures related to using telehealth and long work hours were associated with burnout, while work-life balance and self-compassion may

M. Wasserman (✉)
Graduate School of Education & Psychology, Pepperdine University, Los Angeles, CA, USA
e-mail: melissa.wasserman@pepperdine.edu

J. D. Ford
Ferkauf Graduate School, University of Connecticut School of Medicine, Farmington, CT, USA
e-mail: jford@uchc.edu

A. Lu Steinberg
Private Practice, New York, NY, USA

Ferkauf Graduate School of Psychology, Yeshiva University, The Bronx, USA

Icahn School of Medicine at Mount Sinai, New York, USA

C. R. Figley et al. (eds.), *Pandemic Providers*,
https://doi.org/10.1007/978-3-031-27580-7_7

have protected against burnout (Kotera et al., 2021). A survey of 265 healthcare workers in the southeastern USA that included a sub-set of mental health professionals at four time-points at the end of the first year of the pandemic found that burnout was predicted by experiencing moral injury, depressions symptoms, increased workload, and lack of confidence in support from their organizations' leadership (Dale et al., 2021). As the pressures and uncertainties of the pandemic and the increasing need and demand in the public for scarce mental health services continue a year later, and beyond, the toll taken on mental health professionals' well-being and health is likely to correspondingly grow greater even in periods of apparent recovery from COVID-19.

Thus, while the immediate pressures and traumatic experiences affecting frontline healthcare providers and the general public may ebb and flow, and hopefully will diminish as the pandemic becomes an endemic stressor rather than a prolonged critical incident, the long-term adverse mental health effects of trauma, loss, isolation, and physical and emotional exhaustion caused by the pandemic are likely to become increasingly evident and severe. Correspondingly, the demands and pressures faced by mental health providers and their vulnerability to burnout and psychopathology are more likely to continue to escalate. The workload of those still willing and able to practice will grow, as will their patients' acuity and chronicity—which increases the risk of vicarious or secondary traumatic stress and compassion fatigue as well as burnout. At the very point at which it is most difficult to find the time to be with family, friends, and colleagues, and to engage in avocations and activities that provide a sense of enjoyment and rejuvenation, this is when making that shift to step back and restore work-life balance is most essential.

Psychologists Respond to the Challenge: The Clinician Support Collaborative

Many of the members of the original American Psychological Association Interdivisional COVID-19 Task Force who were psychotherapists quickly noticed the new way we were having to work, staying apart from our clients and colleagues in our own homes and using unfamiliar telehealth technology. Our patients were talking to us about the same issues of compassion fatigue, feeling isolated, coping with loss and uncertainty, fears of contracting the illness, and the added stress of Zoom fatigue and the related technology barriers and crashes. We had to learn to deliver psychotherapy services without the usual in-person cues and relationships, and without the usual contacts with and support from our colleagues. To address the challenges of the shared trauma that we and our patients were navigating, we formed a Work Group and developed a unique drop-in support group for mental health professionals like us that helped us discuss and share ways in which the pandemic has had a global impact, disrupting virtually every aspect of work, personal, family, and social life. While most therapists are trained to keep their own fears and lives out of the therapy room, sharing common issues was an important tool that served to support everyone in the group. The Work Group includes psychologists (in the USA and internationally), with a common goal to identify practical ways to provide psychologists and other mental health professionals and trainees with direct peer support during the pandemic.

Besides providing a forum to share experiences, Work Group members also studied the resources offered online by professional organizations that address mental health issues raised by the pandemic and challenges faced by practitioners as they shifted to telehealth. Overall, psychologists reported that their clients experienced intensified stressors and symptoms, compounded by the threats and disruptions related to the continuing pandemic (Rossi et al., 2021; Litam et al., 2021). The Work Group determined that there was a unique need of mental health professionals that was not being addressed: the critically important personal contact with colleagues for mutual support. Given the enormous demands that we, and our mental health professional colleagues all around the world were facing, we realized that a simple solution was needed to provide a feasible way to enable mental health professionals and trainees to access peer support while we all were moving in and out of a pandemic. Virtual platforms offered the opportunity and vehicle to set up this supportive forum, given social distance and quarantine regulations.

Supportive spaces for mental health clinicians outside the scope of consultation and supervision have always been limited and have been even less available during the pandemic. Yet, secondary traumatic stress is something that continues to impact mental health clinicians and healthcare providers, and the COVID-19 pandemic may have exacerbated already present prevalence rates of vicarious trauma (Aafjes-van Doorn et al., 2020). A grassroots effort was therefore initiated by the Professional Support for Psychologists Work Group in order to build a supportive space for clinicians to join during the pandemic. The rationale for the groups was for mental health clinicians to join and provide mutual support amidst a significant increase in provider stress and burnout as a result of the pandemic. The initiative was named the *Clinician Support Collaborative* (CSC) and was set up by psychologists from around the world, to meet the needs of their fellow mental health professionals and professional trainees. These meetings were offered on an online video platform weekly to mental health clinicians across the world at no cost.

Group procedures were established including developing an online platform for meetings, and interested participants could easily sign up online and choose from the various times offered. To ensure that participants did not mistakenly assume that the meetings provided therapy, announcements describing the CSC clearly stated that the purpose was to bring psychologists and other mental health professionals together to provide peer support in an informal group discussion format. The CSC team members reiterated this crucial description at the outset of each virtual session and were referred to (and referred to themselves) as "facilitators" or "hosts" who led the session and participated on a personal basis as a peer and not as a formal group leader or therapist. The facilitator invited attendees to talk about any professional issues, or personal issues that were affecting their professional practice, that they had encountered in the pandemic. In some cases, the facilitator opened the discussion with a self-disclosure in order to "break the ice" and provide a model (as well as to personally receive support from the other attendees). In other instances, the session began with an attendee immediately volunteering an issue or topic for discussion. Throughout each session, the facilitator modeled a supportive and non-directive approach to interacting and encouraged other attendees to share their experiences without doing any therapeutic intervention. Facilitators ensured that the meeting times offered could accommodate as many time zones as feasible, so participants around the globe could have the opportunity to join in and provide mutual support. Meeting facilitators were referred to as *hosts* to address typical consultation and group dynamics and convey the message that the working group was not offering a therapeutic service, but rather a safe space for clinicians to share and connect with one another in their struggles and experiences of the pandemic. The online scheduling platform where participants would sign up included a disclaimer outlining the rationale, scope, and guidelines for the space and asking participants to agree to these guidelines and parameters prior to enrolling for a meeting time.

The collaborative hosted virtual video sessions on a several-day-per-week basis for mental health professionals (and trainees) to drop in and discuss challenges they were facing as a result of the COVID-19 pandemic. An online event scheduling platform was utilized for outreach and scheduling ease. This link was distributed on flyers and e-mails to different mental health listservs. Participants would sign up on the event scheduling platform where they were also prompted to read a disclaimer about the collaborative meetings. The purpose of providing these sessions using an informal drop-in format was to reduce the real and perceived isolation that we and our mental health colleagues were experiencing due to the total elimination of in-person contact with both our colleagues and our clients—as well as from family and friends. Although virtual contact could not replace those in-person connections, the CSC sessions provided a refreshing and restorative opportunity to see and hear from colleagues and to disclose, reflect on, and give as well as receive support for important concerns and experiences that were affecting our professional and personal lives individually and collectively.

Identified Themes from CSC Meetings

Members of the Work Group served as both hosts and informal facilitators for each session in order to engage participants in spontaneous discussions. Themes surfaced through session discussion, which were congruent with much of the recent research that has been conducted on the impact of COVID-19 on therapist burnout and vicarious trauma, some of which include compassion fatigue/burnout, isolation, managing boundaries, and work-related concerns.

Since mental health providers have been on the frontlines in managing the consequences of the COVID-19 pandemic, providers have experienced the harmful effects of burnout, compassion fatigue, and secondary traumatic stress. Mental health clinicians play a critical role in providing support and relief to those who have experienced an increased need for support because of the pandemic. Mental health providers are now in increased demand and experiencing a heightened level of work pressure, particularly providing teletherapy with patient loads often increasing at a rapid rate (Joshi & Sharma, 2020) and leading to an uptick in compassion fatigue and burnout. *Compassion fatigue* includes the experience of reduced or fatigued capacity for compassion as a direct consequence of the emotional exhaustion of working with others (Figley, 1995, 2002). In mental health clinicians, it may also emerge as constant worry about patient and may be a common reaction for folks who work with highly stressed or traumatized patients. It may also emerge as apathy or decreased bandwidth to empathize or connect with others which may manifest as the experience of emotional numbness. *Burnout* has been identified as the experience of exhaustion or fatigue as a consequence of chronic stress (Maslach, 2003).

Kahill (1988) has identified several categories of symptoms of *professional burnout* including (1) physical symptoms; (2) emotional symptoms; (3) behavioral symptoms; (4) work-related symptoms; and (5) interpersonal symptoms. Physical symptoms include the feeling of exhaustion that so many clinicians within the collaborative groups described as part of the pandemic. This may also emerge as sleep difficulties or possibly even as other somatic symptoms (e.g., headaches, body aches, gastrointestinal symptoms, etc.). Emotional symptoms may include irritability, anxiety, or even a sense of helplessness. Healthcare workers have had to deal with an increased workload and mental and physical exhaustion as a result of the COVID-19 pandemic. Studies have shown that frontline healthcare workers have had to bear the brunt of this, and that they are more likely to experience psychological distress, including challenges with posttraumatic stress and other psychiatric and behavioral health symptomatology (Trumello et al., 2020; Pappa et al., 2020). A recent study also found that healthcare workers who assisted and treated individuals with COVID-19 displayed a positive correlation between self-reported hopelessness and PTSD symptoms (Aguglia et al., 2021). Behavioral health symptoms may include pessimism, cynicism, substance use, or even suicidality. Pandemic burnout-related behavioral symptoms have manifested through increased substance use as a way of coping with the stress and challenges experienced as a result of the COVID-19 pandemic. The Centers for Disease Control and Prevention (2020) reported that 13% of Americans experienced new or increasing substance use in order to cope with the pandemic (Czeisler et al., 2020).

Work-related symptoms are also a part of burnout including poor work performance, absenteeism, or misusing work breaks. Many employees have felt low motivation to engage in daily activities including work-related behaviors. This has been exacerbated by work from home and blurred boundaries between the work and personal aspects of life. Lastly, interpersonal symptoms related to burnout may include isolation and withdrawal and may impact how effectively we communicate and/or connect with others. Undoubtedly, COVID has impacted our interpersonal relationships on every level. The frequency of communication may have decreased, and physical contact was deemed unsafe. Friends, family members, and colleagues were left confused about how safe it would be to be near one another, leaving many feeling alone during times when they may have needed connection the most.

As compassion fatigue plagued the mental healthcare system during the pandemic, clinicians often processed and discussed how secondary traumatic stress impacted so many facets of their lives. Often times, clinicians shared that working with marginalized and unequally affected populations compounded secondary traumatic stress. A participant from the USA who attended several CSC sessions poignantly described how experiencing the intersection of several professional and personal stressors was creating a sense of physical as well as emotional depletion that made every day difficult to face. The professional stressors included being unable to meet in person with clients and vicariously experiencing several clients' distress about their own losses and their sense of that they had been abandoned in their therapy, while also feeling unable to provide them with more than token reassurance and no meaningful solutions to those dilemmas. The attendee also faced the practical problem of having to give up an office space that had been a familiar practice site for many years, while at the same time dealing with a flood of referrals and requests to take on new clients. In the midst of these professional challenges and losses, the attendee also was dealing with chronic health problems that limited mobility and made venturing out of her home frightening due to the risk of potentially catastrophic exposure to the COVID virus. Even walking to the mailbox or taking out the garbage had become a source of anxiety, which was heightened by having neighbors who seemed oblivious to the danger of viral transmission and were callously amused by the attendee's precautions. The attendee also was unable to continue to visit in person with the small group of family members and colleagues who had been a lifeline, and feared becoming perceived by them as a burden and having them cut-off their contact (which already was greatly reduced). The attendee expressed embarrassment initially at disclosing these difficulties and reactions, but this was replaced by a sense of relief when other attendees genuinely empathized and reflected admiration for the courage and resilience these disclosures revealed—for example, one attendee commented, "I don't know if I could handle all that you have on your plate, but it's inspiring to me to hear that you're carrying on and being there for your clients and your family and colleagues in spite of it all. If you can do it, maybe I can too."

A participant from India described doing therapy with a woman who had been sexually victimized and re-victimized, and was being ostracized by her own and her husband's families while also dealing with economic and health problems due to the pandemic. The participant described feeling helpless and incompetent, saying "Nothing I can say will change this woman's life, but there must be something I could do if I had more knowledge as a therapist." The facilitator empathized with the participant's distress, and asked the other attendees if they thought the participant might already be doing some things therapeutically that were going unnoticed but actually were helping this client. Other attendees commented on how they'd found that simply being consistently available and providing an opportunity for clients to have someone on their side to whom they could say things that they couldn't tell anyone else had been a secure base for clients who faced impossible dilemmas like this woman's. They asked the participant why this client continued in therapy, and when the participant had no answer, they suggested spontaneously that it must be because the client felt some important needs were being met or she would not take the precious time (and risk the additional censure from her family) to be in therapy. This led to a group discussion of the value of providing traumatized clients with the experience of relational security, and how important this was for clients who were experiencing multiple traumas and the additional burdens involved in the pandemic. The participant listened carefully, and thanked the group for providing a new perspective that made continuing therapy with this—and other—clients seem possible and worth doing.

Another participant identified how the groups helped them become more attuned to themselves and supported their mindful awareness and acceptance. They described their experience as “a warm hug that we all needed.” They elaborated that the collaborative group sessions “helped me in becoming aware how dissociated I had become with my own body and to getting back in touch with my physical self, and helped also to ease the fear and anxiety housed in my body.…This helped me understand that by being attuned to oneself, we can choose our pace, and decide to move towards acceptance and awareness, just an inch every day.”

Many clinicians discussed experiencing personal and professional *isolation* as they were stripped of their typical day-to-day routines and navigated working from home. Participants often discussed feeling alone in their struggles, like so many during the pandemic leaving limited outlets for self-care and burnout prevention related to social engagement. Those working in group practices and interdisciplinary teams craved their former connections and felt despair in feeling alone while navigating their day-to-day professional responsibilities. Those who engaged in social self-care activities reported a longing to reunite with their support systems in person—which helped them previously manage burnout and vicarious trauma. This only exacerbated isolation that they experienced in other areas of their lives as a result of stay-at-home orders and the COVID-19 pandemic. One participant shared, “the workshops provided a valuable space for me to be present in an alive way also with my colleagues and friends, with some my classmates, some of my seniors, and some unknown yet so familiar in their struggles…I felt held by all of them together, with the promise that we would survive these times.”

Participants often mentioned challenges in *managing work/life boundaries* as they were conducting sessions from home, many of them engaging in teletherapy for the first time. This posed challenges in maintaining therapeutic boundaries within the context of telehealth exacerbated by shared trauma as we all were not only experiencing the pandemic, but also confronting political turmoil, and mass community death. Although tele-counseling has many benefits related to access, it posed some challenges for clinicians who were working from home. Clinicians often mentioned they found it difficult to just “turn off” following the work day. Many spoke of how they benefitted from the commute home after work which provided a natural transition point and routine from work to home life. Given the nature of clinical work and dramatic increase in workload during the pandemic, many clinicians have found the work to be more emotionally demanding which may relate to the increase in Zoom fatigue. This relates to *work-related concerns* which were a theme that also emerged during meetings. Many clinicians questioned whether or not to return to in-person practice in addition to experiencing Zoom fatigue. This led many of the clinicians who joined to discuss and identify how the anxiety of the unknown has impacted so many facets of life. Some shared their questions and internal dialogue related to the decision of whether or not to return to in-person practice and the pros and cons of doing so.

The Experience of Facilitating the Mutual Support Sessions with Colleagues and Trainees

Work Group members shared many observations and personal reactions to facilitating the Clinician Support Collaborative peer support sessions, a sampling of which is offered here. Facilitators were connecting in deep and meaningful ways with one another and with the participants:

> I found the gratitude expressed by virtually every attendee in the support groups that I hosted deeply moving. Just knowing that there are colleagues who not only shared similar emotional reactions to the plethora of pandemic-related professional and personal stressors, but also cared enough to take a genuine interest in each other attendee's experience, seemed almost lifesaving in its impact. Underneath the very professional demeanor and self-effacing demeanor with which we all conducted ourselves in the sessions, there was a deep wellspring of emotion that followed an arc from frustration, loneliness, and discouragement at the outset of the session to a reflective phase of taking stock and reconnecting with core values and a sense of not being alone as the support of other participants began to resonate, and ultimately to a sense of hope and encouragement that often was highlighted by expressions of relief and gratitude. I found myself gradually able, if you'll forgive the cliché—but I mean this sincerely—to actually trust the process. At first, I began the sessions with anxiety, doubting that a brief hour without any set structure could actually be helpful for colleagues who were facing such overwhelming stress. As the sessions proceeded, I "got it"—the comradery of peers is exactly what the doctor ordered. My experience began with a feeling of gratitude that there seemed to be such a clear need, and for the power of the leadership and group that quickly formed. Meeting others in this group was a pleasure, and we talked openly about our experiences during each meeting.

Another facilitator shared the meaningfulness of the groups and how the experiential component in navigating shared trauma was a useful outlet:

> The groups provided much needed support to not only group members, some of whom were isolated in their home offices, or others who were on the very front line in hospitals and other facilities, but to us all. Members shared the impact of political ideologies on ways their friends, family and neighbors were coping, leading to conflicts within their families over exposure and other things. Others experienced profound loss of family members during group meetings. My own experience learning that my Dad contracted COVID19 a few minutes before beginning one drop-in group as a facilitator brought this home to me. My differing role as a facilitator rather than a therapist, lead me to choose to and felt that I could share a bit about my experiences with the group at a later meeting. The heartfelt support of group members was so helpful. These meetings enabled one to experientially feel the pandemic reality, and appreciate the global reality, with its similarities and differences, in a multi-dimensional way, very different from the experience of digesting news reports.

One facilitator shared their experience of how the groups helped contain their own death anxiety and isolation:

> The two meetings I facilitated also contained my own death anxiety, my isolation. In witnessing the grief of my fellow Indians as they expressed their shock, their horror, and their paralysis, I was filled with gratitude. For the first time in a year and a half of working on screen in a country reckoning with its racialized history in which I was interpolated and implicated, I was in a virtual space with familiar names and easily memorizable faces who spoke and understood Hinglish and I found myself connected, not alone.

A facilitator shared how these groups aided in building a more mindful group approach to suffering and shared trauma:

> As a Psychoanalytic Psychotherapist one is trained to work with images of devastation that patients bring. The unprocessed internal devastation is dreamed together with the analyst's mind. When the second wave of Covid hit India, the Psychoanalytic Psychotherapists, were faced with a challenge of unfathomable intensity. Not only were we using our minds to keep our own loved ones alive but we were absorbing the panic and grief from our patients. The devastation of apocalyptic proportions that many visited in their worst nightmares, was now unfolding right in front of their eyes. As we along with our patients watched in horror, the nightmares turned into reality, leaving no space for dreaming or doing psychological work. We felt stuck. We reached out to our colleagues in APA and their response was overwhelming. A group of senior Psychotherapists agreed to open a virtual window for us to breathe. With each of these sessions, our minds felt gathered from the scatter we were experiencing. Our panic found resonance and began to lose its intense hold on us. We realize how absorbing trauma and living trauma had caused us to feel overwhelmed in minds and bodies. The trauma was trapped in various parts of our bodies. We were gently nudged towards movement, dance which gradually loosened up our minds too. There was a space to weep, laugh, share existential angst and mourn one's limits as Psychotherapists. To sum it up, these spaces, restored in us the capacity for negative capability. We felt enabled to move from feeling passively stuck to an active stance of being still.

Another facilitator shared their experience of support and how it is critical to receive help, especially as a helper:

> I am a psychologist-psychoanalyst located in New York City. I specialize in trauma and believed that I had something I could offer my colleagues. And, yes, I felt I was helpful to them. But what I hadn't thought much about at that time was how helpful participating in the Clinicians Collaborative would be to me. When I was most active with this group, I was living in the epicenter of Covid-19 and directly across the street from a makeshift morgue. I was traumatized. While I had friends and colleagues I could readily talk to, it was also helpful to be involved with these meetings. The point is that the people who attended our groups, I believe, felt supported. We helped the helpers to help. In addition, we were helped as well by the groups and by each other.

An unexpected comradery, or what will be referred to as *the meta group*, occurred within the Professional Support for Psychologists Working Group. In the group's administrative meetings, comradeships and connections emerged between working group participants that was often discussed in meetings. Working Group members would share how much they valued the meeting times as they offered ways to connect with other psychologist across the globe and foster meaningful relationships with other clinicians throughout the pandemic. During a time of profound isolation, working group members simultaneously struggled with similar challenges that emerged from the Clinician Support Collaborative groups and were ameliorated by the connections that were built within our own Working Group.

Lessons Learned and Future Directions

There were several challenges in initiating, establishing, and maintaining the collaborative meetings. First, since funding was limited for these groups, we utilized free platforms to manage the administration and outreach efforts related to these meetings. This limited us in terms of technological advancements that we were able to provide. We recommend that larger organizations with a wider range of technological, financial, and administrative resources offer these groups. While Zoom offered the opportunity to come together when social distancing and quarantine prevented in-person engagement, and also enabled global connection, the prevalence of Zoom fatigue increased during the pandemic. Given this, we recommend that groups like this be held in person when feasible to mitigate the impact that Zoom fatigue may have. Zoom fatigue, at times, may have served as a barrier to clinicians joining.

What we learned from listening to our psychologist colleagues in the United States, and then in India, was that encouragement to disengage from work and take time for self-care and personal wellness is appreciated but is not a solution—and could inadvertently increase the sense of personal and professional guilt and failure that is the hallmark of burnout and moral injury. Instead, we were reminded to practice what we preach: that is, to focus instead on the hallmark of psychotherapy. While being careful not to blur boundaries and attempt to therapize our colleagues—or induce them to therapize us—we found that what they, and we, found most restorative was co-creating the psychological safety, support, and space each of us needed for mindful reflection on our feelings (emotional and bodily) and the associated psychological questions, conflicts, and dilemmas that had arisen in our professional and personal lives. This could take the form of sharing a personal experience that was troubling or that had some special personal meaning, or a professional dilemma or case that raised unanswered questions, had a particularly profound vicarious impact, or elicited strong countertransference reactions.

The collaborative group provided a holding environment that enabled every participant—not just the person who was self-disclosing at any particular moment—to reflect more deeply than is possible when taking the responsibility to focus on the patients and provide them with that space in psychotherapy. The non-hierarchical context of the collaborative sessions also freed all of us to be both reflective and supportive without the heavy responsibility of focusing largely on how to best understand and attend to the inner world and best interests of our patients when either doing psychotherapy or participating in a formal clinical supervision/consultation session. The opportunity to flow freely in reflection between the personal and the professional realms made it possible to feel a sense of spontaneity that can go missing—or be replaced by a sense of paradoxical aloneness—in the hours of maintaining the nonjudgmental, emotionally regulated, and other-focused perspective necessary in psychotherapy and psychological assessment.

The sessions with our colleagues in India reflected the varying impact of COVID-19's course, with the impact on different regions varying. India was in the throes of the pandemic in the summer of 2021, as the situation in the USA seemed to have improved. These groups provided an important contrast, due to an interesting combination of the context in which they began and the culture of the participants. Our psychologist colleague in India who had learned of the Clinician Support Collaborative (CSC) took the initiative to request sessions co-hosted by rotating members of the Collaborative and her. Rather than impersonally announcing the meetings to any mental health professional or trainee who was interested, as we had done when we launched the CSC, she intentionally and personally invited a group of psychologists who already were an informal peer support group for one another. We subsequently reflected on how this demonstrated the difference between the individualistic cultural perspective that was evident in our original approach to bringing together our colleagues versus the collectivistic culture and approach adopted by our colleagues in India. These groups also varied from the original ones as they were not only supportive, but also topic driven; topics addressed an overview of trauma, self-care, psychological first aid, secondary traumatic stress, and grief. The group members' familiarity with one another facilitated meaningful, helpful conversation. In all groups the real-life effects of the pandemic had a direct impact on not only group members, but on group process, as members experienced illness and loss, and together spoke of their attempts to navigate this crisis and comfort one another. The geographical distance, coinciding with a period of relative calm in the USA, enabled facilitators to provide a calm holding function for those who participated from India. While both approaches have merit (the more anonymous drop-in groups and the group where participants all worked together and knew each other), the difference in attendance is striking—typically at most two or three participants and only a few who returned multiple times in our original sessions, versus a consistent group of 15–20 colleagues from India in each of those sessions. One challenge of the original groups were that attendees' needs greatly varied, where some experienced the challenges related to loneliness as they were isolated due to health risks and regulations; others were experiencing the challenges of facing the health inequities and incredible needs of many groups and individuals in other health care settings or global regions. Despite these challenges, some members chose to attend regularly most or all of the original group sessions, and expressed gratitude for the opportunity to connect.

Future versions of the CSC could build on and adapt the two approaches with options including closed groups limited to participants who already know one another, or groups composed of some participants who know each other while also inviting others who do not have that prior connection. A key lesson learned is that including a core membership of participants who are joining not just to give and receive support generally but specifically to be with others with whom they share an ongoing connection may be important in order to provide stability and sense of continuity—especially in times such as this pandemic in which instability and discontinuity have become the norm.

Author Note The Professional Support for Psychologists Working Group at the APA Interdivisional Task Force on the Pandemic is represented by Judith Alpert, Tina Balachandran, Julian Ford (co-chair), Ilene Serlin, Arlene Steinberg, and Melissa Wasserman (co-chair). Further details or information on the chapter content are available from the first author upon request. The authors would like to thank all group members for their contributions to the Task Force.

References

Aafjes-van Doorn, K., Békés, V., Prout, T. A., & Hoffman, L. (2020). Psychotherapists' vicarious traumatization during the COVID-19 pandemic. *Psychological Trauma: Theory, Research, Practice, and Policy, 12*(S1), S148–S150. https://doi.org/10.1037/tra0000868

Aguglia, A., Amerio, A., Costanza, A., Parodi, N., Copello, F., Serafini, G., & Amore, M. (2021). Hopelessness and post-traumatic stress symptoms among healthcare workers during the COVID-19 pandemic: Any role for mediating variables? *International Journal of Environmental Research and Public Health, 18*(12), 6579. https://doi.org/10.3390/ijerph18126579

Czeisler, M. É., Lane, R. I., Petrosky, E., Wiley, J. F., Christensen, A., Njai, R., Weaver, M. D., et al. (2020). Mental health, substance use, and suicidal ideation during the COVID-19 pandemic. *Morbidity and Mortality Weekly Report, 69*(32), 1049–1057. https://doi.org/10.15585/mmwr.mm6932a1

Dale, L. P., Cuffe, S. P., Sambuco, N., Guastello, A. D., Leon, K. G., Nunez, L. V., Bhullar, A., Allen, B. R., & Mathews, C. A. (2021). Morally distressing experiences, moral injury, and burnout in Florida healthcare providers during the COVID-19 pandemic. *International Journal of Environmental Research and Public Health, 18*(23), 12319. https://doi.org/10.3390/ijerph182312319

De Kock, J. H., Latham, H. A., Leslie, S. J., Grindle, M., Munoz, S. A., Ellis, L., Polson, R., & O'Malley, C. M. (2021). A rapid review of the impact of COVID-19 on the mental health of healthcare workers: Implications for supporting psychological well-being. *BMC Public Health, 21*(1), 104. https://doi.org/10.1186/s12889-020-10070-3

Figley, C. R. (Ed.). (1995). *Compassion fatigue: Coping with secondary traumatic stress disorder in those who treat the traumatized*. Taylor & Francis Group.

Figley, C. R. (2002). Compassion fatigue: Psychotherapists' chronic lack of self care. *Journal of Clinical Psychology, 58*, 1433–1441. https://doi.org/10.1002/jclp.10090

Joshi, G., & Sharma, G. (2020). Burnout: A risk factor amongst mental health professionals during COVID-19. *Asian Journal of Psychiatry, 54*, 102300. https://doi.org/10.1016/j.ajp.2020.102300

Kahill, S. (1988). Symptoms of professional burnout: A review of the empirical evidence. *Canadian Psychology, 29*(3), 284–297. https://doi.org/10.1037/h0079772

Kotera, Y., Maxwell-Jones, R., Edwards, A. M., & Knutton, N. (2021). Burnout in professional psychotherapists: Relationships with self-compassion, work-life balance, and telepressure. *International Journal of Environmental Research and Public Health, 18*(10), 5308. https://doi.org/10.3390/ijerph18105308

Li, Y., Scherer, N., Felix, L., & Kuper, H. (2021). Prevalence of depression, anxiety and post-traumatic stress disorder in health care workers during the COVID-19 pandemic: A systematic review and meta-analysis. *PLoS One, 16*(3), e0246454. https://doi.org/10.1371/journal.pone.0246454

Litam, S. D. A., Ausloos, C. D., & Harrichand, J. J. S. (2021). Stress and resilience among professional counselors during the covid-19 pandemic. *Journal of Counseling and Development, 99*(4), 384–395. https://doi.org/10.1002/jcad.12391

Maslach, C. (2003). *Burnout: The cost of caring*. Malor Books.

Pappa, S., Ntella, V., Giannakas, T., Giannakoulis, V. G., Papoutsi, E., & Katsaounou, P. (2020). Prevalence of depression, anxiety, and insomnia among healthcare workers during the COVID-19 pandemic: A systematic review and meta-analysis. *Brain, Behavior, and Immunity, 88*, 901–907. https://doi.org/10.1016/j.bbi.2020.05.026

Rolling, J., Mengin, A. C., Palacio, C., Mastelli, D., Fath, M., Gras, A., Von Hunolstein, J. J., Schroder, C. M., & Vidailhet, P. (2021). COVID-19: Mental health prevention and care for healthcare professionals. *Frontiers in Psychiatry, 12*, 566740. https://doi.org/10.3389/fpsyt.2021.566740

Rossi, S., Carbone, R., Pedrelli, E., Artioli, G., Sozzi, A., & Sarli, L. (2021). The experience of the emergency psychologist during the Covid-19 pandemic. *Acta Bio-medica: Atenei Parmensis, 92*(S2), e2021508. https://doi.org/10.23750/abm.v92iS2.12326

Sasaki, N., Asaoka, H., Kuroda, R., Tsuno, K., Imamura, K., & Kawakami, N. (2021). Sustained poor mental health among healthcare workers in COVID-19 pandemic: A longitudinal analysis of the four-wave panel survey over 8 months in Japan. *Journal of Occupational Health, 63*(1), e12227. https://doi.org/10.1002/1348-9585.12227

Sherman, M. D., Sattler, A., Brandenberg, D., & Hooker, S. (2021). Providing psychotherapy in an urban, underserved community during the COVID-19 pandemic. *Journal of Health Care for the Poor and Underserved, 32*(3), 1096–1101. https://doi.org/10.1353/hpu.2021.0115

Trumello, C., Bramanti, S. M., Ballarotto, G., Candelori, C., Cerniglia, L., Cimino, S., Crudele, M., et al. (2020). Psychological adjustment of healthcare workers in Italy during the COVID-19 pandemic: Differences in stress, anxiety, depression, burnout, secondary trauma, and compassion satisfaction between frontline and non-frontline professionals. *International Journal of Environmental Research and Public Health, 17*, 8358. https://doi.org/10.3390/ijerph17228358

Melissa Wasserman is a licensed clinical psychologist and Assistant Professor of Psychology at Pepperdine University's Graduate School of Education & Psychology.

Julian D. Ford is a clinical psychologist and Professor of Psychiatry and Law at University of Connecticut, Director of the Center for the Treatment of Developmental Trauma Disorders and the Center for Trauma Recovery and Juvenile Justice.

Arlene Lu Steinberg is a clinical psychologist in private practice, Adjunct Associate Professor at the Yeshiva University's Ferkauf Graduate School, and Educational Consultant at the Icahn School of Medicine at Mt Sinai.

Chapter 8
International Somatic and Creative Arts Whole Person Approaches

Ilene A. Serlin, Judy Kuriansky, Lori Gill, Lawrence Graber, Hattie Worboys, Amy Li, Patricia Villavicencio Carrillo, and Rita M. Rivera

Introduction

Words alone are not enough to help heal trauma. In this chapter, the authors will focus on the use of nonverbal and symbolic approaches to healing trauma. The authors come from the disciplines of psychology as well as the creative arts therapies, from international locations, and either are artists themselves or use the arts in their therapeutic work. In the first section, we will define whole person approaches

I. A. Serlin (✉)
Serlin Institute of the Healing Arts, San Francisco, CA, USA
e-mail: iserlin@ileneserlin.com

J. Kuriansky
Columbia University Teachers College, New York, NY, USA

L. Gill
Attachment and Trauma Treatment Centre for Healing (ATTCH), St. Catharines, ON, Canada
e-mail: lori@attch.org

L. Graber
Saybrook University, Pasadena, CA, USA

H. Worboys
Body Talks Movement, London, UK

A. Li
Dance4Healing, Mountain View, CA, USA
e-mail: hello@dance4healing.com

P. V. Carrillo
Hospital Clínico San Carlos de Madrid, Madrid, Spain

R. M. Rivera
Duke University, Durham, NC, USA

C. R. Figley et al. (eds.), *Pandemic Providers*,
https://doi.org/10.1007/978-3-031-27580-7_8

and present our mission statement. We then tell our origin story as one of the Work Groups that gathered as part of the APA Interdivisional Task Force on the pandemic. We discuss the work that the group did during the pandemic, focusing on areas of the Arts and Community Healing; Somatic and Mindfulness Approaches; Resilience; Embodied, Creative Practices: Cultivating Body-Nature Resonance; and the Creative and Expressive Arts Therapies. We conclude with Challenges Faced and Lessons Learned.

Mission Statement

Trauma is locked in the body as "speechless terror"; it is a crisis of mortality, meaning, faith and identity, and emotional stuckness (van der Kolk, 2014). Thus, we need modalities that mobilize life energy, express and channel emotions, and strengthen individual and cross-cultural community resilience and connection. Whole person integrative approaches, such as mindfulness and the creative, expressive, and somatic arts therapies, can help participants with the trauma of emergencies face the terror of death and rekindle life force (Carey, 2006; Lev, 2022). They can decrease compassion fatigue and build caregiver regeneration and resilience (Figley, 2002; Serlin, 2007). As humanistic approaches, they focus on strength building, creativity, posttraumatic growth, and growth through adversity (Calhoun & Tedeschi, 1999; Joseph & Linley, 2006; Serlin, 2012).

Origin Story: Personal Account of How the Group Got Started

Ilene Serlin, psychologist and dance movement therapist, leader of the working group and founder of the Serlin Whole Person Integrative Approach

As I write this chapter, I look back on these past 2 years and cannot believe what a journey it has been. After making the emotional and difficult decision to close down my San Francisco office where for 35 years we had built a close collegial community, I had to find a home for all my dear books and possessions. Switching to Zoom and staying home were both a relief and lonely; I missed my friends and colleagues and 35 years of weekly lunches. Then I was diagnosed with thyroid cancer and had surgery and radiation and more isolation. Then our house was flooded, and we spent 4 months in a hotel. The combination of uprootedness, dislocation and disorientation, and claustrophobia was intense.

One measure of stability was our biweekly Zoom calls with the Task Force and our own Work Group. We cared about each other and exchanged creative ways to deal with Zoom fatigue. The other therapists and leaders I met through those Zoom calls were inspiring and supportive and helped me keep my faith in a world gone somewhat crazy.

How did creativity, the arts, and dance help to deal with the trauma from COVID-19?

I began my career as a folk dancer, starting with a trip to Israel when I was 14, and the country itself, Israel, was also 14, having been founded in 1948. At that time, the hope of building a perfect democracy in Israel, and the call back to the land, was greatly appealing to my urban New York adolescent self. In our folk dances, we symbolically picked grapes from the vines and stomped seeds in the earth. Singing and dancing gave us power for motivation and action. During the years of folk dance with the youth group Habonim ("The Builders") and then international folk dance, I felt the enormous power of the arts and movement of the body to create and sustain culture and community. Many years later, I traced my family history back to a village in the Ukraine where dance was part of our religious/ethnic and personal identity. Also, working for years in psychiatric hospitals with backward nonverbal patients with schizophrenia and later with autistic children, I understood the power of nonverbal communication. While teaching in Israel through Lesley University, I experienced the widespread trauma due to recurrent wars and intifadas (Serlin, 2006). Additionally, working with people in China and the Middle East who had experienced trauma, I further understood the power of movement to help people feel, ground, and integrate themselves, find their identities, and express themselves. When fellow psychologists in APA Charles Figley and Maureen O'Landy put out a call for colleagues to join working groups to help process the trauma of COVID-19, I knew that the arts and body could help people deal with the overwhelming trauma from COVID-19. I had to join.

Since most of the Work Groups at that time were focused mostly on populations or specific issues, our group focused on the use of different approaches. To that end, we attracted and invited other psychologists, artists, and organizations that were using the somatic and creative arts to help heal individuals and communities, locally and globally.

The first member who joined from the Task Force, Rita Rivera, a graduate student, was interested in creativity and immediately helped us create a Facebook page and presence on social media, as well as to collect and curate the enormous amount of material that we began to receive on the arts and healing. The next member to join was my colleague from the China Institute of Psychology, Grace Zhou, with whom I had collaborated on creating videos to be used by counselors on their hotlines, and who was training pastoral counselors to work with rural women who experienced domestic violence and abuse. Then, we were joined by Dr. Eleanor Pardess, an Israeli psychologist with whom I had worked in trauma centers; Dr. Vivien Marcow Speiser, in whose program I first worked with trauma in 1986 through Lesley University in Israel; Larry Graber, a graduate student from Saybrook University, dancer, musician, and trauma psychologist with knowledge of rhythm and the body; and Amy Li, a cancer survivor who invented a technology platform through which people could connect and dance with each other and added her support of technology. Through posts that brought physiology and stress reduction techniques to combat Zoom fatigue and physical decline, Dr. Erik Peper from the San Francisco State Department of Holistic Health coached us to better mind/body health and balance.

Weekly posts on Zoom by Lisa Rasmussen created art breaks throughout the day, and Dr. Patricia Villavicencio, an artistic trauma psychologist from Madrid, helped create tool kits on Instagram and collaborative programs with other Work Groups.

Throughout the pandemic, I kept getting news about arts organizations that were using their platforms to heal trauma. As our group kept meeting, we grew to include representatives of these groups. I learned about the groundbreaking work that Johns Hopkins was doing through its new Center for Applied Neuroaesthetics, to establish a new marriage of science and art for the purpose of healing; thus, its director, Susan Magsamen, became part of our group. I had visited the Arts Medicine program at the University of Florida many years ago as they developed ways to bring the arts into the hospital environment and involve the community and asked the director, Dr. Jill Sonke, to join us. Similarly, I had worked with Ping Ho from the UCLArts & Healing and been impressed with their outreach to the community through the arts, so she joined the group and contributed many resources on arts and healing. Dr. Tony Zhou, from the International Association for Creative Arts in Education and Therapy (IACAET), began to host webinars on the arts and trauma featuring creative arts therapists and educators from around the globe.

Our group met weekly and quickly became a support group for all of us. Like the other Work Groups, we were intergenerational and eager to learn from each other. Often, the sessions would begin with one of us leading the others in a short demonstration of our practice, creating a safe container for us to share our own experiences during the ongoing and seemingly endless COVID-19 pandemic. We gave each other feedback and began to prepare a series of tool kits that could be culturally sensitive and reach diverse groups. We cross-linked with other Work Groups as members shared these approaches with other Task Force members and discovered common areas of passion, desire to serve and heal, and mutual collaboration and support. Many of us experienced our group, and the Task Force, with gratitude as it helped us navigate the frighteningly unknown and destabilizing waves of new challenges and losses.

Finally, I turned to another longtime friend and colleague, Dr. Judy Kuriansky, a well-known media psychologist who is also an expert practitioner who contributed her vast intercultural experiences of using healing arts to work with trauma in every region of the world, including in Africa, Haiti, the Middle East, Japan, China, the Caribbean islands, and even Iran. Given her experience also as an award-winning journalist, she is continuing to help with the editing of this chapter.

An enormous amount of activities ensued.

We reached out to our member organizations for weekly posts to help people cope with lockdowns and the traumas of COVID-19. These included arts-based resources to help parents work with children at home, online concerts and gallery exhibits, experiential exercises to develop resilience and compassion, and news about how lockdowns were impacting the emotional and financial lives of artists and community-based organizations. We created and curated podcasts from committee members that provided nature-based, stress reduction, and creative tool kits. We gathered these resources and grouped them into categories that could be shared and disseminated with other mental health professionals. To share and disseminate the materials, we started a Facebook page and Instagram account, sent regular updates to other professional listservs, wrote articles for professional journals and newsletters, created webinars, were interviewed for podcasts, and presented panels at the American Psychological Association and other international meetings (held online https://www.youtube.com/watch?v=XwcUnMrRDtc&t=67s).

Our members were also interviewed by media, and information was shared in classes for psychology students and on other online platforms. We collaborated with the Work Group on Interpersonal Violence to produce weekly roundtable discussions, bringing themes from our expertise such as compassion fatigue and resilience. These roundtable discussions were broadcast live on Zoom and on two Facebook sites and have been viewed by over 600 people.

Our Work Group focused on healing modalities that can help anyone ameliorate trauma from COVID-19. Our art therapists provided activities for parents to do on Zoom with their children, as well as relaxation exercises for stressed parents and working mothers (Potash et al., 2020). In our collaboration with the Interpersonal Violence Group, we taught somatic skills for assertiveness and to increase self-confidence. Also, we taught mindfulness techniques for front-line responders to help with stabilization and decrease burnout and compassion fatigue (Pardess, 2022). We worked with US, Chinese, Israeli, Spanish, and African colleagues to implement trainings and workshops online and with colleagues who could implement these on the ground and to translate practical skill-building materials into other languages. We also disseminated online examples of choreographies and concerts to address cultural loss and build community resilience. We also integrated music videos into workshops and trainings within multiple online resilience-building webinars, with original healing songs like "Hope is Alive" and others written and performed by Judy Kuriansky and her music partner for their workshops and trainings of populations she describes below in this chapter (Parks et al., 2022).

Objectives of Our Work Going Forward

Through our work together in this group, we compiled practical and experiential resources that can be used on online platforms worldwide to address the impacts of trauma. As most of these resources have not been in one place before, we are preparing a means of accessing these for future crises. In addition, we are continuing to create a series of roundtable presentations as well as written materials and tool kits that will be made available at no cost.

Description and Achievements of the Work Group

The following section of this chapter consists of contributions by members of the group describing their work during the COVID-19 pandemic. These are grouped in four areas, the Arts and Community Healing; Somatic and Mindfulness Approaches;

Resilience; Embodied, Creative Practices: Cultivating Body-Nature Resonance; and the Creative and Expressive Arts Therapies.

Arts and Community Healing

by Ilene Serlin

As has been described above, the arts are a particularly effective way for people who cannot express themselves verbally to find symbolic and embodied expression of their suffering and hopes for the future, bringing individual and community change (Carey, 2006; May, 1975; Serlin, 2012). Expressive arts can cross cultures without language barriers and also be easily disseminated on social media; thus, they are powerful tools available to many people at once, reaching whole communities and underserved populations in diverse settings. During the COVID-19 pandemic, many people turned to the arts for comfort, distraction, and healing. Sales for art supplies, musical instruments, knitting stores, and cooking goods surged as people sought to use their hands and bodies to restore a sense of vitality to what was experienced as a disembodied and shrinking world caused by the pandemic.

In this section, we first cover arts organizations that are members of our Work Group and have been sharing abundant arts-based materials throughout the pandemic. Then, we look at how individuals found art to be a significant coping mechanism during this time. We also look at ways in which nonprofessional artists – not the creative arts therapy associations – used art for inspiration and support for people.

Many arts-based organizations are established centers, but the pandemic also spawned new initiatives as the integration of arts into healthcare is a new field proving to be increasingly useful.

Some of these arts-based organizations include the following:

- The Johns Hopkins International Arts and Mind Lab at the Center for Applied Neuroaesthetics, through Executive Director and committee member Susan Magsamen, offered evidence-based art activities to help individuals and families "find new and joyful ways to cope and feel better during this unpredictable time" (https://www.artsandmindlab.org/covid-19-neuro-arts-field-guide/). NeuroArts is an exciting new interdisciplinary field researching how the arts and aesthetic experiences act on the brain and body. The Lab reached out to working mothers who had to deal with childcare during the COVID-19 pandemic, with programs like: "5 Weekend Art Activities to Bust Quarantine Fatigue," using stories for bedtime to boost children's resilience and empathy. To help deal with overwhelming grief and loss, its programs cited brain research to show that art-making can restore meaning and connection with loved ones and even improve immune functioning. Other specialized evidence-based programs offered support to restless teens. Many programs used music for stress reduction and other goals, for example, a jam session increased motivation and cooperation among healthcare workers. At the conference held in a hybrid model, the Center partnered with Ilene Serlin to co-chair a panel for a presentation called *NeuroArts:*

The New Science of the Arts in Health and Well-Being. Panelists, including representatives from the World Health Organization, the National Institutes of Health, and Save the Children Federation, spoke about research and global perspectives. In a surprise appearance, opera singer Renée Fleming introduced a breathing exercise to help with COVID-19 symptoms which affect the respiratory system. Serlin's presentation included a rationale for why the arts heal and a PowerPoint about the development of the Work Group with interviews of group members describing their own work during the pandemic.

- The University of Florida Center for Arts in Medicine provided a robust and quick response to the challenges of the pandemic with resources including a field guide, an arts response repository, and a webinar reply. The arts played a prominent role in allaying the psychological as well as physical impacts of COVID-19 when their Director of Research, Dr. Jill Sonke, also a member of our Work Group, was asked to be part of the Centers for Disease Control's (CDC) project to help children accept the vaccine (https://arts.ufl.edu/sites/creating-healthy-communities/covid-19-arts-response/overview/). The Center, which has funded US $2.1 million for arts and culture-based projects, focuses on public health as well as individual health with webinars like "The Power of Creativity in Public Health: Incorporating Art into Social Change Advocacy." Their perspective of "Creating Healthy Communities: Arts and Public Health in America" created a framework grounded in a social ecological model that includes mechanisms such as self-efficacy, personal and cultural resonance, aesthetic experience, meaning-making, and self-transcendence. Their goals include direct health benefits, increasing health equity and access, creating safe environments, supporting cultural and social change, enriching methods and practices, and strengthening health communication. Working with teachers, students, and interns, the Center has developed action plans to partner with cultural organizations to grow their evidence-based resources locally, both nationally and internationally.
- The integration of arts into healthcare is a new field that is proving to be increasingly useful, giving birth to many new organizations. Another of our committee members, Ping Ho, founded UCLArts & Healing in 2004 (https://uclartsandhealing.org/about-us/). During the pandemic, they created a free, online series to support the resilience of the global community through "social emotional arts" (https://uclartsandhealing.org). Building on the role of creativity in healing, their mission statement is: "to transform lives through creative expression by integrating the innate benefit of the arts with mental health practices for self-discovery, connection, and empowerment." Their programs feature drum circles, partnership programs with the UCLA Integrative Medicine Collaborative, healing poetry, and reimagining learning in post-COVID-19 schools through a creative arts and community-connection lens. They sponsor annual conferences on Creativity and the Arts in Healing and manage a store with hands-on resources with arts activities for community members. They offer a free, online HOPE (Healing Online for People Everywhere) Series, created at the start of the pandemic to support the resilience of our global community, focusing on relevant topics, such as grief, anxiety, trauma, stress management, resilience, connection,

and social justice. Recorded for later viewing, it continues indefinitely as a free monthly offering: https://uclartsandhealing.org/services/community-services/hope-series/. Free downloadable arts activities on this page, including one on responding to trauma in children, are at https://uclartsandhealing.org/free-downloads/. Training programs and scripted manuals for members of the public who wish to offer more extended support to others can be found at *Beat the Odds: Social and Emotional Skill Building Delivered in a Framework of Drumming*.

- Committee co-chair Ilene Serlin created a series of Zoom links that used imagery and movement to teach people about emotional regulation, self-soothing, and creating safe spaces (https://youtu.be/jjy13XQR3aI). Serlin used the online platform of Zoom to help members from the China Institute in Beijing (CIP) soothe family members who were crowded into one room at the beginning of the pandemic (due to lockdowns) and who faced incidents of emotional and physical abuse. Attached is a link to a video that was used in China and with Asian-Americans in the USA: https://youtu.be/nHuI0CU4ezQ. She and committee member Grace Zhou created a series of culturally appropriate movement episodes that told a story from trauma to resilience (https://youtu.be/yrGduYaQDRE).
- The International Association for Creative Arts in Education and Therapy (IACAET) is another new interdisciplinary and international organization using the arts to promote healing during COVID-19. Founded by Work Group member Dr. Tony-Y Zhou, this association "promotes discourse and the development of creative arts in a wide range of fields including education, therapy, healthcare and wellness, performing arts and other allied professions" (https://www.iacaet.org). With a holistic and humanistic perspective, they organized programs like "Movement as a precious tool for self-care" and "Creating 'ME' Space: Space and the flow of ink." Work Group member Vivien Marcow and co-chair Ilene Serlin joined for an "International Conference on Arts and Trauma: From Deconstruction to Reconstruction" (https://www.iacaet.org/event/webinar-international-conversation-on-arts-and-trauma-icat/). A resource guide is listed that provides courses, workshops, and training programs. Their journal, *Creative Arts in Education and Therapy (CAET) – East, West and Global Perspectives*, is an open access international journal sponsored by IACAET and contains articles relevant to the use of the arts to work with COVID-19.
- ARAS, the center for Research in Archetypal Symbolism, put out daily images from international artists called "Art in a Time of Global Crisis: Interconnection and Companionship." In partnership with the Art and Psyche Working Group, they "represent companionship, resilience and hope in the face of threat, fear and struggle" (https://aras.org/special-feature), as shown in Fig. 8.1.
- Daily online art breaks were sent out by other working group members including Lisa Rasmussen (see https://heartsneedart.org/podcast/) and the Boston Arts Consortium for Health with Marcow Speiser https://www.youtube.com/playlist?list=PLLiyTv4bBycrKzcP8nWZXviRLloel0Vk5.

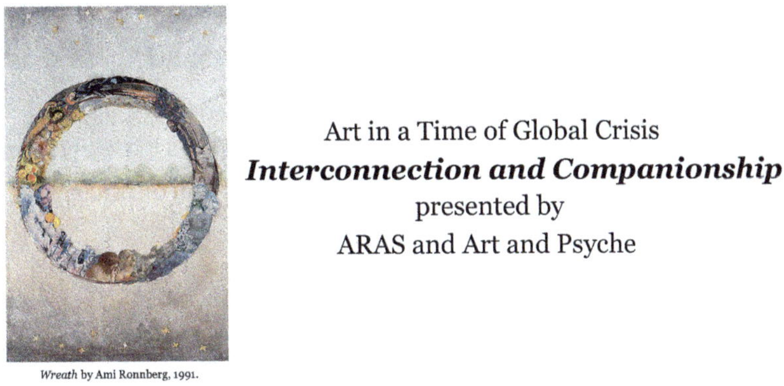

Fig. 8.1 Interconnection and companionship

- Some health professionals and front-line responders, as nurses, used dance to improve resiliency and well-being of staff members (https://www.newsweek.com/nurse-uses-dance-meditation-help-fellow-health-care-workers-cope-during-coronavirus-pandemic-1505068).
- Frontline workers at Unity Health Toronto created a collaborative effort called "The Choreography of Care" in which they connect with each other and with their community (https://youtu.be/kYT-K9FsRMo).
- Psychologists created a special exhibit through the Los Angeles Psychological Association called "Mirrors of the Mind 9: The Psychotherapist as Artist in the time of Coronavirus" (https://www.lacpamirrors.com/#home.html) which gave psychologists an artistic venue to process emotions as COVID-19 caregivers.
- Serlin participated in a panel at the 2021 APA convention on *Exploring Everyday Creativity and Promoting Well-Being: Professionally and Personally* with a PowerPoint on "Crocheting, Crafts and the Problem of Disembodiment during COVID."

Finally, many individual artists contributed their talents to lift the spirits of community members. For example, cellist Yo-Yo Ma gave concerts to soothe anxieties (https://www.boston.com/news/local-news/2021/03/14/after-receiving-his-second-covid-19-shot-yo-yo-ma-staged-an-impromptu-performance-at-mass-clinic/; https://www.youtube.com/watch?v=XqvKDCP5-xE), and opera singers were teaching long-term COVID-19 patients to breathe again (https://edition.cnn.com/2021/07/18/us/therapists-opera-treat-covid-patients/index.html). Cirque du Soleil artists shared their experiences with: QUARANTINE https://www.youtube.com/watch?v=8Cl4yhvmzsk. The world all rocked together to the infectious tune of Jerusalema. Here are Masaka kids dancing in Africa: https://youtu.be/CxM5NnnmZKQ.

Committee members of this group also brought their expertise in art to collaborate with other Work Groups of the Task Force. For example, as described above, they joined the group on Interpersonal Violence to produce a series of weekly roundtables. Some of the arts-based activities included "Cultural Loss and the Use of Traditional Folk Dance to Work with Trauma" and "Creativity." Another member, Dr. Patricia Villavicencio, from Madrid, has worked with children in Uganda and creates games for traumatized children in her own community https://youtu.be/voIHQmSZYBQ. These activities by committee members and in the larger community of artists showed that art became an important tool in the healing of trauma during the pandemic.

Projects by Known Artists

Many individual artists contributed their talents to lift the spirits of community members. For example, cellist Yo-Yo Ma and gave concerts to soothe anxieties (https://www.boston.com/news/local-news/2021/03/14/after-receiving-his-second-covid-19-shot-yo-yo-ma-staged-an-impromptu-performance-at-mass-clinic/; https://www.youtube.com/watch?v=XqvKDCP5-xE), and opera singers were teaching long-term COVID patients to breathe again (https://edition.cnn.com/2021/07/18/us/therapists-opera-treat-covid-patients/index.html). Cirque du Soleil Artists shared their experiences with: QUARANTINE https://www.youtube.com/watch?v=8Cl4yhvmzsk.

Somatic and Mindfulness-Based Interventions

by Lori Gill

Throughout the pandemic the world experienced a global sense of overwhelm and anxiety in constant flux, making it very challenging to maintain balance. This resulted in increased anxiety and depression in individuals of all ages, triggering preexisting underlying trauma experiences, amplifying existing trauma experiences for many people, and creating complex trauma in others (Pressley & Spinazzola, 2020). Key features of trauma include a loss of control, powerlessness, and fear for one's safety. Therapists were also losing their balance and experiencing burnout, physical symptoms, and compassion fatigue. Although many of the COVID-19 circumstances are not within our control, learning to work with controlling what we can (such as our body and mind) are proactive steps we can take toward regaining some semblance of balance.

According to van der Kolk (2014), therapy to achieve change in the stress response pattern is aimed at achieving a balance between the medial prefrontal cortex and the amygdala. Current neuroscience research demonstrates two primary ways of accomplishing this: regulation strategies either from the bottom-up or from the top-down. Top-down regulation involves strengthening self-reflective capacities, increasing the capacity of the medial prefrontal cortex to monitor and appropriately respond to the body's sensations, achieved by awareness training, mindfulness, meditation, and neurofeedback as some key techniques. Bottom-up regulation involves restoring balance to the autonomic nervous system, achieved through learning to regulate physiological reactions through breath, movement, or touch. Since trauma and stress reduce integration of the right and left hemispheres of the brain (Zimmerman & Beaudoin, 2015), the most optimal techniques therefore are integrative, bilaterally stimulating the brain.

Research on compassion fatigue prevention shows that a daily practice is the greatest protective factor. As a result, I encourage you to try some of these practices, notice what works for you, and when and try to find something (or a combination of techniques) you can weave in to a daily practice for your life and work. I invite you to pause and notice your embodied experience (sensations, emotions, shifts), about which you can write, draw, or journal. This action engages the right and the left hemispheres together. It is our hope that this will add more tools to your tool kit, as well as those you support, with the intention of tending to your own healing and promoting wellness. Below is a summary of some techniques and resources our subcommittee has introduced to promote embodied awareness and emotional regulation.

During the Roundtable: Mindfulness Exercises to Practice https://youtu.be/If8o0MYLImY, Hughes spoke about the neuroreceptors built in our brain which are activated without conscious awareness. Working with the vagus nerve by engaging the head, throat, and chest can help brain and nervous system reset and become more grounded. Speakers Dawn Hughes, Erik Peper, and Lori Gill shared various strategies that help accomplish this:

- Singing, toning, humming, and gargling which activates the vagus nerve and tells the brain to refocus while calming the body
- Diaphragmatic breathing with an extended exhale for promoting a sense of calm
- Stretching and intentional movements with the idea of just lovingly moving the body

In another webinar (https://youtu.be/ah-sPEMSDe8), panelists shared strategies for releasing stress and anxiety.

Dr. Michaela Mendelsohn spoke about benefits of movement and exercise (walking, dancing, yoga, running) and utilizing online programs online. Lori Gill shared the "Recognize, Release and Refocus" technique as a tool for shifting affective states:

- *Recognize* – notice what's coming up and acknowledge whether it's an emotion or sensation, press "pause" (symbolically), and just allow those to be there.
- *Release* – release excess energy, tension, sadness, or other feelings through physical discharging/movement (shaking it out, stomping it out, bouncing it out, dancing it out, etc.); through tension-releasing exercises (stretching or bringing awareness to the areas in the body holding the tension or sensations); or through the breath (sighing it out, singing, toning, humming, chanting).
- *Refocus* – once able to reduce the arousal or the intensity of what we are feeling, we are better able to access and utilize higher-order parts of the brain which allow us to see things differently. I invite the use the prompts such as: "Is it true?

Is it real? Is it proportionate? Is this needed here to the same degree now? Especially focus on what is the message you're sending yourself, and what is the message you want to be sending yourself?"

Another panelist, Jamie McHugh, introduced an experiential practice of using the natural world as a way to de-stress by guiding participants through his immersive "7 Days of Beauty" experience (McHugh, 2017). He also provided a prompt of using benevolent touch, taking three breaths and noticing the feedback while considering:

- Am I in a state of distress or eustress?
- Do I just need to take a moment to notice myself, feel myself, and then move on?

He spoke to the power of using our internal implicit resources for cultivating self-nurturance and self-care.

Panelist Ilene Serlin built upon this discussion by noting the heightened need for touch at this time of isolation. In addition to benevolent touch, self-touch can help with grounding and feeling our own presence and existence. She also talked about the need to create safe space and boundaries as a physical enactment. Constricted space accentuates violence, so what to do in a small space if anger is escalating, strengthening boundaries, and saying "no" verbally and nonverbally can bring a sense of security.

Demonstrated activities on the Zoom included:

- Strength – feet on the ground and start with feeling your strength on the ground.
- Tune into the body as great source of information regarding what is happening around you.
- Stay as calm and centered in the face of aggression as possible.
- Centered and balance, pendulating right and left until you find balance again.
- Work with safe space and begin to feel your own bubble.
- Regulate your space and who comes into it and practice close and far.
- Control the boundaries, inviting and pushing away.
- Breathe and fill space with your own self.
- Feel in your body your own voice with authority and strength.

Serlin and McHugh both spoke to the importance of providing our body a day of rest, intentionally unplugging, being present, unfocusing our eyes, and allowing eyes to shift out of overly constricted/focused state. Serlin presented the concept of weaving in the "creation of a healing rhythm in our lives," finding the rhythm between focus and unfocus with intentional shifts such as the following: focus, focus, unfocus; cognitive, cognitive, let it go. She suggested that this healing rhythm in our lives is essential for well-being.

https://youtu.be/ah-sPEMSDe8

In another roundtable, Dr. Eleanor Criswell presented about the use of "Somatics for Humans and Other Animals" describing how powerful animals can be for bringing about a sense of relaxation and unconditional positive regard. However, if animals are unwell or stressed, dysregulation can also be experienced vicariously through them. Therefore, she likes to work with humans and their companion animals to promote conjoint regulation and healing. She also spoke to the process of "pandiculation," by which animals naturally take care of themselves somatically to shift their affective states. Since we, too, are embodied beings, we could all benefit from learning how to do this. See https://youtu.be/mrvCoiEsej0.

Several Work Group members presented at our center's Attachment and Trauma Treatment Centre for Healing's Spring Trauma and Attachment Conference (Gill, 2015). Focusing on embodied practices, Dr. Erik Peper shared tips and resources for reducing and preventing Zoom fatigue and expanded upon in his book, *Tech Stress: How Technology is Hijacking Our Lives, Strategies for Coping, and Pragmatic Ergonomics* (2020). Practical resources we can implement into our day-to-day lifestyle include a stretch break every 15 minutes and using a standing desk and a wedge posture correction cushion. A useful exercise is shifting eye movements to the upper left, right, lower right, and lower left, with mini breaks to gaze off into the periphery – given that our eyes are designed to view distances and the hyper and confined focusing of Zoom places strain on our eyes.

In his workshop, "Inhabiting Ourselves: Embodying Mindfulness and Somatic Self-Care," Jamie McHugh guided us through nourishing and regulating embodied practice activities (see http://somaticexpression.com) including softening the lips and periodically exhaling through the mouth. A soft exhale or sigh can release pressure and reset the nervous system.

Ilene Serlin's workshop on "Trauma-Informed Dance Movement Therapy" engaged participants in spontaneous, playful, and rhythmic movement of the body.

In another webinar in the conference, Lori Gill shared core strategies of our foundational trauma training for the Integrative Trauma and Attachment Treatment Model (ITATM) and provided resources for shifting affective states using mindfulness or somatic resources. Keeping in mind that a moment is all it takes to create a shift, weaving in little shifts that help broaden our window of tolerance can be valuable following trauma and from a compassion fatigue prevention perspective. For more examples, please see https://www.facebook.com/56300169/videos/10101451944583774/, #COVIDIPV #creatingasenseofcalm #broadeningourwindowoftolerence #sensoryresources #windowoftolerence #ATTCH #traumainformed #healingtrauma #attachment, https://youtu.be/ah-sPEMSDe8.

Resilience

by Judy Kuriansky

Resilience is a critical concept in trauma recovery (Nugent et al., 2014) with extensive research and commentaries on the definition, populations who suffer, policy, and applied programs. This section gives an overview of resilience and techniques the section author has used during the COVID-19 period that use somatic and creative arts approaches.

The most common definition of resilience is the ability to "bounce back" after a trauma. According to the American Psychological Association (n.d., 2020), resilience is "the process and outcome of successfully adapting to difficult or challenging life experiences [in the face of adversity, trauma, tragedy, threats, or significant sources of stress] especially through mental, emotional, and behavioral flexibility and adjustment to external and internal demands." This skill can be innate or learned. Factors affecting this adaptation to adversities include personal capacities and coping strategies and available resources.

The approaches described in this chapter and in other chapters throughout this book can all be said to address resilience. The techniques in this section were used in trainings and workshops using expressive arts techniques applied by group member Dr. Judy Kuriansky. These techniques have been extensively applied in interventions around the world worldwide related to other traumas, including natural disasters (e.g., earthquakes, tsunamis, floods, in Haiti, China, Japan, Iran, the USA) and epidemics (HIV, SARS, Ebola, and now COVID-19) (Kuriansky, 2019). They align with the Serlin Whole Person approach (2019) in that they engage cognitive, emotional, and consciousness realms. Also, participants have "fun," which relieves stress from the trauma and facilitates personal growth (Hernik & Jaworska, 2018). While trauma leads to posttraumatic stress, an outcome of these Whole Person-related interventions is the opposite, namely, posttraumatic growth (Calhoun & Tedeschi, 2006) as shown by participants' self-reports.

The toolbox of techniques used here involving expressive arts has been developed over years (Kuriansky, 2008; Kuriansky et al., 2016). These include the "Resilience Ball" (bouncing a ball so hard that it bounces back higher, as a metaphor for recovery and growth from trauma); "My dream" (throwing the ball in the air while announcing one's ambition for the future, to metaphorically experience hope); and the finger lock (interlocking fingers as if glued together to represent personal strength). When paper and colored markers are available, participants sketch a bridge between drawings of a traumatic and a happy experience to show ability to make that transition. A cultural song and dance begins and ends the workshop. Examples included the following.

Democratic Republic of the Congo (DRC) In response to preventing the spread of COVID-19 in a remote African village, a community-based model was implemented consisting of holistic health education, psychosocial support, and myth correction. Women were hired to sew masks, hand-washing stations were installed, and villagers were taught health behaviors (mask wearing, hand-washing, physical distancing) and psychosocial activities (for strength, resilience empowerment, helping, and social connection) (Kuriansky et al., 2022). A unique arts-based feature of the program was originally designed infographics, which visually display healthy physical and psychosocial activities (figures dancing together, breathing in and out, clenching fists for strength). Made in English as well as the local Swahili language, these were distributed widely and posted on walls and fences throughout the village.

Nepal A multistage multistakeholder partnership, also addressing the United Nations global goals, included five webinars on resilience building held over the course of a year and a half during COVID-19 (Khanal & Kuriansky, 2022). Each webinar brought together government, civil society, media, and youth, to shape policy and promote programs to keep the community safe. In each phase, my presentation was not only didactic – teaching about trauma, coping steps to take, and the experience of posttraumatic growth – but also experiential with adaptations of the toolbox techniques both demonstrated and enacted with the registrants and fellow (e.g., like smiling and noting it is impossible for others to not smile back). A phase included a skills-building workshop for staff of a local psychosocial counseling project.

Sierra Leone Communities in this West African developing country faced double trauma when efforts to stave off the COVID-19 pandemic were complicated by an explosion of a tanker leaving hundreds of people dead or burned. In in-person workshops in the country with survivors and their families, I was able to use interactive arts-based activities like tossing yarns to experience interconnectedness and holding pens while circling, sensing community. cohesion.

"Conversations for Change: COVID-19 What's Next?" Day-Long Workshop This day-long workshop during COVID-19 included dance performances acted out on the web platform inviting others to dance in place but experience togetherness. Experiential modules (mediation, movement, expressive writing) (Pennebaker & Evans, 2014) addressed care for oneself and the planet (permaculture, tips for not wasting food) and, again, the United Nations global goals (with lessons of permaculture related to food security).

Chinese Peer Counselor Training for Self-Care and Support Techniques A training for youth volunteering support for other youth involved similar expressive arts activities; participants reported increasing their confidence and ability to help themselves and others during the stress of COVID-19.

China Teacher Training During the pandemic, when returning home to China over a school break, a Chinese student of mine carried out a workshop with selected of my arts-based toolbox techniques with a group of teachers in her hometown, with the teachers reporting great enthusiasm and value in the experience for themselves and their young students.

Resilience Training Two students hosted a webinar on "Our Post-Pandemic Future: The Importance of Cultivating Resilience and Identifying the Key Factors that impact Global & Personal Perceptions of Happiness" including guiding attendees in a mediation, selections from my toolbox techniques, and a guest presentation by the former Ambassador of Iraq to the UN who founded the International Day of Happiness.

Music Videos Given the value of music in healing is extensively documented, two particular songs were played during the webinars and events which align with the themes of love and hope essential for recovery from COVID-19: "One Love" by an African musician and "Hope Is Alive," written by myself and music partner Russell Daisey. To engage experiential elements during online experiences, attendees were invited to fill in activities for stanzas that can be collectively carried out (jump together, wiggle together, hug one another).

Posttraumatic Growth (PTG)

Self-report ratings were made by participants on a scale of "1" (not at all) to "10" (a great deal) for items in questionnaires related to feeling resilient and to PTG and the related experience of "silver linings." In one survey, the mean self-report score of a group of graduate students was high on all three dimensions, respectively, 8.28, 7.7, and 8.25. (Feeling resilient was clarified as "strong" "facing problems and making the best of it," "enduring"). PTG answers revealed self-growth (self-reflection, "doing what I need") and pleasurable activities ("creative time," cleaning clutter, valuing people over celebrity). Similarly, silver linings were self-growth (having time for enjoyable activities, relaxing, mediating reading, cooking, time in nature), enriched relationships (quality time with family and friends), and renewed value on life. Responses during presentations noted above reflected similar themes.

Cultural Competence While culturally sensitivity is always essential, using expressive arts in these interventions that are basically nonverbal suggests their value across diverse cultures as well as viability of replicating these by facilitators of various backgrounds. The universality of the techniques is also noted (Kuriansky, 2019).

Format Certain interactive arts-based techniques are only possible in-person (e.g., tossing different colored yarns to indicate social/community connection), while others can be guided on the online format (deep breathing for "grounding" or smiling into the computer camera to others to unleash pleasurable brain chemicals and emotions).

Technology and the Hybrid Approach

Given restrictions on in-person contact during COVID-19, interventions required pivoting and developing innovations using technological tools, which is itself an art requiring creativity. However, since social contact is shown by research to be crucial in coping with trauma, a hybrid approach has been necessary, combining technological aids with interpersonal activity. Such adaptations – in the growing field of e-mental health – involve many apps, effigies that "communicate," and methodologies like artificial intelligence, virtual reality, and mixed reality which capture interactive in expressive arts innovations (Kuriansky & Kakkattil, 2022) (Fig. 8.2).

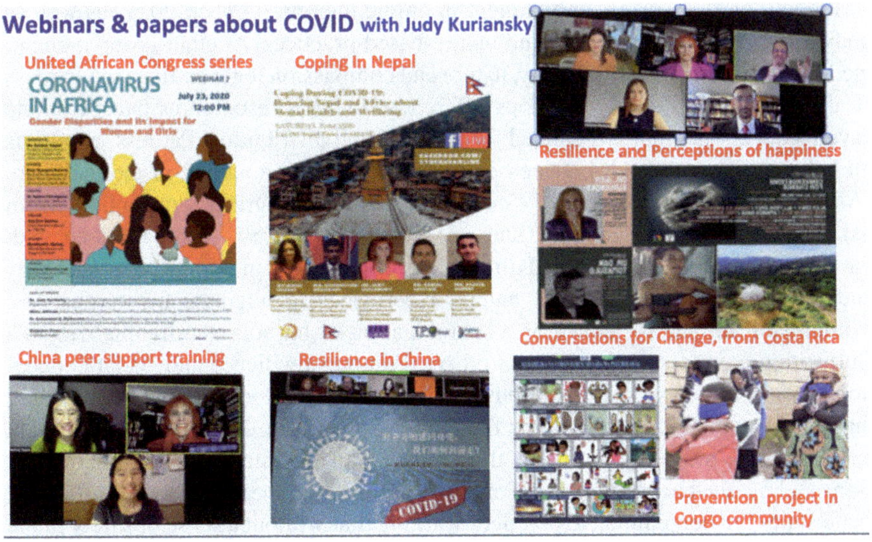

Fig. 8.2 Webinars and papers about COVID with Judy Kuriansky

Embodied, Creative Practices: Cultivating Body-Nature Resonance

by Larry Graber

Nature provides endless opportunities to learn about the cycles of change, life and death, as well as about processes of regeneration. Trauma-related stress is an embodied, relational experience that can impair our ability to build safe relationships with ourselves and others (Porges, 2021). The body's response to trauma is outside conscious control and therefore benefits from body- and arts-based interventions that improve emotional and autonomic balance (van der Kolk, 2014). My professional focus integrates bodily and relational aspects of traumatization with arts and indigenous practices (Graber, 2016, 2017). As a body psychotherapist and trauma specialist, I was invited to join the International Whole Person Work Group to help mobilize online body- and arts-based resources as outreach to the healthcare community. Our Work Group also provided valuable peer support, adding an inoculation against compassion fatigue and vicarious traumatization. The group experience was especially rewarding for its interdisciplinary, international collaboration. I initially served as representative from the Society for Humanistic Psychology of the American Psychological Association to disseminate resources from an existential-humanistic perspective (Bentley, 2022; Frank, 2020; Hoffman, 2021). Humanistic psychology (HP) is a broad human science discipline concerned with core human experiences of creativity, love, relationship, intimacy, spirituality, and existential conditions, such as isolation, connectedness, choice, death, and meaning (Schneider et al., 2015; Serlin & Cannon, 2004). HP advocates a growth-oriented approach to trauma (Serlin et al., 2019), the red thread throughout our Work Group endeavors.

I taught workshops on embodiment in online therapy (Graber, 2021) as well as body, rhythm, imagery, poetry, and nature-based practices. Another group member facilitated workshops on creativity, nature and compassion regeneration (see Pardess et al., 2014). Her Zoom workshops offered an integral resource as part of online psychoeducational tool kits created for international distribution. Pardess' emphasis on balancing compassion between oneself and others is codified in the acronym, "ABCs": *Awareness, Balance, Connection*, which integrates "metaphors from nature, compassionate imagery, and mindfulness practices". I collaborated with Pardess extensively on embodied dimensions of creativity in trauma psychotherapy and led online guided imagery nature experiences to augment her workshops. Compassion fatigue is defined as a "combination of burnout and traumatization". Cultivating compassion for self and others promotes resilience and social connection as an antidote to emotional-physical burnout from lockdowns and recycling threats (Ali et al., 2021; Neff, 2011; Pressley & Spinazzola, 2020). Establishing safe environments, including bodily, is the fundamental first step in Pardess' compassion- and nature-based approach. Porges (2020) echoed the necessity for affirming "safe states" in contemplative practices warning that without a sense of safety in the body (Lakoff & Johnson, 1999) such practices can be counterproductive. Self-compassion also instills a sense of common humanity, the recognition that a person's struggles are part of a larger human experience, reducing a sense of isolation (Neff, 2011). Nature experiences helped to overcome social isolation during the pandemic and instill a sense of wholeness and calm. Compassion fatigue and burnout for healthcare workers have been seriously compromised during COVID-19 who suffer from exposure to a high level of suffering in an overwhelmed healthcare system (Serlin et al., 2013) and from the field of moral injury. Compassion fatigue (Figley, 2002) is an embodied experience, so the expressive arts can promote resilience, generate innovative responses, and enhance compassion satisfaction during pandemics. Existential and humanistic approaches, such as clinical hospitality and existential encounters, can enhance posttraumatic growth and growth through adversity (Joseph & Linley, 2006; Kurter et al., 2016).

Nature's experiential imagery-metaphors imbue cognitive learning (Lakoff & Johnson, 1999) creating embodied templates for healing relationships. For example, the root systems of trees form an elaborate underground fungal network of communication facilitated by chemicals similar to human neurotransmitters (Simard, 2021). Trees transmit intergenerational, inter-tree "wisdom," via these unseen bonds. The implications for human resilience are manifold and may be a reason why nature excursions are associated with health benefits (Hansen et al., 2017; Stier-Jarmer et al., 2021). Pardess (2022) and Pardess et al. (2014) also use poem-making to help integrate nature metaphors with workshop participants' experiences into new healing narratives. Another workgroup member, Jamie McHugh (2017), is a somatic movement therapist and photographer, who created online, contemplative poetry/photo journeys, which help viewers become aware of their embodied connections to nature and themselves.

Expressive writing, such as poetry, has consistently demonstrated physical and mental health benefits (Pennebaker & Evans, 2014). Carroll (2005) notes, "people are frequently moved to write a poem in times of extremity" (p. 161). Gratier and Trevarthen (2008) further emphasize, "poetic stories link many minds in imagined space and time" (p. 124). I developed *Dialogical Poetry™* as a therapeutic tool to give voice to ineffable aspects of traumatization and build empathic resonance in dyads and groups (Graber & Rosemond, 2015). The technique combines poetry writing and creative mythmaking, employing mythical characters and nature symbols in a call-and-response format. With an emphasis on felt experiences, Dialogical Poetry™ bridges the nonverbal and verbal. Anderson (2001) states, "when embodied writing is attuned to the physical senses, it becomes … a path of transformation that nourishes an enlivened sense of presence in and of the world" (p. 83). Poetry dialogues can be facilitated over videoconferencing, phone text, or in-person and thus are a highly versatile method for constructing healing conversations that can be safely embodied and trauma-informed (Zimmerman & Beaudoin, 2015).

My own approach to body and art-based psychotherapy for PTSD was enhanced when Hattie Worboys, a professional dancer and mixed-media movement educator, joined our Work Group in 2021. Worboys' creative teaching style that combines movement and interactive video with children internationally suggested a broad range of mental health and wellness applications in the emerging COVID-19 world. Our collaborative work is aimed at fostering emotional, physical, and social benefits for children and developing dance school curriculum, as well as art-based research on the lived experiences of children and families during COVID-19 and beyond.

Body Talks Movement: Dance as a Restorative Bridge for Children During COVID-19

by Hattie Worboys

"How Body Talks Movement" is an international dance/film program for children that adapted to participants' needs during the pandemic. This section suggests ways it can be developed into the future.

My name is Hattie Worboys. I am an artist, educator, and Director/Founder of Body Talks Movement (BTM). Founded in 2015, BTM is an international participatory dance program that harnesses the healing potential of movement, sound, film, and virtual communication and is designed to reveal the restorative power of movement and the fundamental human need to dance and connect. BTM serves and connects children from mostly disadvantaged communities in the UK and around the world, through an evolving curriculum consisting of dance and video workshops. We aim to empower and give voice to those who feel unheard and marginalized. Dance has been a communal way of honoring the fundamental forces inside us and a form of ritual expression and social bonding for millennia. See: http://hattieworboys.com/.

BTM 2015–2019

After an initial dance exchange between two groups of children in London and New Orleans in 2015, BTM expanded, partnering with local organizations to include children from economically deprived communities in Mumbai, Brazil, Lesvos, Zimbabwe, and Egypt. It became evident that children participating in the workshops were further connecting to their emotions through movement exploration and experiencing deeper body awareness. They were increasing their personal movement vocabulary and becoming further attuned with each other as they danced together.

While working internationally with children living through challenging situations, the program revealed its potential to benefit neurodiverse children and those who had lived through trauma. I found the program helped these children become calmer, more focused, and more confident to express themselves. It allowed them to feel less isolated and develop deeper connections with their peers within their community and others beyond their normal horizons in a creative, nonverbal, and intercultural way. As the children developed an awareness of the "voice" inside their bodies, they seemed to feel recognized, valued, and included in the collaborative creative process. I became interested in collaborating with mental health professionals to explore these benefits further and integrate trauma-informed practices into the program.

BTM Just Before the Pandemic 2019/2020

In the months leading up to the pandemic, I was running a research project of BTM with children in two East London primary schools. Having always run the workshops and film shoots myself, I was in the early stages of developing an inclusive BTM curriculum so that other teachers could run the program to facilitate a wider reach and longer-term benefits for the participants. It was clear that I needed to find a way of identifying and articulating the effective elements that had benefited the participating children to date. I started to make extensive notes after each workshop and gather drawn and written feedback from the participants. Then the real-life workshops had to stop in lockdown.

While researching collaborations between psychology and dance, I was introduced to Dr. Ilene Serlin by Dr. Paula Thomson, a choreographer and psychologist. Dr. Serlin invited me to be part of the International Whole Person Approaches Work Group. Right away, the relevance of my work was recognized, and we started exploring ways to integrate my work with other Work Group projects. It was here that I met Larry Graber, with whom I have been working closely to develop the trauma aware and healing aspects of the program and assemble the BTM program into a more systematic format.

During Lockdown: How BTM Adapted for the Pandemic

During the lockdown I chose to run small workshops with children to increase the intimacy and provide more attention and space to communicate through movement. The format offered a safe space for children to express themselves, to play, and to hear each other. Even though the classes were virtual, the children were able to make connections from their individual homes. These classes contrasted with larger online classes/options by providing more personal attention and space to make meaningful connections. In some cases, children who had previously been intimidated by classmates in live classes felt more at ease to explore their movements and express themselves.

Many children, particularly from lower socioeconomic groups, suffered acute isolation, the feeling of being unheard, a lack of physical activity, an increase in anxiety, and loss of confidence and their desire to socialize. BTM provided participants with an opportunity to connect and express themselves through freestyle movement and video in a more fluid and uninhibited way from their homes. This increases their social connection, personal and interpersonal attunement, and sense of belonging and enhances their confidence in communication skills.

BTM had been connecting children from long-distance locations through movement and video since 2015. Therefore, the global lockdown provided an opportunity to further explore how we can learn to play creatively and communicate virtually in an embodied way through the 2D rectangle of the screen. This opportunity became part of a deeper enquiry into the mental and physical health benefits of explorative movement, attunement, and connection through screens/virtual communication in pandemic. It also was an opportunity to look at the potential of how community can be created through movement and screens (including virtual communication).

Through establishing a safe and permissive space to explore, accept, and even celebrate our own unique qualities through movement, we can then accept and celebrate others' unique qualities, similarities, and differences. Through this, we can discover our universality, form communities, and develop respect for ourselves and each other. Connecting with and really listening to ourselves and others both near and far away from us are life affirming and give meaning. We will continue to develop the potential for these benefits in the BTM program and be flexible and prepared for future pandemic situations.

Future Development

We will bring more movement into the lives of children in the community and school systems. It is also an opportunity to implement community bonding practices and good psychological intentions. BTM will continue to focus on specific issues such as growing polarization between different cultural groups, disintegration of pre-pandemic community structures, and our growing disconnection from

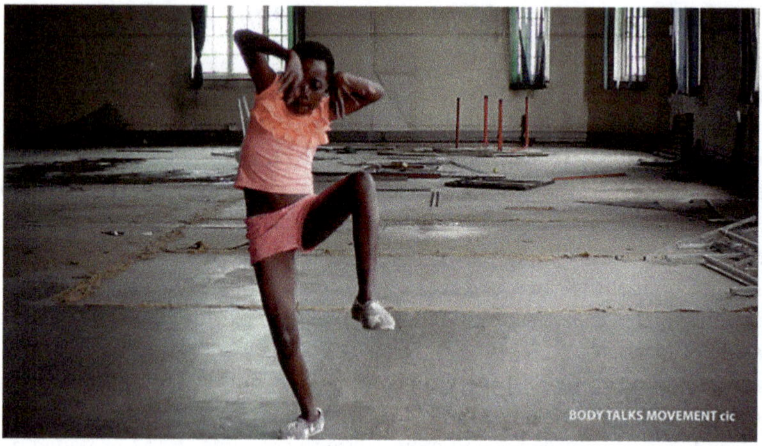

Fig. 8.3 Body Talks Movement

the body's inherent wisdom and healing potential. As we have seen the potential of BTM to lessen our global and inherent tendency of "othering" which became particularly exaggerated in the pandemic, the program will continue to develop methods to build trust in "the other" by providing a space for shared humanity and a more compassionate world view. BTM provides an opportunity to create a global community in pandemic situations that can exist because of the universality of movement. It brings people's very personal experience onto a global platform and highlights our shared suffering, resilience, and "oneness."

In the upcoming months, a team of myself, Larry Graber and Dr. Terry Sweeting, will be working on curriculum development, creating a BTM manual to strengthen resilience and be prepared to respond better in potential future pandemics. Next year, we will run a pilot of the curriculum with a group of children from a traveler community in Somerset, UK, and a group of primarily Bangladeshi children in Newham, London. We'll be exploring how virtual communication through movement and video can create a sense of community and increase well-being. We'll learn more about how it can increase our awareness and sensitivity to our bodies, allowing a more significant connection to ourselves and others and the surrounding environment. We will know how this can translate through screens. BTM will continue to be more flexible and adaptive to meet the needs of children on the frontier of the new COVID-19 world (Fig. 8.3).

Creative and Expressive Arts Therapies

by Ilene Serlin

Creative and expressive arts therapies have many dimensions in common with the healing power of arts in the community and arts medicine. In the arts and community and in arts medicine, practitioners are either medical personnel, community activists, or artists. The creative and expressive arts therapies, on the other hand, are professional organizations with levels of training, supervision, professional ethics, and degrees at the master's level or above. The creative therapies are the oldest, beginning with music therapy that aided brain-damaged soldiers after the war. The therapies include art, music, dance, poetry, psychodrama, and drama. They have separate professional organizations each with its levels of credentialing. For example, I am a BC-DMT, meaning a Board-Certified Dance Movement Therapist. That is equivalent to a BC-RMT, or a Board-Certified Music Therapist. A DMT is a Dance Movement Therapist, equivalent to an RMT, or a music therapist. Dance therapists need at least a master's level of systematic training, plus an internship of about 3000 hours, plus an exam. After receiving the DMT, the student can then go on to apply for the BC-DMT. All the creative arts therapy organizations are working to standardize levels of expertise and professional responsibility. Many creative arts therapists practice as primary therapists and are trained in individual and group therapy. While they have separate professions, they collaborate under the umbrella Creative Arts Therapies Association that also has conferences and collaborations (https://www.nccata.org/). The Expressive Therapies, on the other hand, use the arts in an intermodal way, tracking images and emotions with color, sound, and movement, whatever moves the meaning forward. There is a national and an international association of expressive arts therapists. A growing number are now being trained in trauma-informed work and are supporting relief efforts during COVID-19.

My first challenge came when some psychologists who I supervise through Zoom in China came to sessions with increasing stories of clients experiencing domestic violence. At the beginning of the COVID-19 pandemic, sometimes whole families were quarantined in one room. Tempers flared and emotions were uncontained. So I developed a Zoom video that helped people understand and build inner strength to cope (https://youtu.be/nHuI0CU4ezQ). It involved creating a framework of understanding, grounding in the body and finding inner balance, beginning to explore and expand to the space around the body, feeling and setting boundaries, and creating a safe space. Within that space the person can find ways to both relax and stretch, relieving some of the congestion of quarantine. Moving can feel risky, so the maintenance of a sense of boundaries, control over the boundaries, and balance is essential. With trust, the movement can connect with someone else and become a dialogue.

Because of the great distances, many of the therapists were already using Zoom, and people often used their cell phones to watch videos or talk with their therapists. Hotlines were established through the government and universities so we could put these videos about self-care through movement on those hotlines and reach many people. The China Institute of Psychology asked me to represent them in an International Psychological Forum, and I shared a PowerPoint called Dance Movement Therapy as an Intervention to Work with COVID-19 on May 7, 2021.

Another example is during the time when I was working with the Work Group on Clinician Support Collaborative; one member got a call through a psychoanalytic group in India who needed support during their most critical period of the pandemic. I was one of the ones who offered support, and mine was in asking them to bring their favorite music, slow and fast. We began slowly as they talked of grief. But as the music escalated into traditional Indian rhythms, they grew more energetic and even smiled, more able to face their days.

When I described this experience to my Chinese trainees, they wanted to help. They spontaneously met as a group under the leadership of my assistant Grace Zhou and created their own song and movements that express "From our heart to yours…you are not alone…." https://youtu.be/dpa3mGI5w8Y.

This was an example of how the language of movement is both universal and yet also culturally sensitive. We can cross cultures with simple movements of greeting and support.

What does it mean to be culturally sensitive when working in a different culture? It means not to either try to appropriate or disrespect the other culture. It means approaching with an attitude of what committee member Dr. Eleanor Pardess calls clinical hospitality (Pardess et al., 2014) and cultural humility.

The necessary use of Zoom raises many problematic issues about the lack of embodiment, but it does force attention to the need for the need for tool kits that help people learn simple movements to express grief and move through to recovery. I am involved now with several projects that hope to bring dance into healing tool kits that can be culturally sensitive as well as empowering.

Challenges Faced and Lessons Learned

The arts and experiential trainings play a crucial role in maintaining individual and community health. These interventions can be inexpensive and available to most people and organizations while providing powerful, evidence-based creative solutions to trauma. The pandemic unleashed wellsprings of creative output on social media that were able to help people express emotions and connect across homes and countries during lockdown. Young people today are also unable to either afford therapy or prefer social media, so the genie is out of the box. We look forward to building on these creative new forms of communication for the future.

Authors Note We have no known conflicts of interest to disclose.

Appendices

Art in Communities

Californians for the arts news resources	https://www.californiansforthearts.org/news-resources
Yerba Buena Center for the Arts	https://ybca.org/calendar/
Integrated Care for the Traumatized: A Whole Person Approach by I.A. Serlin, S. Krippner, & K. Rockefeller, Eds., Reviewed by Andrew M. Bland	https://www.millersville.edu/psychology/files/bland/blandtrauma.pdf
Review of *Whole Person Healthcare by Ilene Serlin* by Ed Lundeen	https://www.ileneserlin.com/wp-content/uploads/2022/05/Book-review-Whole-Person-Healthcare.jpg
Art in a Time of Global Crisis: Interconnection and Companionship by ARAS and the Art and Psyche Working Group	https://aras.org/special-feature
The awe of being alive	https://aeon.co/essays/to-feel-the-awe-of-living-learn-to-live-with-terror-and-wonder
Daria Abreu Feraud from Cuba joins Sharon in Mexico for a Concert on Facebook	facebook.com/sharon.katz.2000
Creating Healthy Communities: Arts + Public Health in America, COVID-19 Arts Response Overview	https://arts.ufl.edu/sites/creating-healthy-communities/covid-19-arts-response/arts-covid-19-response/
COVID-19 NeuroArts Field Guide	https://www.artsandmindlab.org/covid-19-neuro-arts-field-guide/
Worried About Closed Schools and Learning Loss? The Arts Can Help	https://www.artsandmindlab.org/worried-about-closed-schools-and-learning-loss-the-arts-can-help/
"One Day" sung in Arabic, Hebrew and English, Haifa, February 14, 2018	https://www.youtube.com/watch?v=XqvKDCP5-xE
Spiegel im Spiegel for Cello and Piano (Arvo Pärt)	https://www.youtube.com/watch?v=FZe3mXlnfNc
Boston Arts Consortium for Health, May 1, 2020	https://www.youtube.com/playlist?list=PLLiyTv4bBycrKzcP8nWZXviRLloel0Vk5
One Day in Jordan, Ilene Serlin, PhD	https://www.youtube.com/watch?v=7XlVetyP70U
Kensington and Chelsea Music Society: A musical message, May 2020	https://youtu.be/VeHQZ1yuT_s
Hotline for Mandarin Speakers	https://drive.google.com/drive/folders/1bULPROoBMUqST_35BYJFdFEDS2_1zWyu
COVID-19 Phone Call by Dr. Ani Kalayjian	https://www.youtube.com/watch?v=oRekOIeSZ34
What Comes After the Global Pandemic? An Emotional, Ecological and Spiritual Transformation by Dr. Ani Kalayjian	

Everybody Must Stay Home – Bob Dylan Coronavirus Parody	https://youtu.be/ErFN7Y7qnLg
Quarantine: Through The Eyes of Cirque du Soleil Artists	https://www.youtube.com/watch?v=8Cl4yhvmzsk
How to Engage the Arts to Build COVID-19 Vaccine Confidence	https://www.cdc.gov/vaccines/covid-19/vaccinate-with-confidence/art.html
Creative Approaches to COVID-19 Vaccination to Unite the Arts and Sciences	https://www.cdc.gov/vaccines/covid-19/vaccinate-with-confidence/art.html
Center for Arts in Medicine COVID resources	https://arts.ufl.edu/sites/creating-healthy-communities/covid-19-arts-response/arts-covid-19-response/
NeuroArts Blueprint: Advancing the Science of Arts, Health, and Wellbeing	https://www.artsandmindlab.org/resource/neuroarts-blueprint-advancing-the-science-of-arts-health-and-wellbeing/
Mirrors of the Mind 9: The Psychotherapist as Artist in the time of Coronavirus	https://www.lacpamirrors.com/#home.html
Mirrors Gallery Books	https://www.lacpamirrors.com/#about/about_books.html
After receiving his second COVID-19 shot, Yo-Yo Ma staged an impromptu performance at Mass. clinic	https://www.boston.com/news/local-news/2021/03/14/after-receiving-his-second-covid-19-shot-yo-yo-ma-staged-an-impromptu-performance-at-mass-clinic
Hear Me Roar	https://www.bchcreativearts.org/blog/hear-me-roar
What Happens in the Brain When People Make Music Together?	https://neurosciencenews.com/music-collaberation-brain-18607/
International Arts + Mind Lab	https://www.artsandmindlab.org/?mc_cid=cee506ec94&mc_eid=43b3112353
Opera singers are teaching long-term Covid-19 patients to breathe again	https://www.cnn.com/2021/07/18/us/therapists-opera-treat-covid-patients/index.html
Art is Moving: Joy's Story	http://artismoving.org/stories/joy/
Center for Arts in Health newsletter, July 2021	https://mailchi.mp/arts.ufl.edu/newsletterjuly2021-8022846?e=b2c7b8707a
Art is Moving: Take an Art Break!	http://artismoving.org
Creating Healthy Communities: Arts + Public Health in America	https://arts.ufl.edu/sites/creating-healthy-communities/resources/arts-public-health-core-outcomes-set-briefing-paper
Creating Healthy Communities 2022	https://arts.ufl.edu/sites/creating-healthy-communities/collaboration/2022-convening/
Art & Covid-19 Repository	https://response.arts.ufl.edu/art-and-covid-19-repository
The Role of the Performing Arts in Improving and Maintaining our Well-being during & post-COVID Pandemic	https://drive.google.com/file/d/1y4ngU7ju5ZFzS8ypTmNLVDj8B0aMR2Hd/view?usp=sharing link to pdf

Generating youth dialogue through the literary arts: A citywide youth health collaboration in the U.S.	https://drive.google.com/file/d/1PPrZinVvnQ0dVkzoWAEKRqRxmN1yjSTf/view?usp=sharing
The Choreography of Care	https://youtu.be/kYT-K9FsRMo
University of Florida Center for the Arts in Medicine: Engaging Arts & Culture for COVID-19 Vaccine Confidence	https://www.vaccinate.arts.ufl.edu
University of Florida Center for the Arts in Medicine: Creating Healthy Communities	https://arts.ufl.edu/sites/creating-healthy-communities/resources/arts-public-health-core-outcomes-set-briefing-paper/
University of Florida Center for the Arts in Medicine: Arts + Public Health Response	https://response.arts.ufl.edu
Masaka Kids Africana Dancing to Jerusalema	https://www.youtube.com/watch?v=TH4V-yHbJXk
Promote Solidarity and a Culture of Peace to Combat Stigma and Conflict during the Pandemic Recovery	https://drive.google.com/file/d/1Ia2SVtP447mmaxvrmEHyM8glQg_bzXLY/view?usp=sharing
Creating Healthy Communities 2022	https://arts.ufl.edu/sites/creating-healthy-communities/collaboration/2022-convening/
Engaging Arts & Culture for Covid-19 Vaccine Confidence: Arts Response Repository and Field Guides	https://www.vaccinate.arts.ufl.edu
Arts for the Health of It, presented by Hearts Need Art	https://heartsneedart.org/podcast
Los Angeles County Psychological Association, Mirrors of the Mind: The Psychotherapist as Artist (3 volumes)	https://app.thebookpatch.com/BookStoreResults?search=Mirrors%20of%20the%20mind
Ilene Serlin and Grace Zhou, Heart Dance, a COVID Cross-cultural Dialogue	https://www.youtube.com/watch?v=yrGduYaQDRE
Ecological Consciousness During Times of Global Pandemic	https://youtu.be/aC8XQ2Z_YGE
Dr. Ani Kalayjian's Poetry Series: Please Call God	https://www.youtube.com/watch?v=LJdxy8VF1Mo
Dr. Ani Kalayjian's Poetry Series: Love Will Prevail	https://www.youtube.com/watch?v=406kaBbCqZo
Dr. Ani Kalayjian's Poetry Series: The Other Side of Love	https://www.youtube.com/watch?v=cvz4qz7JTDs
Dr. Ani Kalayjian's Poetry Series: Let Love Transform You	https://www.youtube.com/watch?v=AiAWuCxeORE
Dr. Ani Kalayjian's Poetry Series: COVID-19 Phone Call	https://www.youtube.com/watch?v=oRekOIeSZ34
Serlin, I. (2022). Dance movement therapy: Crossing cultural and professional bridges. *Body, Movement and Dance in Psychotherapy, 18*(1), 75–85.	https://doi.org/10.1080/17432979.2021.2021988

Whole Person Care for Traumatized: Building Resiliency & Self-Care in Response to the Coronavirus	https://www.youtube.com/watch?v=nHuI0CU4ezQ
Dance movement therapy in Beijing	https://www.youtube.com/watch?v=l9ijMORiBXI
A Whole Person Approach to Working with Trauma and Building Resilience	https://link.springer.com/article/10.1007/s10465-020-09335-6
Accelerating the Field of Neuroaesthetics (a short video by Susan Magsamen)	https://youtu.be/GcFed72v0p8
How to Engage the Arts to Build COVID-19 Vaccine Confidence: Creative Approaches to COVID-19 Vaccination to Unite the Arts and Sciences	https://www.cdc.gov/vaccines/covid-19/vaccinate-with-confidence/art.html
NeuroArts Blueprint: Advancing the Science of Arts, Health, and Wellbeing	https://www.artsandmindlab.org/wp-content/uploads/2021/12/NeuroArtsBlue_Vol2_ExSumReport_v24spreads.pdf
Creating Healthy Communities: Arts + Public Health in America, COVID-19 Arts Response Overview	https://www.artsandmindlab.org/wp-content/uploads/2021/12/NeuroArtsBlue_Vol2_ExSumReport_v24spreads.pdf
Hattie Worboys: Body Talks Movement	http://hattieworboys.com
Pelias, R. J. (2021). Contact and the 2020 pandemic: A poetic autoethnography. *International Review of Qualitative Research, 14*(2), 358–364.	https://doi.org/10.1177/1940844721991081
Wyatt, J. (2021). Three lockdown poems. *International Review of Qualitative Research, 14*(2), 365–367.	https://doi.org/10.1177/1940844720974105
Carless, D. (2021). What can a song bring? Balancing out the picture in pandemic. *International Review of Qualitative Research.*	https://doi.org/10.1177/19408447211049529
Callahan, J. L. (2022). Introduction to the special issue on pandemic impacts. *American Psychological Association, 32*(1), 1–2.	https://doi.org/10.1037/int0000282
Kidd, A. (2022). Therapists facing masks: A qualitative study of the nature of relationships between masks and relational depth. *Counselling and Psychotherapy Research, 00*, 1–15.	https://doi.org/10.1002/capr.12517
Engelen, M., & Shechter, A. (2022). Living the data: Reflections on living and working during the Covid-19 pandemic. *Psychodynamic Practice, 28*(1), 85–93.	https://doi.org/10.1080/14753634.2021.2022304
Newsletters and websites	https://drive.google.com/drive/folders/1xurkTP09dZbBVmWpB1mgnD_BSGxFkk6r

Outside Inside Plein Air Project	https://docs.google.com/document/d/1MgVnRvPcRmm55X6AwwC6YKNvrdNaZapD/edit#heading=h.gjdgxs
Beishi University hotline service terminated, long-distance consultation started	https://mp-weixin-qq-com.translate.goog/s/KKVhiot3-qfklk1SmVxzUQ?_x_tr_sl=auto&_x_tr_tl=en&_x_tr_hl=en&_x_tr_pto=wapp
The Future of Healing: Shifting From Trauma Informed Care to Healing Centered Engagement	https://ginwright.medium.com/the-future-of-healing-shifting-from-trauma-informed-care-to-healing-centered-engagement-634f557ce69c
Yo-Yo Ma Tells Story Behind His Cello Performance At Vaccination Center	https://www.youtube.com/watch?v=8t9-SvRv2zg
Songs of Comfort and Hope—Yo-Yo Ma and Kathryn Stott	https://www.youtube.com/watch?v=UDV0qXQ0_7c&list=OLAK5uy_kGR3mbeS0JAqwyGREDkqFtiEXg5-uFn1k
UCLA Arts & Healing HOPE: Healing Online for People Everywhere	https://uclartsandhealing.org/services/community-services/hope-series/
UCLA Arts & Healing Free Downloads	https://uclartsandhealing.org/free-downloads/
Beat the Odds: Social and Emotional Skill Building Delivered in a Framework of Drumming	https://uclartsandhealing.org/services/professional-development/beat-the-odds-drumming-program/
Social Emotional Arts on a Shoestring: Supportive Art, Movement, Music, and Writing for Individuals and Groups in Any Setting	https://uclartsandhealing.org/services/professional-development/social-emotional-arts-on-a-shoestring/
Certificate Program in Social Emotional Arts	https://uclartsandhealing.org/services/professional-development/social-emotional-arts-cert-program/
Dance for All: Social and Emotional Learning through Creative Movement	https://uclartsandhealing.org/services/professional-development/dance-for-all-program/
The Key Role the Arts and Humanities play	https://www.linkedin.com/feed/update/urn:li:ugcPost:6945737878014427136

Lori Gill

Relaxation Place	Video	Attachment and Trauma Treatment Centre for Healing	https://www.youtube.com/watch?v=UfBw5p7WK9o&t=24s
Tapping Through Intense Emotions	Video	Attachment and Trauma Treatment Centre for Healing	https://www.youtube.com/watch?v=9IZP1TEVIes
Understanding Affect Regulation Working with the Window of Tolerance	Video	Attachment and Trauma Treatment Centre for Healing	https://www.youtube.com/watch?v=omy_po9gszc

Mindfulness as a way to cope with COVID-19-related stress and anxiety	https://drive.google.com/file/d/1ULkml32wIEPg5Mv6Op4XVur9cWvzjk2j/view?usp=sharing
Garcia, E., Di Paolo, E. A., & De Jaegher, H. (2022). Embodiment in online psychotherapy: A qualitative study. *Psychology and Psychotherapy: Theory, Research and Practice, 95*, 191–211.	https://doi.org/10.1111/papt.12359
Rathenau, S., Sousa, D., Vaz, A., & Geller, S. (2022). The effect of attitudes toward online therapy and the difficulties perceived in online therapeutic presence. *Journal of Psychotherapy Integration, 32*(1), 19–33.	https://psycnet.apa.org/record/2021-95011-001
Dance, Creative Arts, and Somatic Therapies in the Healing of Trauma by Dr. Ilene Serlin, a Review of *The Body Keeps the Score: Brain, Mind, and Body in the Healing of Trauma* by Bessel A. van der Kolk	https://www.researchgate.net/publication/282447745_Dance_Creative_Arts_and_Somatic_Therapies_in_the_Healing_of_Trauma
COVID Coach for iPhone, a free mobile app to provide resources and enhance emotional support during the pandemic	https://apps.apple.com/app/apple-store/id1504705038
COVID Coach for Android, a free mobile app to provide resources and enhance emotional support during the pandemic	https://play.google.com/store/apps/details?id=gov.va.mobilehealth.ncptsd.covid
Move Better, Feel Better Summit	https://courses.futurelifenow-online.com/summit-2020-day-4/

Sensorimotor Psychotherapy COVID-19 Resources	https://sensorimotor.pages.ontraport.net/covid-19-news
Creative Therapy Umbrella, Episode # 30 – Embodiment, Collaboration, and Social Trauma, with Dr. Amber Gray, Ph.D., MPH, MA, BC-DMT, LPCC, NCC	https://creativetherapyumbrella.com/2020/03/26/30-embodiment-collaboration-and-social-trauma-with-dr-amber-gray-ph-d-mph-ma-bc-dmt-lpcc-ncc/
Emotional Well-Being and Coping During COVID-19	https://psychiatry.ucsf.edu/coronavirus/coping
Nurse Uses Dance, Meditation To Help Fellow Health Care Workers Cope During Coronavirus Pandemic by Katherine Fung	https://www.newsweek.com/nurse-uses-dance-meditation-help-fellow-health-care-workers-cope-during-coronavirus-pandemic-1505068
The New School at Commonweal	https://tns.commonweal.org
Dr. Danny Brom: Post traumatic stress disorder in Israel, May, 2015	https://www.youtube.com/watch?v=42fblBpJ3Z8
Creativity, Resilience, and Healing Trauma: Dr. Serlin interviews Eleanor Pardess at SELAH Israel Crisis Management Center, Tel-Aviv, Israel, May 18, 2015	https://www.youtube.com/watch?v=IN26HNdH2Pg&feature=youtu.be
COVID-19 Guided Imagery and Music (GIM) Self-Help Resource	https://www.youtube.com/watch?v=ssKIjeGY_Lg
Online Open Studio 05 – A Postcard to Myself by Lefika La Phodiso	https://youtu.be/QUjd32SoIcg
Grief Resource Guide	www.covidgriefresources.com
What The History of Pandemics Can Teach Us About Resilience	https://www.nytimes.com/2021/04/01/health/pandemics-plague-history-resilience.html
Physical inactivity is associated with a higher risk for severe COVID-19 outcomes: a study in 48 440 adult patients	https://bjsm.bmj.com/content/55/19/1099
Clean the air with plants	https://peperperspective.com/2021/03/22/clean-the-air-with-plants/
Avoid Zoom fatigue, be present and learn	https://drive.google.com/file/d/1SAodsWPHLnR3IiVhQ9CNZDDm9SRRZ_oR/view?usp=sharing
Reduce Stress, Anxiety, and Negative Thoughts with Somatics	https://drive.google.com/file/d/1yP5TQqEjEx1jpkot1gD6YB97VnoNna5m/view?usp=sharing
Increase Productivity, Decrease Procrastination, and Increase Energy	https://drive.google.com/file/d/1V63yjgqwpy05xydSQbR8-Nk4EeT0tnnr/view?usp=sharing

Reactivate your second heart	https://peperperspective.com/2021/06/14/reactivate-your-second-heart/
Conscious Visionary Nurses on the Edge of Evolution by Mary Rockwood Lane	https://nursescholars.kaiserpermanente.org/conscious-visionary-nurses-tele-summit/
Somatic expression: Body Wisdom for Modern Times by Jamie McHugh	http://www.somaticexpression.com/calendar.html
Embodied Resilience by Ilene Serlin	https://drive.google.com/file/d/1YXwCkCUqqSv7yfmhERtUFG6iAmF5cHMF/view?usp=sharing
A breath of fresh air: Breathing and posture to optimize health	https://peperperspective.com/2022/04/03/a-breath-of-fresh-air-breathing-and-posture-to-optimize-health/
Camille B. Wortman, Jessica Gregory & Andrew Wortman, *Grief Resource Guide*	https://www.covidgriefresources.com/wp-content/uploads/Grief-Resource-Guide-3-5-2022.pdf
Erik Peper et al., Avoid Zoom Fatigue, Be Present and Learn	https://www.neuroregulation.org/article/view/21206/13976
The Peper Perspective: Clean the air with plants	https://peperperspective.com/2021/03/22/clean-the-air-with-plants/
UCL Reports: COVID-19 Social Study weekly reports	https://www.covidsocialstudy.org/results
Sallis, R., et al. (2021). Physical inactivity is associated with a higher risk for severe COVID-19 outcomes. *British Journal of Sports Medicine, 55*(19), 1099–1105.	https://pubmed.ncbi.nlm.nih.gov/33849909/
Embodiment in Online Therapy	https://docs.google.com/presentation/d/1OBk5p4PJNitsbJMTVAf%2D%2Dyk6curqpfPT
Mindfulness & Somatics	*See folder Mindfulness, Self Compassion and COVID*
Compassionate goals, prosocial emotions, and prosocial behaviours during the COVID-19 pandemic	https://drive.google.com/file/d/1w1KFaa6Mm-pfRa7YPjHgZDv6PjzbBT9N/view?usp=sharing
Coping with COVID-19 – Longitudinal analysis of coping strategies and the role of trait mindfulness in mental well-being	https://drive.google.com/file/d/18_vNg99lnNKEiGfRsLHgnVE8JPhVsZ0D/view?usp=sharing
Mindfulness moments for clinicians in the midst of a pandemic	https://drive.google.com/file/d/1ZuHXV_sFEKxUIB5fNOWjaKJ00lUhCfFi/view?usp=sharing
Buffering Traumatic Reactions to COVID-19	https://psycnet.apa.org/record/2022-45143-001
Freedom of movement with the Alexander Technique	https://peperperspective.com
Somatic Expression: Body Wisdom for Modern Minds by Jamie McHugh	http://www.somaticexpression.com

Tuber, S., Da Costa, R., Eidman, J., Feldman, H., & Hadar, O. (2022). Dialectical reflections on the advantages and disadvantages of tele-play therapy. *Journal of Infant, Child, and Adolescent Psychotherapy, 21*(1), 19–26.	https://doi.org/10.1080/15289168.2022.2043058
Vanhooren, S., Grosemans, A., & Breynaert, J. (2022). Focusing, the felt sense, and meaning in life. *Person-Centered & Experiential Psychotherapies, 21*(3), 250–268.	https://doi.org/10.1080/14779757.2022.2028660
Javier Bartos, L., Pilar Posadas, M., & Krägeloh, C. (2022, February 17). Perceived benefits of a remote yoga and mindfulness program for student musicians during COVID-19. *The Humanistic Psychologist.*	https://doi.org/10.1037/hum0000277
Vanhooren, S., Grosemans, A., & Breynaert, J. (2022). Focusing, the felt sense, and meaning in life. *Person-Centered & Experiential Psychotherapies, 21*(3), 250–268.	https://doi.org/10.1080/14779757.2022.2028660
Garcıa, E., Di Paolo, E. A., & De Jaegher, H. (2022). Embodiment in online psychotherapy: A qualitative study, British Psychological Society. *Psychology and Psychotherapy: Theory, Research and Practice, 95*, 191–211.	https://drive.google.com/drive/u/1/folders/1iZJyd8aqKHokHk9moaFiSYkpskd7fnzp

Kuriansky

Tsai, J., & Morissette, S. B. (2022). Introduction to the special issue: Resilience and perseverance for human flourishing. *Psychological Trauma: Theory, Research, Practice, and Policy, 14*(S1), S1–S3.	https://doi.org/10.1037/tra0001215
Aafjes-van Doorn, K., Békés, V., Prout, T. A., & Hoffman, L. (2020). Psychotherapists' vicarious traumatization during the COVID-19 pandemic. *Psychological Trauma: Theory, Research, Practice, and Policy, 12*(S1), S148–S150.	https://psycnet.apa.org/record/2020-37319-001
Ashby, J. S., Rice, K. G., & Kira, I. A. (2022). The relationship of COVID-19 traumatic stress, cumulative trauma, and race to posttraumatic stress disorder symptoms. *Journal of Community Psychology, 50*(6), 2597–2610.	https://doi.org/10.1002/jcop.22762
Blanc, J., Briggs, A. Q., Seixas, A. A., Reid, M., Jean-Louis, G., & Pandi-Perumal, S. R. (2021). Addressing psychological resilience during the coronavirus disease 2019 pandemic: A rapid review. *Current Opinion in Psychiatry, 34*(1), 29–35.	https://doi.org/10.1097/YCO.0000000000000665
Bozdağ, F., & Ergün, N. (2021). Psychological resilience of healthcare professionals during COVID-19 pandemic. *Psychological Reports, 124*(6), 2567–2586.	https://doi.org/10.1177/0033294120965477
Burke-Garcia, A., Johnson-Turbes, A., Mitchell, E. W., Verlenden, J. M. V., Puddy, R., Mercado, M. C., Nelson, P., Rabinowitz, L., Xia, K., Wagstaff, L., Feng, M., Caicedo, L., & Tolbert, E. (2021). How right now? Supporting mental health and resilience amid COVID-19. *Traumatology, 27*(4), 399–412.	https://europepmc.org/article/pmc/pmc8967147
Calder, A. J., Novak, L. F., & Lane, A. (2020). We're all going crazy now: How the COVID-19 pandemic can promote more compassionate clinical perspectives. *Journal of Humanistic Psychology*.	https://doi.org/10.1177/0022167820938615
Carbajal, J., Ponder, W. N., Whitworth, J., Schuman, D. L., Galusha, J. M., Carbajal, J., Ponder, W. N., Whitworth, J., & Donna, L. (2021). The impact of COVID-19 on first responders' resilience and attachment. *Journal of Human Behavior in the Social Environment, 32*(6), 781–797.	https://doi.org/10.1080/10911359.2021.1962777
Cook, L. L., Zschomler, D., Biggart, L., & Carder, S. (2020). The team as a secure base revisited: Remote working and resilience among child and family social workers during COVID-19. *Journal of Children's Services, 15*(4), 259–266.	https://doi.org/10.1108/JCS-07-2020-0031
Diane, S., Litam, A., Ausloos, C. D., & Harrichand, J. J. S. (2021). Stress and resilience among professional counselors during the COVID-19 pandemic. *Journal of Counseling & Development, 99*(4), 384–395.	https://doi.org/10.1002/jcad.12391

Ergu, N. (2021). Psychological resilience of healthcare professionals during COVID-19 pandemic. *Psychological Reports, 124*(6), 2567–2586.	https://doi.org/10.1177/0033294120965477
Huang, Y.-L., Li, Z.-W., Kung, Y.-W., & Su, Y.-J. (2022). The facilitating role of dispositional mindfulness in the process of posttraumatic growth: A prospective investigation. *Psychological Trauma: Theory, Research, Practice, and Policy, 14*(S1), S174	https://psycnet.apa.org/record/2022-03794-001
Jones, P. J., & McNally, R. J. (2022). Does broadening one's concept of trauma undermine resilience? *Psychological Trauma: Theory, Research, Practice, and Policy, 14*(S1), S131–S139.	https://drive.google.com/file/d/1cdSITQWW5vcufCa7r3nUW1f_ToPqeLOJ/view
Kira, I. A., Shuwiekh, H. A. M., Ashby, J. S., Elwakeel, S. A., Alhuwailah, A., Sous, M. S. F., Baali, S. B. A., Azdaou, C., Oliemat, E. M., & Jamil, H. J. (2021). The impact of covid-19 traumatic stressors on mental health: Is covid-19 a new trauma type. *International Journal of Mental Health and Addiction*. Advance online publication.	https://pubmed.ncbi.nlm.nih.gov/34248442/
Buchanan, G. J. R., Ballard, J., Fatiha, N., Song, S., & Solheim, C. (2022). Resilience in the system: COVID-19 and immigrant- and refugee- serving health and human service providers. *Families, Systems, and Health, 40*(1), 111–119.	https://pubmed.ncbi.nlm.nih.gov/34807638/
Killgore, W. D. S., Taylor, E. C., Cloonan, S. A., & Dailey, N. S. (2020). Psychological resilience during the COVID-19 lockdown. *Psychiatry Research, 291*(May), 113216.	https://doi.org/10.1016/j.psychres.2020.113216
Lissoni, B., Del Negro, S., Brioschi, P., Casella, G., Fontana, I., Bruni, C., & Lamiani, G. (2020). Promoting resilience in the acute phase of the COVID-19 pandemic: Psychological interventions for intensive care unit (ICU) clinicians and family members. *Psychological Trauma: Theory, Research, Practice, and Policy, 12*, 105–107.	https://doi.org/10.1037/tra0000802
Munroe, M., Al-Refae, M., Chan, H. W., & Ferrari, M. (2022). Using self-compassion to grow in the face of trauma: The role of positive reframing and problem-focused coping strategies. *Psychological Trauma: Theory, Research, Practice, and Policy, 14*(S1), S157.	https://pubmed.ncbi.nlm.nih.gov/34735189/
Manchia, M., Gathier, A. W., Yapici-Eser, H., Schmidt, M. V., De Quervain, D., Van, T., Bisson, J. I., Cryan, J. F., Howes, O. D., Pinto, L., Van Der Wee, N. J., Domschke, K., Branchi, I., & Vinkers, C. H. (2022). The impact of the prolonged COVID-19 pandemic on stress resilience and mental health: A critical review across waves. *European Neuropsychopharmacology, 55*, 22–83.	https://doi.org/10.1016/j.euroneuro.2021.10.864
Mannarini, T., Fedi, A., Rizzo, M., & Zhao, J. (2021). The potential of psychological connectedness: Mitigating the impacts of COVID-19 through sense of community and community resilience. *Journal of Community Psychology, 50*(5), 2273–2289.	https://doi.org/10.1002/jcop.22775

Nuttman-Shwartz, O. (2015). Shared resilience in a traumatic reality: A new concept for trauma workers exposed personally and professionally to collective disaster. *Trauma, Violence, and Abuse, 16*(4), 466–475.	https://doi.org/10.1177/1524838014557287
Prieto-Ursúa, M., & Jódar, R. (2020). Finding meaning in hell. The role of meaning, religiosity and spirituality in posttraumatic growth during the coronavirus crisis in Spain. *Frontiers in Psychology, 11*, 567836.	https://www.frontiersin.org/articles/10.3389/fpsyg.2020.567836/full
Prime, H., Wade, M., & Browne, D. T. (2020). Risk and resilience in family well-being during the COVID-19 pandemic. *American Psychologist, 75*(5), 631–643.	https://doi.org/10.1037/amp0000660
Rolin, S. N., Flis, A., & Davis, J. J. (2022). Work coping, stress appraisal, and psychological resilience: Reaction to the COVID-19 pandemic among health care providers. *Psychology & Neuroscience, 15*(2), 131–146.	https://pesquisa.bvsalud.org/global-literature-on-novel-coronavirus-2019-ncov/resource/pt/covidwho-1331374?lang=en
Rosen, B., Preisman, M., Hunter, J., & Maunder, R. (2020). Applying psychotherapeutic principles to bolster resilience among health care workers during the covid-19 pandemic. *American Journal of Psychotherapy, 73*(4), 144–148.	https://doi.org/10.1176/APPI.PSYCHOTHERAPY.20200020
Shklarski, L., Abrams, A., & Bakst, E. (2021). Navigating changes in the physical and psychological spaces of psychotherapists during Covid-19: When home becomes the office. *Practice Innovations, 6*(1), 55–66.	https://psycnet.apa.org/record/2021-07055-001
Tsai, J., & Morissette, S. B. (2022). Introduction to the special issue: Resilience and perseverance for human flourishing. *Psychological Trauma: Theory, Research, Practice, and Policy, 14*(S1), S1–S3.	https://doi.org/10.1037/tra0001215
Yang, M. (2020). Resilience and meaning-making amid the COVID-19 epidemic in China. *Journal of Humanistic Psychology, 60*(5), 662–671.	https://doi.org/10.1177/0022167820929215

Body Talks Movement

Hope for abdominal discomfort	https://peperperspective.com/
Comfort After Crisis by Jonathan Curiel	https://www.sfgate.com/health/article/Comfort-after-crisis-It-may-take-weeks-to-get-2877695.php
Collective Trauma and Existential Anxiety by Robert Stolorow	https://www.huffpost.com/entry/collective-trauma-and-exi_b_680945
Exercise in Times of Global Pandemic: Soul-Surfing by Dr. Ani Kalayjian	https://www.youtube.com/watch?v=nk-aedntLWs
Islands of Security: Promoting Resilience & Growth	https://www.pardess.info/islands-of-security-promoting-resilience-growth-presentation-for-a-p-a-covid-taskforce/
Compassion Regeneration: Nature as a Resource for Staff Support	https://www.pardess.info/compassion-regeneration-nature-as-a-resource/
Posttraumatic Growth as a Process and an Outcome: Vexing Problems and Paradoxes Seen From the Perspective of Humanistic Psychology by Stephen Joseph	https://doi.org/10.1037/hum0000156
Trauma-Focused Presence by Anthony Cameron	https://doi.org/10.1177/0022167819880653
The Case for Existential (Spiritual) Psychotherapy by Kirk J. Schneider	https://doi.org/10.1007/s10879-014-9278-8
The President's Column by Dr. Ilene Serlin in The San Francisco Psychologist	http://www.union-street-health-associates.com/articles/SFPA-summer-2009-president%27s-column.pdf
Posttraumatic Growth: Whole Person Approaches to Working With Trauma by Dr. Ilene Serlin	http://www.union-street-health-associates.com/articles/post_traumatic_growth.pdf
Working with Trauma in Israel: Lessons for America	http://www.union-street-health-associates.com/articles/national_psychologist.pdf
The existential basis of trauma by Neil Thompson and Mary Walsh	https://www.tandfonline.com/doi/abs/10.1080/02650531003638163?journalCode=cjsw20
Invisible Losses: Secondary Trauma, Survivor Guilt and Moving Through the COVID-19 Crisis by Michael W. Rabow, MD & David Bullard, PhD	https://meri.ucsf.edu/blog/invisible-losses-secondary-trauma-survivor-guilt-and-moving-through-covid-19-crisis

Stanley Krippner: Advocate for Healing Trauma by Ilene Serlin and Erika Hansen. In Jeannine A. Davis & Daniel B. Pitchford (Eds.), Stanley Krippner: A Life of Dreams, Myths, and Visions	http://www.union-street-health-associates.com/articles/a-life-of-dreams-myths-and-visions.pdf
Integrated Care for the Traumatized, a Whole-Person Approach by Ilene Serlin, Stanley Krippner, and Kirwan Rockefeller	https://www.tandfonline.com/doi/abs/10.1080/17432979.2020.1724194?journalCode=tbmd20
Kinaesthetic Imagining by Ilene Serlin. In B.E. Thompson & R.A. Neimeyer (Eds.), Grief and the expressive therapies: Practices for creating meaning	http://www.union-street-health-associates.com/articles/kinesthetic-imagining-2014.pdf
The courage to move by Ilene Serlin. In S. Schwartz, V. Marcow Speiser, P. Speiser, & M. Kossak (Eds.), The arts and social change: The Lesley University experience in Israel	http://www.union-street-health-associates.com/articles/courage-to-move1.pdf
Global Resilience Summit	https://www.globalresiliencesummit.org
Live Whole Health: Self-care episode #8 – Compassion	https://www.blogs.va.gov/VAntage/73950/live-whole-health-self-care-episode-8-compassion/
Emerging from the Coronavirus	https://www.nytimes.com/interactive/2021/04/05/us/coronavirus-pandemic.html
Jewish hospital chaplains are on the pandemic's spiritual front line	https://www.jweekly.com/2021/02/16/jewish-hospital-chaplains-are-on-the-pandemics-spiritual-front-line
What Existentialists Can Teach Us About COVID-19 by Kirk J. Schneider Ph.D.	https://www.psychologytoday.com/us/blog/awakening-awe/202005/what-existentialists-can-teach-us-about-covid-19
The many facets of trauma by Makenna Berry	https://www.saybrook.edu/blog/2011/10/21/10-21-11/
Blues, Trauma, Existential Vulnerability by Robert D Stolorow PhD	https://www.psychologytoday.com/us/blog/feeling-relating-existing/201204/blues-trauma-existential-vulnerability
Psychoanalysis Meets Existentialism: Robert Stolorow on Trauma and Authenticity by Carlo Strenger	https://www.psychologytoday.com/us/blog/homo-globalis/201104/psychoanalysis-meets-existentialism-robert-stolorow-trauma-and
Existential Anxiety and Traumatic Stress in Adolescents by Carl Weems, PhD	https://istss.org/public-resources/trauma-blog/2016-september/existential-anxiety-and-traumatic-stress-in-adoles
Emotional Well-Being and Coping During COVID-19	https://psych.ucsf.edu/coronavirus/coping
"Epidemics and Society" Review: Hiding From Life to Stay Alive by Felipe Fernández-Armesto	https://www.wsj.com/articles/epidemics-and-society-review-hiding-from-life-to-stay-alive-11587764677

Whole Person Psychology: Embodiment and Humanistic Psychology	https://www.youtube.com/watch?v=qu2GFoFYwM4
The New York Times: What the History of Pandemics Can Teach Us About Resilience	https://www.nytimes.com/2021/04/01/health/pandemics-plague-history-resilience.html
Cultivating Creativity & Compassion: COVID-19 as a Transformative Opportunity	https://www.pardess.info/cultivating-self-compassion-creativity-covid-19-as-a-transformative-opportunity/
Compassion Regeneration: Nature as a Resource for Staff Support	https://www.pardess.info/islands-of-security-promoting-resilience-growth-presentation-for-a-p-a-covid-taskforce/
Cultivating Creativity & Compassion: COVID-19 as a Transformative Opportunity	Cultivating Creativity & Compassion: COVID-19 as a Transformative Opportunityhttps://www.pardess.info/cultivating-self-compassion-creativity-covid-19-as-a-transformative-opportunity/
Compassion Regeneration: Nature as a Resource for Staff Support	https://www.pardess.info/islands-of-security-promoting-resilience-growth-presentation-for-a-p-a-covid-taskforce/
Embodiment in Online Therapy	https://docs.google.com/presentation/d/1OBk5p4PJNitsbJMTVAf%2D%2Dyk6curqpfPT
Additional papers may be found in the folder Compassion Fatigue and Arts for Healing	https://drive.google.com/drive/folders/10uoDeGGM44F5uYzo-kzsGsyIvl00j3p9?usp=sharing
Ali, D. A., Figley, C. R., Tedeschi, R. G., Galarneau, D., & Amara, S. (2021). Shared trauma, resilience, and growth: A roadmap toward transcultural conceptualization. *Psychological Trauma: Theory, Research, Practice, and Policy, 15*(1), 45–55.	https://psycnet.apa.org/record/2021-55324-001
Mendenhall, T. (2021). We are in this together: Maintaining our health care teams' wellness during challenging times. *Families, Systems, and Health, 39*(3), 541–543.	https://psycnet.apa.org/doiLanding?doi=10.1037%2Ffsh0000650
Smith-Macdonald, L., Lusk, J., Lee-Baggley, D., Bright, K., Laidlaw, A., Voth, M., Spencer, S., Cruikshank, E., Pike, A., Jones, C., & Bremault-Phillips, S. (2022). Companions in the abyss: A feasibility and acceptability study of an online therapy group for healthcare providers working during the COVID-19 pandemic. *Frontiers in Psychiatry*, 12(January), 1–13.	https://doi.org/10.3389/fpsyt.2021.801680

Whitt-Woosley, A., Sprang, G., & Eslinger, J. (2022). The impact of COVID-19 and experiences of secondary traumatic stress and burnout. *Psychol Trauma, 14*(3), 507–515.	https://psycnet.apa.org/record/2022-33825-003
Hoffman, L. (2021). Existential–humanistic therapy and disaster response: Lessons from the COVID-19 pandemic. *Journal of Humanistic Psychology, 61*(1), 33–54.	https://journals.sagepub.com/doi/full/10.1177/0022167820931987
Bland, A. M. (2020). Existential givens in the COVID-19 crisis. *Journal of Humanistic Psychology, 60*(5), 710–724.	https://doi-org.ezprimo1.idc.ac.il/10.1177/0022167820940 1
Counted, V., Pargament, K. I., Bechara, A. O., Joynt, S., & Cowden, R. G. (2022). Hope and well-being in vulnerable contexts during the COVID-19 pandemic: Does religious coping matter? *The Journal of Positive Psychology, 17*(1), 70–81.	https://doi-org.ezprimo1.idc.ac.il/10.1080/17439760.2020.1832247
Cénat, J. M., Noorishad, P.-G., Blais-Rochette, C., McIntee, S.-E., Mukunzi, J. N., Darius, W. P., Broussard, C., Morse, C., Ukwu, G., Auguste, E., & Menelas, K. (2020). Together for hope and resilience: A humanistic experience by the vulnerability, trauma, resilience and culture lab members during the covid-19 pandemic. *Journal of Loss and Trauma, 25*, 643–648.	https://www.tandfonline.com/doi/full/10.1080/15325024.2020.1774704
Morrill, Z. (2021). Introduction to the COVID-19 second special issue. *Journal of Humanistic Psychology, 61*(2).	https://doi.org/10.1177/0022167820966412
Whitt-Woosley, A., Sprang, G., & Eslinger, J. (2022). The impact of COVID-19 and experiences of secondary traumatic stress and burnout. *Psychological Trauma, 14*(3), 507–515.	https://doi.org/10.1037/tra0001183
Companions in the abyss: A feasibility and acceptability study of an online therapy group for healthcare providers working during the COVID-19 pandemic. *Frontiers in Psychiatry*, 12(January), 1–13.	https://doi.org/10.3389/fpsyt.2021.801680
Addressing the Psychological and Emotional Impact of the COVID-19 Pandemic for Children, Families and Healthcare Staff	https://www.healthcaretoolbox.org/covid19
Sustaining the Well-Being of Healthcare Personnel during Coronavirus and other Infectious Disease Outbreaks	https://www.cstsonline.org/assets/media/documents/CSTS_FS_Sustaining_Well_Being_Healthcare_Personnel_during.pdf
US Dept of Veteran Affairs, National Center for PTSD, Managing Health Care Workers' Stress Associated with the COVID-19 Virus Outbreak	https://www.ptsd.va.gov/covid/COVID_healthcare_workers.asp
Schwartz Center for Compassionate Healthcare, Caring for Yourself & Others During the COVID-19 Pandemic: Managing Healthcare Workers' Stress	https://istss.org/ISTSS_Main/media/Documents/Schwartz-Center-Watson-SFA-Final-PDF.pdf
AMA, Monitor and Assess the Well-Being of Your Physicians and Care Teams	https://clinician.health/%E2%80%8E

Center for the Study of Traumatic Stress, COVID-19 Pandemic Response Resources	https://www.cstsonline.org/resources/resource-master-list/coronavirus-and-emerging-infectious-disease-outbreaks-response
National Center for PTSD Coronavirus (COVID-19) Resources for Managing Stress	https://www.ptsd.va.gov/covid/index.asp
Journal of Traumatic Stress, Virtual Special Issue: Resilience and Recovery in the Era of the COVID-19 Pandemic	https://istss.org/education-research/jts/jts-virtual-special-issues/virtual-issue-resilience-and-recovery
Session recording from the ISTSS 35th Annual Meeting, Resilience in Perilous Times: Pathways to the Future	https://istss.org/education-research/online-learning/free-recordings#Resilience
Mayo Clinic Proceedings, Strategies for Resiliency of Medical Staff During COVID-19	https://www.mayoclinicproceedings.org/article/S0025-6196(20)30722-9/fulltext
ISTSS Webinar, Responding to the COVID-19 Pandemic: Toolkit for Emotional Coping for Healthcare Staff	https://istss.org/public-resources/covid-19-resources#For-Healthcare-Workers
Covid Resources Uploaded by Eleanor Pardess	https://drive.google.com/drive/folders/10uoDeGGM44F5uYzo-kzsGsyIvl00j3p9
2022 Covid Resources, Humanistic	https://drive.google.com/drive/u/1/folders/1iZJyd8aqKHokHk9moaFiSYkpskd7fnzp
Embodiment in Online Therapy	https://docs.google.com/presentation/d/1OBk5p4PJNitsbJMTVAf%2D%2Dyk6curqpfPT
Arts for Healing in the Face of Covid	https://drive.google.com/drive/folders/1vXBo7aV9llBYTAecPuepZDc6XN9EQVYw
Webinar on Emotion as Gateway to the Anomalous	https://mindgains.org/
Covid Resources Task Force	https://www.dropbox.com/sh/ltwtih27kuoome1/AABG8FKBIM8T1aJxW028v4zPa?dl=0
Cultivating resilience in the context of Covid	https://drive.google.com/drive/folders/1rlJzHk2DeFL8Kzd7n13M02tYLnQvw6_K
Behrends, A., Müller, S., & Dziobek, I. (2012). Moving in and out of synchrony: A concept for a new intervention fostering empathy through interactional movement and dance. *The Arts in Psychotherapy, 39*, 107–116.	https://doi.org/10.1016/j.aip.2012.02.003

Bernieri, F., Reznick, J. S., & Rosenthal, R. (1988). Synchrony, pseudosynchrony, and dissynchrony: Measuring the entrainment process in mother-infant interactions. *Journal of Personality and Social Psychology*, *54*(2), 243–253.	https://liberalarts.oregonstate.edu/sites/liberalarts.oregonstate.edu/files/psychology/research/bernieri_reznick_and_rosenthal_1988_synchrony_pseudosynchrony_and_dissynchrony.pdf
Callier, D. M., & Hill, D. C. (2021). Autoethnography that moves the soul: Activating the creative in troubled times. *International Review of Qualitative Research, 14*(2), 283–287.	https://doi.org/10.1177/1940844720974106
Decety, J., & Meyer, M. (2008). From emotion resonance to empathic understanding: A social developmental neuroscience account. *Development and Psychopathology, 20*(4), 1053–1080.	https://doi.org/10.1017/S0954579408000503
Dissanayake, E. (2008). If music is the food of love, what about survival and reproductive success? *Musicae Scientiae, 12*(Suppl. 1), 169–195.	https://www.researchgate.net/publication/258173165_If_music_is_the_food_of_love_what_about_survival_and_reproductive_success
Fraenkel, D. (1983). The relationship of empathy in movement to synchrony, echoing, and empathy in verbal interactions. *American Journal of Dance Therapy, 6*, 31–48.	https://link.springer.com/article/10.1007/BF02579518
Frank, R. (2016). Moving experience: Kinaesthetic resonance as relational feel. In M. Spagnuolo Lobb, N. Levi, & A. Williams (Eds.), *Gestalt therapy with children: From epistemology to clinical practice* (pp. 87–99). Istituto di Gestalt HCC Italy.	https://psycnet.apa.org/record/2016-46244-003
Frank, R. (2020). Developing presence online. *The Humanistic Psychologist, 48*(4), 369–372.	https://doi.org/10.1037/hum0000208
Fuchs, T. (2012). The phenomenology of body memory. In S. C. Koch, T. Fuchs, M. Summa, & C. Müller (Eds.), *Body memory, metaphor and movement* (pp. 9–22). John Benjamins.	https://doi.org/10.1075/aicr.84.03fuc
Fuchs, T. (2017a). Collective body memories. In C. Durt, T. Fuchs, & C. Tewes (Eds.), *Embodiment, enaction, and culture: Investigating the constitution of the shared world* (pp. 333–352). MIT Press.	https://doi.org/10.7551/mitpress/10799.003.0023
Fuchs, T., & De Jaegher, H. (2009). Enactive intersubjectivity: Participatory sense-making and mutual incorporation. *Phenomenology and the Cognitive Sciences, 8*, 465–486.	https://link.springer.com/article/10.1007/s11097-009-9136-4

Fuchs, T., & Koch, S. C. (2014). Embodied affectivity: On moving and being moved. *Frontiers in Psychology, 5*, 508.	https://doi.org/10.3389/fpsyg.2014.00508
Gallagher, S., & Lindgren, R. (2015). Enactive metaphors: Learning through full-body engagement. *Educational Psychology Review*, *27*(3), 391–404.	https://doi.org/10.1007/s10648-015-9327-1
Gallagher, S., & Payne, H. (2014). The role of embodiment and intersubjectivity in clinical reasoning. *Body, Movement and Dance in Psychotherapy: An International Journal for Theory, Research and Practice, 10*(1), 68–78.	https://doi.org/10.1080/17432979.2014.980320
Gordon, I., Gilboa, A., Cohen, S., & Kleinfeld, T. (2020a). The relationship between physiological synchrony and motion energy synchrony during a joint group drumming task. *Physiology & Behavior, 224*, 113074.	https://doi.org/10.1016/j.physbeh.2020.113074
Gordon, I., Gilboa, A., Cohen, S., Milstein, N., Haimovich, N., Pinhasi, S., & Siegman, S. (2020b). Physiological and behavioral synchrony predict group cohesion and performance. *Scientific Reports, 10*(1), 8484.	https://doi.org/10.1038/s41598-020-65670-1
Hübl, T., & Avritt, J. J. (2020). *Healing collective trauma: A process for integrating our intergenerational and cultural wounds.* Sounds True.	https://www.amazon.com/Healing-Collective-Trauma-Integrating-Intergenerational/dp/1683647378
Johnson, M. (2017). *Embodied mind, meaning, and reason: How our bodies give rise to understanding*. University of Chicago Press.	https://press.uchicago.edu/ucp/books/book/chicago/E/bo27035179.html
Malloch, S. N. (1999). Mothers and infants and communicative musicality. *Musicae Scientiae*, *3*(Suppl. 1), 29–57.	https://doi.org/10.1177/10298649000030S104
Malloch, S., & Trevarthen, C. (Eds.). (2009a). *Communicative musicality: Exploring the basis of human companionship*. Oxford University Press	https://www.amazon.com/Communicative-Musicality-Exploring-basis-companionship/dp/0199588724
Malloch, S., & Trevarthen, C. (2018). The human nature of music. *Frontiers in Psychology, 9*, 1680.	https://doi.org/10.3389/fpsyg.2018.01680
Mayo, O., & Gordon, I. (2020). In and out of synchrony—Behavioral and physiological dynamics of dyadic interpersonal coordination. *Psychophysiology, 57*(6), e13574.	https://doi.org/10.1111/psyp.13574
Orkand, S. C. (2020). Dance/movement as resilience, unity and community in Rwanda: Shared experience over difference. *American Journal of Dance Therapy, 42*(1), 5–15.	https://doi.org/10.1007/s10465-020-09325-8
Osborne, N. (2009). Music for children in zones of conflict and post-conflict: A psychobiological approach. In S. Malloch, & C. Trevarthen (Eds.), *Communicative musicality: Exploring the basis of human companionship* (pp. 545–564). Oxford University Press.	https://www.amazon.com/Communicative-Musicality-Exploring-basis-companionship/dp/0199588724

Ramseyer, F., & Tschacher, W. (2011). Nonverbal synchrony in psychotherapy: Coordinated body movement reflects relationship quality and outcome. *Journal of Consulting and Clinical Psychology, 79*(3), 284–295.	https://doi.org/10.1037/a0023419
Rolef Ben-Shahar, A. (2012). The relational turn and body psychotherapy IV. Gliding on the strings that connect us: Resonance in relational body psychotherapy. *International Body Psychotherapy Journal: The Art and Science of Somatic Praxis, 11*(1), 12–24.	https://www.ibpj.org/issues/articles/Rolef%20Ben-Shahar%20-%20The%20Relational%20Turn%20and%20Body%20Psychotherapy.pdf
Sheets-Johnstone, M. (1999a). Emotion and movement: A beginning empirical-phenomenological analysis of their relationship. *Journal of Consciousness Studies, 6*(11–12), 259–277.	https://philpapers.org/rec/SHEEAM
Sheets-Johnstone, M. (2011a). Embodied minds or mindful bodies? A question of fundamental, inherently inter-related aspects of animation. *Subjectivity, 4*(4), 451–466.	https://doi.org/10.1057/sub.2011.21
Spagnuolo Lobb, M. (2020). Gestalt therapy during coronavirus: Sensing the experiential ground and "dancing" with reciprocity. *The Humanistic Psychologist, 48*(4), 397–409.	https://doi.org/10.1037/hum0000228
Tanaka, S. (2015). Intercorporeality as a theory of social cognition. *Theory & Psychology, 25*(4), 455–472.	https://doi.org/10.1177/0959354315583035
Tortora, S. (2006). *The dancing dialogue: Using the communicative power of movement with young children*. Paul H. Brookes.	https://www.suzitortora.com/publication/2017/9/11/the-dancing-dialogue-using-the-communicative-power-of-movement-with-young-children-2006
Trevarthen, C. & Malloch, S. (2000). The dance of wellbeing: Defining the musical therapeutic effect. *Norwegian Journal of Music Therapy, 9*(2), 3–17.	https://www.researchgate.net/publication/249064480_The_Dance_of_Wellbeing_Defining_the_Musical_Therapeutic_Effect
Vanaerschot, G. (1997). Empathic resonance as a source of experience-enhancing interventions. In A. C. Bohart, & L. S. Greenberg (Eds.), *Empathy reconsidered: New directions in psychotherapy* (pp. 141–165). American Psychological Association.	https://psycnet.apa.org/doi/10.1037/10226-006
Shorer, M., & Leibovich, L. (2020). Young children's emotional stress reactions during the COVID-19 outbreak and their associations with parental emotion regulation and parental playfulness. *Early Child Development and Care*. Advanced Online Publication.	https://doi.org/10.1080/03004430.2020.1806830

Bray, P. (2010). A broader framework for exploring the influence of spiritual experience in the wake of stressful life events: Examining connections between post-traumatic growth and psycho-spiritual transformation. *Mental Health, Religion and Culture*, *13*, 293–330.	https://pubmed.ncbi.nlm.nih.gov/21948147/
Bray, P. (2013). Bereavement and transformation: A psycho-spiritual and post-traumatic growth perspective. *Journal of Religion and Health 52*(3), 890–903.	https://doi.org/10.1007/s10943-011-9539-8
Courtois, C. A. (2017). Spiritual challenges resulting from trauma: Implications for inclusive psychotherapy. In S. N. Gold (Ed.), *APA handbook of trauma psychology: Foundations in knowledge* (Vol. 1, pp. 559–572). American Psychological Association.	https://doi.org/10.1037/0000019-028
Abram, D. (1996). *The spell of the sensuous: Perception and language in a more-than-human world.* Vintage.	https://www.amazon.com/Spell-Sensuous-Perception-Language-More-Than-Human/dp/0679776397
Andrews, T. (2010). *Animal speak: The spiritual & magical powers of creatures great and small.* Llewellyn Publications.	https://www.amazon.com/Animal-Speak-Spiritual-Magical-Creatures-ebook/dp/B007GAYNLY
Atkinson, R. (1995). *The gift of stories: Practical and spiritual applications of autobiography, life stories and personal mythmaking*. Bergan & Garvey.	https://www.amazon.com/Gift-Stories-Applications-Autobiography-Mythmaking/dp/089789443X
Bouse, K., J. (2019). *Neo-shamanism and mental health.* Palgrave Macmillan.	https://doi.org/10.1007/978-3-030-31911-3
Cajete, G. A. (2017). Children, myth and storytelling: An Indigenous perspective. *Global Studies of Childhood, 7*(2), 113–130.	https://doi.org/10.1177/2043610617703832
Dunlea, M. (2019). *BodyDreaming in the treatment of developmental trauma: An embodied therapeutic approach.* Routledge.	https://www.amazon.com/BodyDreaming-Treatment-Developmental-Trauma-Therapeutic/dp/0367025930
Etherington, K. (Ed.). (2003). *Trauma, the body and transformation: A narrative inquiry*. Jessica Kingsley.	https://www.amazon.com/Trauma-Body-Transformation-Narrative-Inquiry/dp/1843101068
Feinstein, D., & Krippner, S. (2008). *Personal mythology: Discovering the guiding stories of your past—creating a vision for your future*. Energy Psychology Press.	https://www.amazon.com/Personal-Mythology-Psychology-Your-Evolving/dp/0874774837
Hansen, M. M., Jones, R., & Tocchini, K. (2017). Shinrin-Yoku (Forest Bathing) and nature therapy: A state-of-the-art review. *International Journal of Environmental Research and Public Health*, *14*(8), 851.	https://doi.org/10.3390/ijerph14080851
Harjo, J. (2021). *Poet warrior: A memoir.* Norton.	
Hart, T. (2003). *The secret spiritual world of children*. New World Library.	https://www.amazon.com/Secret-Spiritual-World-Children-Breakthrough/dp/1930722192

Kalsched, D. (2013b). *Trauma and the soul. A psycho-spiritual approach to human development and its interruption.* Routledge.	https://www.amazon.com/Trauma-Soul-psycho-spiritual-development-interruption/dp/0415681464
Lincoln, V. (2000). Ecospirituality: A pattern that connects. *Journal of Holistic Nursing, 18*(3), 227–244.	https://journals.sagepub.com/doi/10.1177/089801010001800305
Ross, S. L. (2020). *The map to wholeness: Real-life stories of crisis, change, and reinvention—Your guide through the 13 phases of transformation*. North Atlantic Books.	https://www.amazon.com/Map-Wholeness-Real-Life-Reinvention-Your-Transformation/dp/1623173825
Rust, M.-J. (2020). *Towards an ecopsychotherapy*. Confer Books.	https://www.amazon.com/Towards-Ecopsychotherapy-Mary-Jane-Rust/dp/1913494128
Simard, S. (2021). *Finding the mother tree: Discovering the wisdom of the forest.* Knopf Doubleday.	https://www.amazon.com/Finding-Mother-Tree-Discovering-Wisdom/dp/052565609X
Slattery, D. P. (2000). *The wounded body: Remembering the markings of flesh*. SUNY.	https://sunypress.edu/Books/T/The-Wounded-Body
Slattery, D. P. (2012). *Riting myth, mythic writing: Plotting your personal story*. Fisher King Press.	https://www.tandfonline.com/doi/abs/10.1080/00332925.2012.731924
SunWolf. (2004). Once upon a time for the soul: A review of the effects of storytelling in spiritual traditions. *Communication Research Trends, 23*(3), 3–19.	http://cscc.scu.edu/trends/v23/v23_3.pdf
Vaughan-Lee, L. (Ed.), (2013). *Spiritual ecology: The cry of the earth, a collection of essays.* The Golden Sufi Center.	https://www.amazon.com/Spiritual-Ecology-Earth-Llewellyn-Vaughan-Lee/dp/1941394140
Wohlleben, P. (2021). *The heartbeat of trees: Embracing our ancient bond with forests and nature* (J. Billinghurst, Trans.). Greystone Books.	https://www.amazon.com/Heartbeat-Trees-Embracing-Ancient-Forests/dp/1771646896

Somatic and Creative Arts Therapies

Celebrating Creative Arts Therapies and Child Life Services	https://www.bchcreativearts.org/blog
To the core	https://aeon.co/essays/art-like-loss-can-shock-us-into-our-authentic-self
Art Therapy in Pandemics: Lessons for COVID-19 by Jordan S. Potash, Debra Kalmanowitz, Ivy Fung, Susan A. Anand, and Gretchen M. Mille	https://doi.org/10.1080/07421656.2020.1754047
Life, death and transformation: Keep moving by Fulya Kurter, Elcin Bicer, Elyan Aysoy, and Ilene Serlin	https://doi.org/10.1386/jaah.7.1.107_1
Responding to natural and manmade disaster with dance movement therapy by Ilene Serlin	https://doi.org/10.1386/jaah.9.2.203_1
Healing Intergenerational Trauma with Dance Movement Therapy by Ilene Serlin, PhD, BC-DMT	https://traumapsychnews.com/2017/05/healing-intergenerational-trauma-with-dance-movement-therapy/
Embodiment in Existential/Humanistic Psychology in China by Dr. Ilene Serlin	http://www.apadivisions.org/division-32/publications/newsletters/humanistic/2018/07/art-embodiment.aspx
Expressive and Creative Arts Therapies by Kim A. Bella and Ilene A. Serlin	https://doi.org/10.1002/9781118591277.ch29
Dance/Movement Therapy, Edited by Irving B. Weiner & W. Edward Craighead in The Corsini Encyclopedia of Psychology, Volume 4	https://www.amazon.com/Corsini-Encyclopedia-Psychology-4/dp/0470170239
Finding Ground in the Swirl with Ambar Gray	https://soundcloud.com/sharon-weil/finding-ground-in-the-swirl-with-amber-gray
Dance to Health Volunteer Evaluation Report 2019	https://dancetohealth.org/volunteer-evaluation-report-2019/
Dance to Health, Phase 1 roll-out "test and learn" evaluation report	https://ae-sop.org/wp-content/uploads/sites/63/2020/06/AESOP-Dance-to-Health-Phase-1-Overall-evaluation-Report-April-2020-FINAL.pdf
Tend Your Orchard, Cece Carpio and Miguel "Bounce" Perez of Trust Your Struggle	https://ybca.org/event/tend-your-orchard
Where the Hell is Matt? 2012	https://www.youtube.com/watch?v=Pwe-pA6TaZk
Whole Person Care for the Traumatized: Building Resiliency and Self-Care in Response to the Coronavirus [China Hotline]	https://youtu.be/nHuI0CU4ezQ
Ilene Serlin: How to Learn the Secrets of the Body in Dance Movement Therapy & Know Yourself Better	https://www.youtube.com/watch?v=4Qst9wunB3U&feature=youtu.be

Dance Movement Therapy, Beijing, China	https://www.youtube.com/watch?v=l9ijMORiBXI
Haka Dance with Dr. Ilene Serlin, PhD, BC-DMT	https://www.youtube.com/watch?v=ocDL6RXjRTw
Spiral Dance with Ilene Serlin	https://www.youtube.com/watch?v=wLpLFk3qBhw
Creative Arts Therapies in Palliative Care and Late Old Age	https://docs.google.com/forms/d/e/1FAIpQLSfjqwPGsJ6U4AV2AQf-ymHCIWAuKLUANblTkCeQZSQre_iVzg/viewform
Waking up the bear: Dance/movement therapy group model with depressed adult patients during COVID-19 2020	https://library.psychology.edu/wp-files/uploads/2020/12/Waking-up-the-Bear-Sheerie-Lotan-Mesika.pdf
Arts and Therapy in the Time of the Pandemic	https://sites.edgehill.ac.uk/rcaw/2020/05/27/online-international-event/
Screen–bridges: dance movement therapy in online contexts	Garcia-medrano, S., & Garcia-medrano, S. (2021). Screen–bridges: Dance movement therapy in online contexts contexts.*Body, Movement and Dance in Psychotherapy, 16*(1), 65–73. https://doi.org/10.1080/17432979.2021.1883741
Coping with the Covid-19 lockdown through dance movement therapy	Re, M. (2021). Isolated systems towards a dancing constellation: Coping with the Covid-19 lockdown through a pilot dance movement therapy tele-intervention.*Body, Movement and Dance in Psychotherapy, 16*(1), 9–19. https://doi.org/10.1080/17432979.2021.1879934
	See 2020-21 references to scholarly papers regarding the use of arts for healing The use of arts for healing -Publications during COVID (2020-1)
The Arts in Psychotherapy Tele-psychodrama therapy during the COVID-19 pandemic	Biancalani, G., Franco, C., Silvia, M., Moretto, L., Orkibi, H., Keisari, S., & Testoni, I. (2021). Tele-psychodrama therapy during the COVID-19 pandemic: Participants' experiences.*The Arts in Psychotherapy, 75*(July), 101836.
Shifting to tele-creative arts therapies during the COVID-19 pandemic	Feniger-Schaal, R., Orkibi, H., Keisari, S., Sajnani, N. L., & Butler, J. D. (2022). Shifting to tele-creative arts therapies during the COVID-19 pandemic: An international study on helpful and challenging factors.*The Arts in Psychotherapy, 78*(February), 101898.
Creative Adaptability: Conceptual Framework, Measurement, and Outcomes in Times of Crisis	https://www.frontiersin.org/articles/10.3389/fpsyg.2020.588172/full
Creative Adaptability and Emotional Well-Being During the COVID-19 Pandemic	Orkibi, H., Ben-Eliyahu, A., Reiter-Palmon, R., Testoni, I., Biancalani, G., Murugavel, V., & Gu, F. (2021). Creative adaptability and emotional well-being during the COVID-19 pandemic: An international study.*Psychology of Aesthetics, Creativity, and the Arts.*

Tuber, S., Da Costa, R., Eidman, J., Feldman, H., Hadar, O., Kaur, N., Zanotti, P., Schulder, T., & Tocatly, K. (2022). Dialectical reflections on the advantages and disadvantages of tele-play therapy. *Journal of Infant, Child, and Adolescent Psychotherapy, 21*(1), 19–26.	https://doi.org/10.1080/15289168.2022.2043058
The Arts and COVID-19: A Time of Danger and Opportunity?	https://sites.edgehill.ac.uk/rcaw/2020/04/29/the-arts-and-covid-19-a-time-of-danger-and-opportunity/
Art Therapy in Pandemics: Lessons for COVID-19	https://www.tandfonline.com/doi/full/10.1080/07421656.2020.1754047
Whole Person Care for Traumatized: Building Resiliency & Self-Care in Response to the Coronavirus by Dr. Ilene A. Serlin	https://youtu.be/nHuI0CU4ezQ
Dance movement therapy in Beijing by Dr. Ilene A. Serlin	https://www.youtube.com/watch?v=l9ijMORiBXI&feature=youtu.be
Ilene Serlin interviewed by Dr. Mark Yang, Beijing Center for Training and Education Beijing, China May 10, 2018	https://www.youtube.com/watch?v=qu2GFoFYwM4&feature=youtu.be
Trauma-Informed Practices and Expressive Arts Therapy Institute	https://www.trauma-informedpractice.com
Braus, M., & Morton, B. (2020). Art therapy in the time of COVID-19. *Psychological Trauma: Theory, Research, Practice, and Policy, 12*(S1), S267–S268.	https://psycnet.apa.org/record/2020-37310-001
Expressive Arts Therapy, Trauma-Informed Online Learning Courses with Cathy Malchiodi	https://www.trauma-informedpractice.com/online-live-courses

References

Several books released during the pandemic are excellent resources for helpers and those seeking to learn more about trauma, wellness, and becoming more embodied. Here are a few of our favorites: *The Whole-Person Approach to Integrated Health Care*; *Trauma and Expressive Arts Therapy: Brain, Body, and Imagination in the Healing Process*; and *Becoming Safely Embodied: A Guide to Organize Your Mind, Body and Heart to Feel Secure in the World.* A wealth of resources also available on social media platforms are Transforming the Experience-Based Brain, International Whole Person Approaches (COVID WG), COVID IPV, and ATTCH Niagara Caring Community Connections. The Attachment and Trauma Treatment Centre for Healing's wide variety of trauma-informed mindfulness and emotional regulation resources to promote embodied awareness, wellness, and stress reduction is available on their YouTube channel. The Mindful Living Collective is an excellent resource offering free groups and programs like conscious connection circles that provide an opportunity to connect to others in a meaningful way. Jamie McHugh provides resources inviting an immersive sensory and embodied experience on his site http://somaticexpression.com.

Ali, D. A., Figley, C. R., Tedeschi, R. G., Galarneau, D., & Amara, S. (2021). Shared trauma, resilience, and growth: A roadmap toward transcultural conceptualization. *Psychological Trauma: Theory, Research, Practice, and Policy, 15*(1), 45–55. Advance online publication. https://doi.org/10.1037/tra0001044

American Psychological Association. (n.d.). *APA dictionary of psychology*. https://dictionary.apa.org/resilience

Anderson, R. (2001). Embodied writing and reflections on embodiment. *The Journal of Transpersonal Psychology, 33*(2), 83–98.

Bentley, P. G. (2022). Compassion practice as an antidote for compassion fatigue in the era of COVID-19. *Journal of Humanistic Counseling, 61*, 1–16. https://doi.org/10.1002/johc.12172

Calhoun, L. G., & Tedeschi, R. G. (1999). *Facilitating posttraumatic growth: A clinician's guide*. Erlbaum.

Calhoun, L. G., & Tedeschi, R. G. (2006). *Handbook of post-traumatic growth: Research and practice*. Psychology Press.

Carey, L. (Ed.). (2006). *Expressive and creative arts methods for trauma survivors*. Jessica Kingsley.

Carroll, R. (2005). Finding the words to say it: The healing power of poetry. *Evidenced-Based Complementary and Alternative Medicine, 2*(2), 161–172. https://doi.org/10.1093/ecam/neh096

Figley, C. R. (Ed.). (2002). *Treating compassion fatigue*. Brunner-Routledge.

Frank, R. (2020). Developing presence online. *The Humanistic Psychologist, 48*(4), 369–372. https://doi.org/10.1037/hum0000208

Gill, L. (2015). *Integrative Trauma and Attachment Treatment Model® (ITATM) manual: Sensory regulation to integrate the brain, mind, and body*.

Graber, L. M. (2016). Embodiment, music, and music making: A body arts whole person approach to trauma. In I. Serlin (Chair), *Embodiment: Roots of humanistic psychology*. Workshop presented at the 9th Annual Conference of the Society for Humanistic Psychology (American Psychological Association, Division 32), San Francisco, CA.

Graber, L. M. (2017). The rhythms of life & healing: Sound, rhythm & movement. In I. A. Serlin, M. B. Leventhal, & L. M. Graber (Eds.), *Healing international populations through movement*. Workshop presented at the Expressive Therapies Summit: Creativity and the Arts in Healing, Los Angeles, CA.

Graber, L. M. (2021). *Embodiment in online therapy*. Interpersonal Violence (IPV) Roundtables: APA COVID-19 Task Force IPV Workgroup.

Graber, L. M., & Rosemond, K. V. (2015). *Embodiment and cultural expressions of trauma and healing: Transformation through body poetry and embodied writing*. Workshop presented at the 12th International Erickson Congress, Phoenix, AZ.

Gratier, M., & Trevarthen, C. (2008). Musical narrative and motives for culture in mother-infant vocal interaction. *The Journal of Consciousness Studies, 15*(10–11), 122–158.

Hansen, M. M., Jones, R., & Tocchini, K. (2017). Shinrin-Yoku (Forest Bathing) and nature therapy: A state-of-the-art review. *International Journal of Environmental Research and Public Health, 14*(8), 851. https://doi.org/10.3390/ijerph14080851

Hernik, J., & Jaworska, E. (2018). The effect of enjoyment on learning. In J. Hernik & E. Jaworska (Eds.), *Proceedings of INTED2018 conference* (pp. 508–514). IATED Academy. https://doi.org/10.21125/inted.2018.1087

Hoffman, L. (2021). Existential–humanistic therapy and disaster response: Lessons from the Covid-19 pandemic. *Journal of Humanistic Psychology, 61*(1), 33–54. https://doi.org/10.1177/0022167820931987

Joseph, S., & Linley, P. A. (2006). Growth following adversity: Theoretical perspectives and implications for clinical practice. *Clinical Psychology Review, 26*, 1041–1053.

Khanal, S., & Kuriansky, J. (2022). Promoting resilience in the Nepali community in response to the COVID-19 pandemic: A multistage multistakeholder partnership addressing goals of the United Nations 2030 Agenda. In J. Kuriansky & P. Kakkattil (Eds.), *Resilient health: Leveraging technology and social innovations to transform healthcare for COVID-19 recovery and beyond*. Elsevier.

Kuriansky, J. (2008). A clinical toolbox for cross-cultural counseling and training. In U. P. Gielen, J. G. Draguns, & J. M. Fish (Eds.), *Principles of multicultural counseling and therapy* (pp. 295–330). Taylor and Francis/Routledge.

Kuriansky, J. (2019). Expressive arts for helping children heal in crisis and disaster. In I. A. Serlin, S. Krippner, & K. Rockefeller (Eds.), *Integrated health care for the traumatized: A whole person approach*. Rowman & Littlefield.

Kuriansky, J., & Kakkattil, P. (Eds.). (2022). *Resilient health: Leveraging technology and social innovations to transform healthcare for COVID-19 recovery and beyond*. Elsevier.

Kuriansky, J., Polizer, Y., & Zinsou, J. (2016). Children and Ebola: A model resilience and empowerment training and workshop. In J. Kuriansky (Ed.), *The psychosocial aspects of a deadly epidemic: What Ebola has taught us about holistic healing* (pp. 175–214). ABC-CLIO/Praeger.

Kuriansky, J., Bazibuhe, J. M., Cullimore, B., Vossen, D., Kikuni, L., Imani, F., Tapper, G., Evans, S., Ray, E., & da Cruz, L. (2022). Responding to COVID-19 in the Democratic Republic of the Congo: A community-based model of holistic health education, psychosocial support, and myth correction. In J. Kuriansky & P. Kakkattil (Eds.), *Resilient health: Leveraging technology and social innovations to transform healthcare for COVID-19 recovery and beyond*. Elsevier.

Kurter, F., Bicer, E., Aysoy, E., & Serlin, I. (2016). Life, death and transformation: Keep moving. *Journal of Applied Arts & Health, 7*(1), 107–116.

Lakoff, G., & Johnson, M. (1999). *Philosophy in the flesh: How the embodied mind challenges the western tradition*. Basic Books.

Lev, M. (2022). *Artmaking resilience: Reflections on art-based research of bereavement and grief*. Creative Arts in Education and Therapy (CAET), pp. 126–138. Retrieved from https://caet.inspirees.com/caetojsjournals/index.php/caet/article/view/379

May, R. (1975). *The courage to create*. Bantam Books.

McHugh, J. (2017). *Embodying nature, becoming ourselves: A somatic-expressive journey*. http://www.somaticexpression.com/articles/EmbodyingNature.html

Neff, K. D. (2011). *Self-compassion*. William Morrow.

Nugent, N. R., Sumner, J. A., & Amstadter, A. B. (2014). Resilience after trauma: From surviving to thriving. *European Journal of Psychotraumatology, 5*, 25339. https://doi.org/10.3402/ejpt.v5.25339. PMID: 25317260; PMCID: PMC4185140.

Pardess, E. (2022). *Cultivating creativity & compassion: COVID-19 as a transformative opportunity.* Pardes 2022 Cultivating Creativity & Compassion – COVID-19.

Pardess, E., Mikulincer, M., Dekel, R., & Shaver, P. (2014). Dispositional attachment orientations, contextual variations in attachment security, and compassion fatigue among volunteers working with traumatized individuals. *Journal of Personality, 82*(5), 355–366. https://doi.org/10.1111/jopy.12060

Parks, S., Kuriansky, J., & Koch, P. (2022). Confronting the crisis of COVID-19: Evolution of a model for preservation of people and the planet. *International Perspectives in Psychology, 11*(3), 188–196. https://doi.org/10.1027/2157-3891/a000053

Pennebaker, J. W., & Evans, J. (2014). *Expressive writing: Words that heal*. Idyll Arbor.

Peper, E., Harvey, R., & Faass, N. (2020). *Tech stress: How technology is hijacking our lives, strategies for coping, and pragmatic ergonomics*. North Atlantic Books.

Porges, S. W. (2020). The COVID-19 pandemic is a paradoxical challenge to our nervous system: A polyvagal perspective. *Clinical Neuropsychiatry, 17*(2), 135–138. https://doi.org/10.36131/CN20200220

Porges, S. W. (2021). *Polyvagal safety: Attachment, communication, self-regulation*. Norton.

Potash, J., Kalmanowitz, D., Fung, I., Anand, S., & Miller, G. (2020). Art therapy in pandemics: Lessons for COVID-19. *Journal of the American Art Therapy Association, 37*(2), 105–107. https://doi.org/10.1080/07421656.2020.1754047

Pressley, J., & Spinazzola, J. (2020). *Coping strategies for complex trauma survivors contending with the coronavirus (COVID-19) pandemic*. Retrieved from https://www.complextrauma.org/wp-content/uploads/2020/04/Complex-Trauma-Resource-9-Joseph-Spinazzola.pdf

Schneider, K. J., Pierson, J., & Bugental, J. T. (Eds.). (2015). *The handbook of humanistic psychology: Theory, research, and practice* (2nd ed.). SAGE Publications.

Serlin, I. (2006). The use of the arts to work with trauma in Israel. *The San Francisco Psychologist*, 8–9.

Serlin, I. A. (2007). *Whole person healthcare* (3 volumes). Praeger.
Serlin, I. A. (2012). The courage to move. In S. Schwartz, V. Marcow Speiser, P. Speiser, & M. Kossak (Eds.), *The arts and social change: The Lesley University experience in Israel* (pp. 117–125). Porat Books.
Serlin, I. A., & Cannon, J. (2004). A humanistic approach to the psychology of trauma. In D. Knafo (Ed.), *Living with terror, working with trauma: A clinician's handbook* (pp. 313–331). Jason Aronson.
Serlin, I., Figley, C., & Pardess, R. (2013). *Developing resiliency: Compassion fatigue and regeneration*. American Psychological Association.
Serlin, I., Krippner, S., & Rockefeller, K. (Eds.). (2019). *Integrated care for the traumatized*. Rowman & Littlefield.
Simard, S. (2021). *Finding the mother tree: Discovering the wisdom of the forest*. Knopf Doubleday.
Stier-Jarmer, M., Throner, V., Kirschneck, M., Immich, G., Frisch, D., & Schuh, A. (2021). The psychological and physical effects of forests on human health: A systematic review of systematic reviews and meta-analyses. *International Journal of Environmental Research and Public Health, 18*(4), 1770. https://doi.org/10.3390/ijerph18041770
van der Kolk, B. (2014). *The body keeps the score: Brain, mind and body in the healing of trauma*. Penguin Books.
Zimmerman, J., & Beaudoin, M. (2015). Neurobiology for your narrative: How brain science can influence narrative work. *Journal of Systemic Therapies, 34*(2), 59–74. https://doi.org/10.1521/jsyt.2015.34.2.59

Ilene A. Serlin, Ph.D, BC-DMT, psychologist, dance therapist, Fellow APA, Past-Pres.SF Psych. Assoc., Past-Pres. Society of Humanistic Psychology of APA, (Gen. Ed.) *Whole Person Healthcare*, (Co-Ed) *Integrated Care for the Traumatized.* International teacher and trainer.

Judy Kuriansky, Ph.D., represents NGOs at UN, first responder in disasters worldwide, award-winning TV reporter and radio call-in advice talk host, author many books including Israeli-Palestinian conflict, Technology and Social Innovations for post-COVID-19 recovery.

Lori Gill, RP, MACP, CTIC, founder Attachment and Trauma Treatment Centre for Healing and the creator of the Integrative Trauma and Attachment Treatment Model (ITATM)®. Trauma and Attachment Therapist, International Trainer, Consultant, & Subject Matter Expert.

Lawrence Graber, MA, CBBP, psychotherapist in Santa Monica, CA specializing in arts and body-based psychotherapy for posttraumatic stress, couple therapy, clinical hypnosis, medical psychology, dance and creative arts. Certified body psychotherapist in Biodynamic Psychology.

Hattie Worboys, Founder, Artistic Director of Body Talks Movement C.I.C. Artist, educator focusing on choreography, movement research, video/sound art, creating participatory, inclusive multi-disciplinary, creative workshops, video-art-installation and film.

Amy Li, Founder of Dance4Healing, a behavior-centered telehealth social venture leading telehealth into physical rehabilitation. A graduate from Singularity University, on the board of directors of Humanity+.

Patricia Villavicencio Carrillo, Ph.D, Health psychologist and Clinical Psychologist Specialist at Hospital Clinico San Carlos de Madrid, associate professor at the Department of Clinical Psychology of Complutense University of Madrid, coordinator of the Uganda EMDR team.

Rita M. Rivera, M.S., CTP, Chair American Academy of Clinical Psych-Division of Graduate Students (AACP-DGS), Student Rep APA's Society of Group Psychology and Group Psychotherapy (Div. 49), Past Chair of the Florida Psych Assoc Graduate Students (FPAGS).

Chapter 9
International Student Collaborations on COVID-19

Rita M. Rivera, David Benitez, Gabriel L. Medianero Araúz, and Tarah Coppolino

International Student Collaborations on COVID-19 Through the Higher Education

The Higher Education Work Group is part of the COVID-19 Psychology Task Force, which was established by 14 divisions of the American Psychological Association. The Higher Education Work Group is the only division of the Task Force that is completely led by psychology students and trainees. As students, clinicians, and researchers, members of the Higher Education Work Group were initially drawn to the COVID-19 Psychology Task Force due to the APA's reputation as the leading psychological organization in the country, if not the world. Hence, members sought to collaborate with APA-affiliated divisions and organizations to support initiatives that empower and improve, strengthen, and advance the student community amid the coronavirus crisis.

R. M. Rivera (✉)
Duke University, Durham, NC, USA

D. Benitez
Department of Clinical Psychology, Albizu University, Miami, FL, USA

G. L. Medianero Araúz
Department of Psychology, Universidad de Panama, Panama City, Panama

T. Coppolino
Department of Psychology, William James College, Newton, MA, USA

C. R. Figley et al. (eds.), *Pandemic Providers*,
https://doi.org/10.1007/978-3-031-27580-7_9

The Higher Education Working Group Origin Story

Before COVID-19, students already experienced stress and were vulnerable to various mental health issues such as anxiety and depression. It became clear that the pandemic heightened many preexisting issues and presented new challenges. The review of public health research reveals that it rarely captures the effects of worldwide events on students, so the Higher Education Work Group decided to elevate psychology student voices to understand how COVID-19 impacted and continues to affect students' educational pursuits.

The Higher Education Work Group was established in the spring of 2020 after a group of psychology students and trainees became part of the larger APA Interdivisional COVID-19 Task Force. The Higher Education WG proceeded to establish social media platforms, particularly a Facebook group and an email listserv that was the primary means of communication between members. During 2020, the group met regularly, about twice a month, and worked to identify their main initiatives. The first chair of the Higher Education Work Group was Rita M. Rivera, who also led efforts to develop the group. In January of 2022, David Benitez became co-chair with Ms. Rivera, and in March 2022, Gabriel Medianero joined the leadership team as the Representative for International Affairs. Ms. Tarah Coppolino, who has been one of the group's original members since its formation in 2020, transitioned from student to early career professional in 2021. As such, Ms. Coppolino serves as the ECP representative of the work group.

A scholar-activist lens, rooted in equity and social justice, informed the following initiatives:

- Promoting individual and community physical health and well-being. Students under significant stress are susceptible to neglecting their health as they fulfill their academic and personal responsibilities. The added stress of trying to meet educational requirements, such as practicum hours, while many institutions were closed to outsiders, made education more difficult. We openly advocated for community care efforts that foster overall well-being and resilience among students. The group has utilized social media to promote tools and resources tailored for students of different backgrounds, as well as provide support to encourage physical and emotional wellness as we all experience the pandemic.
- Academic and institutional justice. COVID-19 continues to have deleterious consequences in the academic world. Students encounter many obstacles that can hinder their education, academic success, professional development, and careers. These included residence halls that closed when universities went online requiring new housing; new methods of learning using Zoom, Blackboard, Canvas, and other digital platforms; difficulty in obtaining sufficient internet or computer access; and lack of available tutorials or study groups. The lack of informal learning or access to professors limited students' ability to develop important contacts for future job recommendations. We tried to identify possible solutions to ameliorate social injustices and diminish the pandemic's impact on students' education.

- Research as a social justice tool. The working group gathered information from graduate psychology students across the United States to assess their concerns and needs during the initial stages of the COVID-19 pandemic. Preliminary analyses suggest that students reported concerns regarding transitioning back to face-to-face instruction, financial resources, and fulfilling graduation requirements on time (e.g., practicum and internship hours, defending dissertations, course completion). Students also expressed concern regarding lack of accommodations from their institutions, practicum/internship sites, and academic programs.

Mission Statement

The Higher Education Work Group is comprised of student leaders across the country. We are dedicated to build on the strengths and resiliency of the student and trainee community and to provide resources and support during and after the COVID-19 pandemic.

Gathering Resources

Resources for each initiative were gathered through the American Psychological Association (APA) student campus ambassador Facebook group, APA Divisions listservs/newsletters, and multiple psychological associations, including the Florida Psychological Association Graduate Students (FPAGS) Division, the National Latinx Psychological Association (NLPA), the Hispanic Neuropsychological Society (HNS), the Interamerican Society of Psychology (SIP), and the Global Student Psychology Committee (GSPC). Novel uses of technology helped us recruit new members through an online poll for those interested in the group on the American Psychological Association student campus ambassador Facebook page. We used teleconferencing order to meet and communicate with other members. Gathering and emailing resources were done through listservs, and a Facebook page was created to keep up to date with other members.

Social Media Social networks became critical during the pandemic to inform (as well as misinform) the public. Mental health professionals and educators used platforms such as Facebook, Instagram, Twitter, and LinkedIn to provide resources and guide individuals during COVID-19 times. These platforms also allowed mental health professionals and trainees to disseminate information and resources that they themselves developed. As such, members of the Higher Education agreed that use of social media was vital for the WG to access and distribute resources.

National and International Psychological Associations and Organizations Members of the Higher Education WG also hold membership in several psychological organizations and societies. These include the American Psychological Association (APA) and the American Psychological Association Division of Graduate Students (APAGS), as well as the following APA Divisions: the Society for General Psychology (Div. 1); the Society for the Teaching of Psychology (Div. 2); the Society for Behavioral Neuroscience and Comparative Psychology (Div. 6); the Society for Personality and Social Psychology (Div. 8); the Society for the Psychological Study of Social Issues (SPSSI); the Society of Clinical Psychology (Div. 12); Educational Psychology (Div. 15); the Society of Counseling Psychology (Div. 17); the Society for Military Psychology (Div. 19); Adult Development and Aging (Div. 20); the Society for the Advancement of Psychotherapy (Div. 29); the State, Provincial and Territorial Psychological Association Affairs (Div. 31); the Society for the Psychology of Women (Div. 35); the Society for the Psychology of Religion and Spirituality (Div. 36); the Society for Health Psychology (Div. 38); the Society for Clinical Neuropsychology (Div. 40); the American Psychology-Law Society (Div. 41); the Society for the Psychology of Sexual Orientation and Gender Diversity (Div. 44); the Society for the Psychological Study of Culture, Ethnicity and Race (Div. 45); the Society for the Study of Peace, Conflict and Violence (Div. 48); the Society of Group Psychology and Group Psychotherapy (Div. 49); the Society of Addiction Psychology (Div. 50); International Psychology (Div. 52); the Society of Clinical Child and Adolescent Psychology (Div. 53); the Society for Prescribing Psychology (Div. 55); and Trauma Psychology (Div. 56).

Members were also affiliated and leaders of other psychological associations, including the Hispanic Neuropsychological Society (HNS), the National Latinx Psychological Association (NLPA), the American Academy of Clinical Psychology (AACP), the Interamerican Society of Psychology (SIP), the Global Student Psychology Committee (GSPC), the Florida Psychological Association (FPA), the North Carolina Psychological Association (NCPA), the Illinois Psychological Association (IPA), the American Rehabilitation Counseling Association (ARCA), the National Academy of Neuropsychology (NAN), the American Congress of Rehabilitation Medicine (ACRM), and the International Honor Society in Psychology (Psi Chi). As such, the membership of the WG was able to access and distribute resources through the social media pages of diverse organizations both in the United States and across the globe.

Developing and Disseminating Resources

Throughout the past years, members of the Higher Education Working Group collaborated with one another, as well as with other students, trainees, early career professionals, and professionals in psychology and mental health. Several products were developed and disseminated by the membership of the WG. The most significant are as follows.

Publications The membership of the Higher Education Working Group produced a wide array of articles on diverse topics pertaining to the COVID-19 impact on education. Several members used their collaborations to voice their concerns for the well-being of mental health professionals and students training amid the coronavirus pandemic (Benitez & Rivera, 2022b; Medianero et al., 2021a, 2022c; Rivera, 2021d, e, i, j; Rivera & Benitez, 2021; Rivera et al., 2022b). Some contributions were used to emphasize the significant role that trainees play in the advancement of the field of psychology (Benitez & Rivera, 2022a, d; Medianero et al., 2021b; Rivera, 2021m; Rivera & Benitez, 2020; Rivera et al., 2022b). Several of the leaders and members of the Higher Education Working Group also wrote pieces on their efforts in leading and developing student branches of psychological organizations, including the Florida Psychological Association Graduate Students (FPAGS) Division and the American Academy of Clinical Psychology-Division of Graduate Students (AACP-DGS) (Benitez & Rivera, 2022a, c; Rivera, 2021m; Rivera & Benitez, 2020). Furthermore, members also collaborated on research and articles that promoted psychological strategies for overall well-being and to reduce adverse psychological effects brought by the pandemic (Rivera, 2020a, c, 2021a, b, g, k, l; Rivera & Benitez, 2022). In addition, some articles were translated into different languages (Rivera, 2020b) or originally written in Spanish and later translated to English (Rivera et al., 2021d). Information on these articles can be accessed online through the links provided in Table 9.1.

Conference Presentations Members of the Higher Education Working Group presented their research at several international psychological conferences, including the American Psychological Convention and the Regional Congress of the Interamerican Society of Psychology. Members used these platforms to advocate for the psychological well-being of healthcare workers during the pandemic (Coppolino & Rivera, 2021), to highlight the COVID-19 impact on education throughout the globe (Medianero et al., 2022a), to promote proper training of telepsychology for psychology students (Medianero et al., 2022b), to raise awareness on the impact of the pandemic on international students in the United States (Rivera, 2021c), and to discuss ways educational programs could support students during the crisis (Rivera, 2021h; Rivera et al., 2021b, c). Some conventions recorded these presentations; recordings, posters, and papers of these professional presentations can be accessed online through the links provided in Table 9.2. Members of the working group further presented their research at Spanish-speaking conventions, such as the 2021 Interamerican Congress of Psychology in Puerto Rico, as well as at their local institutions across the United States and Latin America.

Roundtables and Webinars Members of the Higher Education Working Group participated in roundtables and webinars sponsored by several organizations, including the American Psychological Association's Division of International Psychology (Div. 52), the Global Student Psychology Committee (GSPC), the Psychology Coalition at the United Nations (PCUN), the Interamerican Society of Psychology, the Student Division of the International Association of Applied

Table 9.1 Publications

Author(s)	Title and link	Description
Benitez and Rivera (2022a)	Predoctoral Residency: Professional Psychology and Intern Clinicians – Link available	In this article, psychology student leaders seek to encourage the empowerment of interns/predoctoral residents as part of the very advancement of our discipline as an integral, irreplaceable healthcare profession
Benitez and Rivera (2022b)	Psychology Trainees May Not Be Allowed to Practice What They Preach – Link available	This article emphasizes an urgent need for clinical research focused on burnout among psychology students
Benitez and Rivera (2022d)	The Mental Health Primary Care Disconnect – Link available	This article highlights the value of integrating mental health within primary care settings
Medianero et al. (2022c)	Group Therapy in a COVID-19 Era: Strengthening Training for Psychology Students – Link available	Psychology student clinicians and leaders in group psychotherapy argue the need to augment students' preparation in group psychotherapy
Rivera (2020a)	Coronavirus Pandemic: A Trigger for Survivor's Guilt? – Link available	This article focuses on describing how the coronavirus pandemic can trigger survivor guilt. The author highlights the psychological and physiological symptomatology of this syndrome and provides strategies and interventions that can be applied to reduce these effects
Rivera (2020c)	The Psychology of Problem-Solving Amid the Coronavirus Pandemic – Link available	This article provides an overview of problem-solving strategies and how these can be implemented amid the pandemic
Rivera (2021a)	Benefits of virtual psychotherapy groups for students during COVID-19 – Link available	The author argues how virtual psychotherapy groups can serve as support systems for students during pandemic times while also adhering to safety regulations
Rivera (2021b)	Celebrating minority mental health awareness month amidst the COVID-19 pandemic – Link available	The author encourages mental health providers to reflect and listen to the needs of minority populations
Rivera (2021d)	COVID-19 Pandemic: Considerations for the study and practice of psychology – Link available	The author highlights the importance of collaboration between mental health providers both in practice and in the education of trainees and student clinicians
Rivera (2021g)	Fostering emotional regulation by practicing self-compassion – Link available	The author discusses the benefits of practicing self-compassion and ways to do so
Rivera (2021j)	Strategies for Psychology Students Experiencing Imposter Syndrome – Link available	This article provides strategies that can aid psychology students move past negative feelings and cope with imposter syndrome
Rivera (2021k)	The Lethal COVID-19 Pandemic Forges Resilience for Life – Link available	The author notes reflections individuals continued to contemplate a year after the declaration of COVID-19

(continued)

Table 9.1 (continued)

Author(s)	Title and link	Description
Rivera (2021l)	The Link Between Nutrition and Mental Health – Link available	This article highlights research findings between nutrition and mental health
Rivera (2021m)	The value of student membership: Supporting the next generation – Link available	The author discusses recommendations for faculty members, academics, professionals, and members interested in supporting the future generation of psychology
Rivera and Benitez (2020)	Clinicians in Training and the RxP Movement – Link available	The authors argue that as clinicians in training, it is imperative for graduate students to remain informed about initiatives that impact not only their field of study and future career but also the populations they serve
Rivera and Benitez (2021)	The Future of Mental Health Care Is Burning Out – Link available	The article conveys how student-clinicians and early career professionals are experiencing burnout and are susceptible to challenges and distress brought by COVID-19
Rivera and Benitez (2022)	Self-Care Practices for Your Daily Routine – Link available	Self-care can take many forms, but at its most basic level, it entails taking care of yourself physically, psychologically, and emotionally. This article provides self-care practices individuals can incorporate in their daily routines
Rivera et al. (2022b)	Disaster Management Amidst COVID-19: Fostering Competencies Among Psychology Trainees – Link available	This article provides strategies that can be incorporated to improve training in emergency and disaster management for psychology students
Articles in Spanish		
Medianero et al. (2021a)	Creación de vínculos educativos y colaborativos entre pares: Aprendiendo de la pandemia del Coronavirus a través del diálogo y la diversidad – Link available	Psychology students share their experiences amid the pandemic, particularly the development of collaborations between trainees across different countries
Medianero et al. (2021b)	Experiencias positivas durante la pandemia o derivadas de ésta. Formación en telepsicología: Una necesidad para nuestra profesión – Link available	During the COVID-19 lockdowns, telehealth boomed as a way to maintain care and assistance in one of the most complex times in recent history. The authors reflect on the need for telepsychology training.
Rivera (2021e)	COVID-19 y síndrome del impostor: ¿La pandemia agrava el fenómeno para los estudiantes? – Link available	The author discusses how because of the pandemic, students have encountered many obstacles that can hinder their education, academic success, professional development, careers, and, most importantly, their physical and psychological well-being
Rivera et al. (2021d)	Relación entre mentores profesionales y estudiantes: Consideraciones ante el COVID-19 – Link available	This article highlights ways faculty members and academic mentors can support students and trainees during the pandemic

Table 9.2 Conference presentations

Author(s)	Title and link	Description
Coppolino and Rivera (2021)	Art therapy & self-efficacy: The role of burnout among healthcare workers battling COVID-19 – Link available	Results from this systematic review revealed that art therapy techniques can help reduce feelings of burnout across healthcare workers
Rivera (2021c)	COVID-19 impact on international students in the US – Link available	In this symposium, PsyD candidate and international student Rita M. Rivera discusses several ways in which the pandemic affected international students pursuing their education in the United States
Rivera (2021h)	Imposter syndrome: Supporting students during the COVID-19 pandemic	In this symposium, PsyD candidate and international student Rita M. Rivera discusses evidence-based strategies for helping students experiencing imposter syndrome
Rivera et al. (2021c)	Factors that influence the relationship between mentors and students: The impact of COVID-19 in higher education and mentorship	Student leaders from the Interamerican Psychological Society [Sociedad Interamericana de Psicología] present their findings on the role of mentorship in students' academic success and emotional well-being
Conference presentations in Spanish		
Medianero et al. (2022a)	Impacto del COVID-19 en la educación de Panamá, Honduras, y El Salvador [COVID-19 Impact in the education of Panama, Honduras, and El Salvador]	Findings of this systematic review showed that the pandemic increased illiteracy rates in El Salvador, Panama, and Honduras. Individuals from low and medium socioeconomic continue to face obstacles in their activities educational in these nations
Medianero et al. (2022b)	Consideraciones en telepsicología desde la experiencia estudiantil [Considerations for the use of telepsychology: Perspective of student clinicians]	In this symposium, psychology student clinicians discuss the use of telepsychology amid the COVID-19 pandemic and the importance of implementing proper training in psychology programs

Psychology, and the Asociación IberoAmericana de Neurociencias y Psiquiatría. Members also participated in webinars sponsored by several academic institutions, including Albizu University-Miami Campus, Albizu University-San Juan Campus, the Universidad Tecnológica de El Salvador, and the Universidad de Panama. At some of these events, members highlighted the impact of the COVID-19 pandemic on student populations (Rivera, 2021f), the value of student-led collaborations (Aganan et al., 2022; Rivera, 2022a, c), and the role of psychology trainees in the internalization of psychology (Rivera et al., 2021a, 2022a). Recordings of some of these roundtables and webinars can be accessed from Table 9.3.

Table 9.3 Roundtables and webinars

Author(s)	Title and link	Description
Aganan et al. (2022)	Advocacy, Community Engagement, and Social Change: Perspectives from Student Leaders Across the Globe – Link available	Student leaders of the International Council of Psychologists (ICP), the Global Student Psychology Committee (GSPC), APA Division 52 (International Psychology), the Psychology Coalition at the United Nations (PCUN), and Division 15 (Student Division) of the International Association of Applied Psychology (IAAP) discuss their advocacy efforts and initiatives focused on social change
Rivera et al. (2021a)	International Psychology: Students at the United Nations – Link available	International Psychology and United Nations leaders discuss different opportunities for student involvement in the UN and international activities
Rivera et al. (2022a)	Student Leadership in International Psychology: Perspectives from Across the Globe – Link available	Student leaders of the APA's Division 52, APA's Division 48, Division 15 of the International Association of Applied Psychology (IAAP), the European Federation of Psychology Students' Associations (EFPSA), and the Interamerican Society of Psychology (SIP) share their experiences on the globalization of psychology
Roundtables and webinars in Spanish		
Rivera (2021f)	El impacto de la pandemia por COVID-19 en estudiantes universitarios [The impact of the COVID-19 pandemic in college students]	PsyD candidate and international psychology student leader Rita M. Rivera discusses different ways the coronavirus pandemic affected life for college populations
Rivera (2022b)	Prevención del Burnout en estudiantes y profesionales de psicología [Burnout among psychology professionals and trainees] – Link available	PsyD candidate and Honduran psychotherapist Rita M. Rivera discusses burnout among mental health care providers amid the COVID-19 pandemic
Rivera (2022d)	Trastorno de Duelo Prolongado [Prolonged Grief Disorder] – Link available	PsyD candidate and Honduran psychotherapist Rita M. Rivera presents an overview of the latest addition to the DMS-V-TR, Prolonged Greif Disorder

Key Areas

When developing research and disseminating resources, the Higher Education Working Group focused on several areas related to the impact of the pandemic on education. The following are the key areas of interest.

Educational Inequalities

The psychological impact of COVID-19 has not been fully evaluated, and this includes the effect the pandemic had on higher education. Throughout the world, governments and local authorities established lockdowns and social distancing measures to prevent the transmission of the virus. Although online modalities made it possible for many trainees to continue their education, transitioning to virtual learning, also known as e-learning, was not an option for student populations across the globe. This transition, as well as the disruption of education, led to other effects, such as delay of course completion, postponement of graduation ceremonies, and issues transitioning to the workforce. Overall, academic resources were not distributed equally before the pandemic, and the COVID-19 crisis further impacted this disadvantage. Research has indicated that BIPOC students were much more impacted by educational inequality, further placing these trainees at higher risk of experiencing mental health conditions like depression and anxiety (Dorn et al., 2022; Simon, 2021).

At-Risk Student Populations

Although COVID-19 was a global crisis, some populations were more prone to experiencing challenges that placed them at higher psychological risk. Some of these included the following.

Scholarship students These trainees relied on social programs and/or sports or artistic scholarships to fund their studies. During the pandemic, most of these programs were suspended or completely canceled. In some circumstances, these funds were never relocated to students, or trainees were not able to meet the scholarship requirements (i.e., play sports games, perform their art in public shows) during the lockdowns. We learned of this initially through anecdotal evidence from members of our WG who were directly affected or who knew peers who were impacted by the loss of scholarships and funding programs. Universities and higher education institutions where our members were enrolled during the pandemic experienced suspension of sports and artistic scholarships, as well as funding opportunities like work-study positions and on-campus employment used as tuition reimbursement.

Low-income students This population faced further challenges brought by the socioeconomic implications of the pandemic. Some of the issues faced included unemployment and/or loss of income, experienced by either the student themselves or their family members. Trainees reported several issues, including food insecurity, difficulties accessing places to study (i.e., libraries, study rooms, laboratories, and offices) and study materials and resources (i.e., printing services, books, and reference materials), closure of dorms and residence halls, inability to travel home to see family and loved ones, and barriers accessing healthcare (i.e., medications, doctor's appointments, and medical services, including mental health aid). Students reported that prior to the pandemic, universities and higher education institutions offered many programs that provided some of these basic resources to trainees, including food stamps and coupons, free healthcare and sanitary products, and sliding scale fees for medical appointments. Nevertheless, many of these programs and services were suspended during COVID-19, further exacerbating these needs, particularly for low-income students.

Students that lived in remote areas In some countries, such as Honduras and Panama, there is remote access where individuals do not have access to electricity or power or a reliable internet connection. Students in these circumstances may not have been able to transition to online learning or may have experienced challenges when connecting to their virtual courses. In most of these cases, trainees chose to take a leave of absence and continue their studies until courses were offered in person. Nonetheless, there were some students who reported dropping out of their programs. Few students who chose to continue their studies despite these barriers were connected with resources, particularly the contact information of public town hall settings where they could access free, reliable internet connection. Still, in these cases, students had to travel long distances and also risk the possibility of contracting COVID-19.

Students as caregivers Trainees who also hold roles as their family caregivers face several additional challenges. For instance, for this population, COVID-19 stress may be more intense as they have to take sanitary precautions to avoid risking their loved ones from infection. For example, one of our members from Latin America reported their mother was sick with cancer and undergoing chemotherapy during the pandemic. This member noted they felt very "stressed" and "nervous" about leaving their home, contracting the virus, and getting their mother sick. The member often referred to themselves as "responsible" for their mother's well-being, which included minimizing all risk of infection and, thus, staying at home as much as possible.

Furthermore, students who had or lived with children may have experienced additional stressors as they faced the transition to virtual education. During the pandemic, children themselves needed assistance to complete their coursework, as well as supervision from their parents and caregivers. Trainees who were in this predicament may have prioritized their children's education before their own. For instance, one of our members chose to take a leave of absence from their master's during the COVID-19 pandemic to support their child better and homeschool them. They acknowledged it was "incredibly difficult" to continue their own studies while also homeschooling their child and tending to their parental responsibilities.

Students with disabilities and/or preexisting health conditions These populations may have not had their disabilities taken into consideration in the virtual setting or during the transition to e-learning. In addition, lockdowns and other regulations may have exacerbated their anxiety, distress levels, and behavioral issues. Members of our WG who had preexisting health conditions reported experiencing high levels of stress and anxiety when they were expected to complete practicum rotations at high-risk settings, such as medical centers and hospitals. Often, these trainees felt they were choosing between completing their coursework and caring for their health.

Students with dysfunctional families Trainees that lived with or were exposed to dysfunctional families may have been subject to increased stress levels during the COVID-19 lockdowns. This was the case for members exposed to domestic and/or interpersonal violence, family members with substance use/abuse, and parents in the process of separating or divorcing during the pandemic.

Challenges Faced and Lessons Learned

Our work group faced lessons concerning the recruitment of members, issues of retention and scheduling difficulties due to different time zones, and students' busy schedules. Moreover, many of our members transitioned from students to early career professionals or maintained both professional and trainee status. Throughout the past years, we learned how to use new technology to facilitate communication. Technological advances allowed trainees and students throughout the globe to continue their education and has fostered international exchange of knowledge and experience. However, these changes and advances brought new advantages, as well as challenges, many which we continue to explore and evaluate. We also acknowledge that there are many students who have been unable to transition to online modalities or returned to in-person schooling. Many of these new advances were accessible only to those that have the resources to make the transition to virtual learning. Thus, we affirmed the importance of having structures in place that support students should pandemics continue, or new ones develop.

Moreover, our members and leaders learned the value of student engagement, leadership, and advocacy. Despite facing significant barriers and challenges, trainees worldwide continued leading research, mentored and supported each other, advocated for themselves and the populations they served, and were at the healthcare frontlines of the pandemic. Students learned firsthand the value of peer support as oftentimes they were able to identify and implement solutions to issues impacting their educational institutions and student communities. Trainees also became leaders in many organizations where spaces had been traditionally and historically reserved only for advanced professionals in the field. Through their leadership, students showcased their skills, actively contributing to societies and communities and impacting their professions. All of this work led advanced professionals to recognize students and trainees as colleagues that share unique knowledge and experiences and novel perspectives needed for the development of their profession. Students were not just invited to the table, but they also actively led the conversation and sought to expand it.

The Higher Education Work Group recognizes that students and trainees are often considered the future of their professions. We invite professionals and higher education institutions to continue supporting trainees as, through the pandemic, we have learned that students are key stakeholders in the advancement of their professions, with much of the contributions occurring in the present.

Author Note We have no known conflicts of interest to disclose.

References

Aganan, J., Campos, K., Page, D., Rivera, R. M., & Kwizera, R. (2022). *Advocacy, community, engagement, and social change: Perspectives from student leaders across the globe.* Invited presentation as part of the International Council of Psychologists, APA Division 52, IAAP's Division 15, and the Global Student Psychology Committee Collaborative Webinar, United States.

Benitez, D., & Rivera, R. M. (2022a). Predoctoral residency: Professional psychology and intern clinicians. *The Florida Psychologist, Spring 2022*, 16. https://cdn.ymaws.com/www.flapsych.com/resource/resmgr/publications/FPA_Spring_2022_final.pdf

Benitez, D., & Rivera, R. M. (2022b). Psychology trainees may not be allowed to practice what they preach. *Psychology Today*. https://www.psychologytoday.com/us/blog/physio-and-psych/202202/psychology-trainees-may-not-be-allowed-practice-what-they-preach

Benitez, D., & Rivera, R. M. (2022c). The American Academy of Clinical Psychology-Division of Graduate Students. *Bulletin of the American Academy of Clinical Psychology, Summer 2022.*

Benitez, D., & Rivera, R. M. (2022d). The mental health primary care disconnect. *The Florida Psychologist, Winter 2021*, 14.

Coppolino, T., & Rivera, R. M. (2021). *Art therapy & self-efficacy: The role of burnout among healthcare workers battling COVID-19* [Poster session]. American Psychological Association Convention.

Dorn, E., Hancock, B., Sarakatsannis, J., & Viruleg, E. (2022). *COVID-19 and learning loss—Disparities grow and students need help.* McKinsey & Company. https://www.mckinsey.com/industries/public-and-social-sector/our-insights/covid-19-and-learning-loss-disparities-grow-and-students-need-help

Medianero, G., Balva, D., Atherley, A., Gómez-Henao, J., & Majul, S. (2021a). Creación de vínculos educativos y colaborativos entre pares: Aprendiendo de la pandemia del Coronavirus a través del diálogo y la diversidad. *SIP Bulletin, 109*, 55–57.

Medianero, G., Rivera, R. M., & Balva, D. (2021b). Experiencias positivas durante la pandemia o derivadas de ésta. Formación en telepsicología: Una necesidad para nuestra profesión. *Sociedad Interamericana de Psicología Boletín, 109*, 34–35.

Medianero, G., Rivera, R. M, & Mejia, E. (2022a). *Impacto del COVID-19 en la educación de Panamá, Honduras, y El Salvador (COVID-19 Impact in the education of Panama, Honduras, and El Salvador)* [Poster session]. Congreso Regional de la Sociedad Interamericana de Psicología (SIP), Chile.

Medianero, G., Rivera, R. M., & Balva, D. (2022b). *Consideraciones en telepsicología desde la experiencia estudiantil (Considerations for the use of telepsychology: Perspective of student clinicians).* [Conference session]. XII Encuentro Internacional de Estudiantes de Psicología, Cuba.

Medianero, G., Rivera, R. M., & Balva, D. (2022c). Group therapy in a COVID-19 era: Strengthening training for psychology students. *The Group Psychologist, 32*(1). https://www.apadivisions.org/division-49/news-events/psychology-student-training

Rivera, R. M. (2020a). Coronavirus pandemic: A trigger for survivor's guilt? *Latinx Psychology Today, 7*(1). https://www.nlpa.ws/assets/docs/newsletters/FALL2020.pdf
Rivera, R. M. (2020b). Public education in Honduras: How the COVID-19 pandemic exacerbated an on-going educational crisis. *Trauma Psychology News (APA Division 56), 15*(3), 14–15. https://traumapsychnews.com/2020/11/public-education-in-honduras-how-the-covid-19-pandemic-exacerbated-an-on-going-educational-crisis/
Rivera, R. M. (2020c). *The psychology of problem-solving amid the coronavirus pandemic*. Psi Chi, The International Honor Society in Psychology. https://www.psichi.org/blogpost/987366/357099/The-Psychology-of-Problem-Solving-Amid-the-Coronavirus-Pandemic#.X3u812hKjIW
Rivera, R. M. (2021a). Benefits of virtual psychotherapy groups for students during COVID-19. *The Group Psychologist, 31*(1). https://www.apadivisions.org/division-49/publications/newsletter/group-psychologist/2021/03/virtual-group-benefits
Rivera, R. M. (2021b). *Celebrating minority mental health awareness month amidst the COVID-19 pandemic*. Society of Counseling Psychology-American Psychological Association Division 17. https://www.div17.org/connect%2D%2D-celebrating-minority-mental-health-awareness-month-amidst-covid-19
Rivera, R. M. (2021c). *COVID-19 impact on international students in the US* [Symposium session]. Division 52-International Psychology COVID-19 Taskforce: An international, multifaceted, collaborative initiative at the American Psychological Association Convention, United States.
Rivera, R. M. (2021d). *COVID-19 pandemic: Considerations for the study and practice of psychology*. Revista Desde Adentro, 7ma Edición, 17. https://infocentral.albizu.edu/wp-content/uploads/2021a/11/revista-7th-Edition-HD1.pdf
Rivera, R. M. (2021e). COVID-19 y síndrome del impostor: ¿La pandemia agrava el fenómeno para los estudiantes? *International Psychology Bulletin (APA Division 52), Spring 2021*. http://div52.net/ipb-2021-25-2/
Rivera, R. M. (2021f). *El impacto de la pandemia por COVID-19 en estudiantes universitarios [The impact of the COVID-19 pandemic in college students]*. Invited presentation as part of the Día del Psicólogo, Universidad Tecnológica de El Salvador (UTEC), El Salvador.
Rivera, R. M. (2021g). Fostering emotional regulation by practicing self-compassion. *The Florida Psychologist, Summer 2021*, 6.
Rivera, R. M. (2021h). *Imposter syndrome: Supporting students during the COVID-19 pandemic* [Symposium session]. Division 52-International Psychology Hospitality Suite Student Program at the American Psychological Association Convention, United States.
Rivera, R. M. (2021i). International and multidimensional perspectives on the impact of COVID-19 (IMPACT-C19). *International Psychology Bulletin (APA Division 52), Summer 2021*. http://div52.net/ipb-2021-25-3/#collaborations
Rivera, R. M. (2021j). Strategies for psychology students experiencing imposter syndrome. *Florida Psychologist, Spring 2021*, 12.
Rivera, R. M. (2021k). The lethal COVID-19 pandemic forges resilience for life. *Psychology Today*. https://www.psychologytoday.com/us/blog/psychological-trauma-coping-and-resilience/202103/the-lethal-covid-19-pandemic-forges
Rivera, R. M. (2021l). The link between nutrition and mental health. *Albizu Magazine, Fall 2021*. https://magazine.albizu.edu/the-link-between-nutrition-and-mental-health/
Rivera, R. M. (2021m). The value of student membership: Supporting the next generation. *Florida Psychologist, Fall 2021*, 10–11.
Rivera, R. M. (2022a). *El líder y la diversidad cultural [Leadership and cultural diversity]*. Invited presentation as part of the Leadership Week at Albizu University, Puerto Rico.
Rivera, R. M. (2022b). *Prevención del burnout en profesionales y estudiantes de psicología [Burnout among psychology professionals and trainees]*. Invited presentation as part of the Psychology Week sponsored by the Asociación de Estudiantes de Psicología de Panama, the Global Student Psychology Committee, the Interamerican Psychology Society, IAAP's Division 15, the Panamanian Association of Psychologists, and the Asociación IberoAmericana de Neurociencias y Psiquiatría, Universidad de Panama, Panama.

Rivera, R. M. (2022c). *The value of student-led research throughout the history of psychology.* Invited keynote address as part of the Albizu University-6th Annual South Florida Student Research Symposium, United States.
Rivera, R. M. (2022d). *Trastorno de Duelo Prolongado [Prolonged Grief Disorder].* Invited presentation as part of the Asociación de Estudiantes de Psicología de Panama, Universidad de Panama, Panama.
Rivera, R. M., & Benitez, D. (2020). Clinicians in training and the RxP movement. *Florida Psychologist, Fall 2020*, 7–9.
Rivera, R. M., & Benitez, D. (2021). The future of mental health care is burning out. *Psychology Today*. https://www.psychologytoday.com/us/blog/physio-and-psych/202107/the-future-mental-health-care-is-burning-out
Rivera, R. M., & Benitez, D. (2022). Self-care practices for your daily routine. *Albizu University's Magazine*. https://magazine.albizu.edu/self-care-practices-for-your-daily-routine/
Rivera, R. M., Kalayjian, A., Clopton, N., Congress, E., Novikova, I., Osborn, S., & Kuriansky, J. (2021a). *International Psychology: Students at the United Nations*. Invited presentation as part of the APA Division 52 and The Psychology Coalition at the United Nations (PCUN) Collaborative Webinar, United States.
Rivera, R. M., Ramírez, J. G., & Echeverri, M. F. (2021b). *¿De qué diversidad hablamos? La labor del docente en la formación del estudiante* [Symposium session]. Congreso Interamericano de Psicología, Puerto Rico.
Rivera, R. M., Ramírez, J. G., & Echeverri, M. F. (2021c). *Factors that influence the relationship between mentors and students: The impact of COVID-19 in higher education and mentorship* [Symposium session]. Division 52-International Psychology Hospitality Suite Student Program at the American Psychological Association Convention, United States.
Rivera, R. M., Ramírez, J. G., Echeverri, M. F., & Jiménez, F. (2021d). Relación entre mentores profesionales y estudiantes: Consideraciones ante el COVID-19. *Sociedad Interamericana de Psicología Boletín, 109*, 32–33.
Rivera, R. M., Altungy, P., Beckman, S., Ghanim, D, Henao, J. G., Couwet, D., & Balva, D. (2022a). *Student leadership in international psychology: Perspectives from across the globe.* Invited presentation as part of the APA Division 52, IAAP's Division 15, EFPSA, and SIP Collaborative Webinar, United States.
Rivera, R. M., Medianero, G., Benitez, D., Balva, D., & Kekesi, E. K. (2022b). Disaster management amidst COVID-19: Fostering competencies among psychology trainees. *International Association of Emergency Managers Bulletin, 39*(6), 23–26.
Simon, C. (2021). *How COVID taught America about inequity in education.* The Harvard Gazette. https://news.harvard.edu/gazette/story/2021/07/how-covid-taught-america-about-inequity-in-education/

Rita M. Rivera, M.S., CTP, Chair American Academy of Clinical Psych-Division of Graduate Students (AACP-DGS), Student Rep APA's Society of Group Psychology and Group Psychotherapy (Div. 49), President of the Global Student Psychology Committee, Past Chair of the Florida Psych Assoc Graduate Students (FPAGS).

David Benitez, M.S., Vice-Chair American Academy of Clinical Psych-Division of Graduate Students (AACP-DGS), Student Rep APA's Society for Prescribing Psychology (Div. 55), Past Chair of the Florida Psych Assoc Graduate Students (FPAGS), President of AU Neuropsychology Society, President of AU Division of Clinical Psychopharmacology.

Gabriel L. Medianero Araúz Ambassador of J. of Science Policy and Governance (JSPG), AmbassadorLatin America (Students and Early Career Psych) of International Assoc. of Applied Psychology, Latin America International Regional Coordinator of Society for Community Research and Action.

Tarah Coppolino, M.A. SMART certified mental health counselor and school-based program intake coordinator at the Community Counseling of Bristol County in Taunton, Massachusetts, member of the American Counseling Association and the American Art Therapy Association.

Part III
Lessons Learned

Given the lack of information when it began, and the shocking, "unprecedented" way this virus so quickly turned our worlds upside down, we learned many lessons that we hope our readers will take away. We write about them in this part. Here are a few:

A battle with a virus has no easy win. Just when you think the virus is going to succumb to social distancing or mask wearing, it mutates, and another version survives. Changing projections and conflicting advice were sent by national and local institutions. Politicians pointed fingers and created false and self-serving narratives. Nonetheless, the most effective way to fight the virus is to follow the science, not the politicians.

Children need the social stimulation of being with their peers and learning consistent with their developmental needs. Homeschooling is neither a substitute for regular school nor a substitute for regular teachers. We learn, of course, that working mothers are not properly prepared to be full-time teachers as well as full-time wives and mothers.

Humans are social beings and need to be with other humans in meaningful relationships. In-person relationships are important but contact over the internet can be a positive temporary solution for many people. The use of Zoom opened new possibilities of connection, and the use of the arts helped cross-cultural barriers. On the other hand, isolation, especially among the older adults, was exacerbated by COVID lockdown and sometimes led to despair.

People need to grieve their losses. Sometimes grieving losses collectively with the experiences and complexities of caring friends and family. This collective grief happens often with others who have also experienced grief and losses. Those who could not visit their loved ones in hospitals or complete a mourning process, however, may have had more complex and unresolved grief.

We psychologists and other mental health professionals went through this existential crisis together. With the support of each other or just being together (even over zoom) made it easier to bear. Those of us on the Task Force as well as the therapists who volunteered with one or more of the Working Groups noticed it: How being in the crisis together changed our way of doing therapy and bringing more egalitarian and transparent relationships. This transformed the "crisis" into an historic and inspiring effort.

In the chapter on telehealth, we describe how the mental health workforce that was initially resistant to delivering services via digital technologies rose to the occasion, developing new ways to reach the people who needed us. Many still craved the personal touch, but others were relieved to not having to travel to offices. Instead, delivering or receiving psychotherapy in homes, cars, or other private spaces reduced stress and sometimes provided new windows into people's lives. Once the barriers to insurance and payment were removed, the mental health industry underwent enormous changes that appear to be here to stay. Chapter 10 is a description of various ways of using technology to reach people.

Despite the closing of universities and research institutions, research continued and even flourished during the 3 years when the world was in various stages of being shut down. Chapter 11 describes the incredible network of researchers who connected around the world to share their studies using the internet for connection. This permitted those students working on theses and dissertations to complete their work with consultation from other scholars. Conferences went online and then found new hybrid formats. Interestingly, many of the findings were used immediately to help in the healing process as we began to come out of the most dangerous period. We discovered similarities among our international colleagues and experienced our global interconnectedness.

The final Chap. 12 pulls together many of the important lessons learned during this 3-year journey by the organizers of this inspiring group of mental health practitioners and researchers. Reflecting on the impact of these 3 years on ourselves, we understand how important our connection with each other and in our group the others was as we moved through the unknown. We made lifelong friendships and new professional colleagues as we survived those trials and tribulations put before us. We learned from each other and from those who we were helping. Our lives have been forever changed.

Chapter 10
Telepsychology and Digital Therapeutics

Lenore E. A. Walker

The ability to perform psychotherapy and psychological assessment using digital technology began long before the COVID-19 pandemic, but there was a great deal of resistance from many psychotherapists to treat patients using these devices. Concerns were about possible lack of privacy, confidentiality, the perception that the therapeutic alliance would be compromised, and the lack of nonverbal communication cues. However, when the World Health Organization (WHO) declared COVID-19 a global pandemic and the world went into lockdown mode in 2020, depression, anxiety, and posttraumatic stress rose quickly. Many psychotherapists responded by quickly by pivoting to treating patients using audio- and videoconferencing with various forms of digital instruments, especially smartphones and computers. Data already had suggested that telehealth could be as effective as in-person therapy (Poletti et al., 2020), with as good a therapeutic relationship (Etzelmuller et al., 2018), and could increase affordable care in rural and underserved areas (Tuerk et al., 2018). As we reviewed how the various groups worked during the pandemic, it became apparent that technology and the world of the internet opened new ways for psychologists to function (Brooks et al., 2020; Wind et al., 2020). Surprisingly, many psychologists described they liked using telehealth and staying at home rather than delivering services in person at their offices. Many patients have stated similar preferences. The use of telepsychology during this period remedied some of the health inequities in parts of the population around the world who previously were not able to access psychotherapy, for example, older adults (Shrira et al., 2020), people with chronic physical illness (Hacker et al., 2021), and those experiencing domestic abuse and family violence (Usher et al., 2020). The lack of training and technical difficulties has been an obstacle to more widespread use of telepsychotherapy (Tuerk et al., 2018; Poletti et al., 2020). However, telepsychology is not

L. E. A. Walker (✉)
Nova Southeastern University College of Psychology, Davie, FL, USA
e-mail: walkerle@nova.edu

C. R. Figley et al. (eds.), *Pandemic Providers*,
https://doi.org/10.1007/978-3-031-27580-7_10

appropriate for all psychotherapy clients. For example, in a sample of creative art therapists who asked how COVID-19 had impacted their work, the largest group (45%) were still seeing their clients, while 31% were not. The reason most cited for termination was that the clients did not want to meet online (Feniger-Schaal et al., 2020).

Systematic study and recommendations for the ethical use of technology had not yet caught up with the pace with which their use was mandated by the pandemic. The practitioners we worked with struggled with new issues such as licensure and insurance coverage across state and country borders. Guidelines for an ethical and best practice use of telepsychology needed to be reviewed. Therefore, our Task Force undertook a review of telepsychology that we describe here. In this chapter we cover definitions of telepsychology, how it may be performed, guidelines for its use, special areas of concern including ethical standards and legal issues, and results of studies of its efficacy for consumers and psychotherapists. The definition of telepsychology according to the APA Guidelines for the Practice of Telepsychology[1] is:

> …the provision of psychological services using telecommunication technologies. Telecommunication is the preparation, transmission, communication, or related processing of information by electrical, electromagnetic, electromechanical, electro-optical, or electronic means (Committee on National Security Systems, 2010). Telecommunication technologies include but are not limited to telephone, mobile devices, interactive videoconferencing, email, chat, text, and internet (e.g. self-help websites, blogs, and social media). These communications may be in writing, or include images, sounds or other data. These communications may be synchronous with multiple parties communicating in real time (e.g. interactive videoconferencing, telephone) or asynchronous (e.g. email, online bulletin boards, storing and forwarding information).
>
> Technologies may augment traditional in person services (e.g., psychoeducational materials online after an in-person therapy session), or be used as stand-alone services (e.g. therapy or leadership development provided over videoconferencing). Different technologies may be used in various combinations and for different purposes during the provision of telepsychology services. For example, videoconferencing and telephone may also be used for direct service while email and text is used for non-direct services (e.g. scheduling). Regardless of the purpose, psychologists strive to be aware of the potential benefits and limitations in their choices of technologies for particular clients in particular situations. (P. 3)

In the almost 3 years since our working groups have been providing consultation and materials to psychologists and other mental health professionals, the use of telepsychology has expanded, laws have been modified to accommodate interstate provision, and guidelines for its use in practice have been promulgated. Third-party payors for mental health services have continued paying although still on a temporary basis even after the pandemic crisis was considered over. The public health emergency (PHE) declaration by the US government has just been renewed in October 2022, suggesting the relaxed rules put in place during COVID-19 will continue for some time. Our experience working with practitioners is that telecommunication technologies present both opportunities to work with patients who otherwise would be unable to attend in-person treatment and challenges that include

[1] https://apa.org/practice/guidelines/telepsychology (2013)

confidentiality issues, burdensome state regulations, and technology failures. At the same time, the opportunity to provide additional interventions to augment treatment using APPs or other tools became much more available, especially with development by both commercial vendors and government-sponsored groups, such as the US Department of Defense and US Department of Veterans Affairs.

The COVID-19 emergency spurred the US Congress to add a section waiving certain requirements under telehealth, for patients to receive services in their own homes with fewer restrictions (*Coronavirus Preparedness and Response Supplemental Appropriations Act, 2020*).[2] For those using Medicare, similar waivers occurred under the guidelines issued by the *Centers for Medicare & Medicaid Services*[3] (CMS, 3/17/2020). The law and its regulations made it possible for patients to receive services in their own homes or any healthcare facility during the PHE (public health emergency), suspending the requirements for previously approved sites. It also permitted providers to provide services from their own homes. However, providers still must be licensed in their jurisdiction. We discuss the problems with interjurisdictional regulation later in this chapter. Interestingly, providers originally were required to use smartphones or computers that had both audio and video components that allowed for two-way, real-time communication. This ruled out telephone-only sessions, which later has also become permissible for reimbursement. At the same time, the US Department of Health and Human Services relaxed its HIPPA requirements so that audio and visual technologies that were not in compliance (such as Skype, FaceTime, and others) could be used during the emergency. Once these new US government regulations were in place, other insurance companies and third-party payors followed.

Issues Around Beginning Practice

As might be expected, most practitioners did not have much experience around conducting psychotherapy sessions outside of their offices. Thus, for most there was a steep learning curve for both technology and clinical practice areas. The stay-at-home mandate applied to those who were in private offices or clinics at first. Shortly afterwards, as hospitals became overloaded with acutely ill COVID-19 patients, many who worked in hospitals were also advised to stay at home, especially if their patients were in outpatient settings where digital devices were available. Mental health apps were being developed and recommended both to augment treatment and, in some places where treatment with a provider was not possible, as a standalone intervention. There has not been sufficient research to determine the effectiveness of apps by themselves. The VA has suggested it is better than no intervention,

[2] https://www.congress.gov/bill/116th-congress/hoU.S.e-bill/6074/text

[3] https://www.cms.gov.newsroom/fact-sheets/medicare-telemedicine-health-care-provider-fact-sheet.

which was the alternative during the emergency period for some. As we found with professionals in many of the working groups, there were often more questions than answers for practitioners as they began changing from in-person to telephone or computer platforms. By year two, many psychotherapists had closed their offices and reported they preferred working at home. Today, during year three, many psychotherapists state they do not have plans to reopen their offices, although others have gone back.

Choosing which platform to use was an initial issue as many new commercial platforms became available shortly after the lockdown. New names became part of the lexicon; Zoom, Doxy.me, and VSee joined the more familiar Skype and FaceTime. Decisions had to be made to determine if providers or patients had sufficient bandwidth to support a particular program. Younger patients and providers were able to adapt to these technologies much faster than those who were older. Although there was concern that patients would not have the requisite technology, it became clear that most had access at least to a smartphone on which to connect to audio or video sessions with the therapist. In fact, more people who wanted services were able to connect to technology than attend in-person sessions. Most practitioners reported that their office hours filled up quickly and, by year two, could not accept new clients.

At the same time, new technology-only services were begun by various commercial companies. Psychologists who worked for these companies were guaranteed at least 25 hours of services by some companies, although payment was at or below the amount that many might earn in independent practice. Nonetheless, many new therapists were able to set up practices in their own homes, working for these entities, who provided clients for them. Prior to the pandemic, there had been an attempt by large corporations such as Walmart or Amazon to set up brief walk-in psychotherapy services. They too switched to telepsychology during the pandemic. Concern has arisen that in many of these corporations, credentials of their providers are not matching the needs of the clients they are being asked to treat. In fact, there is a growing concern that the corporatization of psychotherapy is beginning to occur, like the takeover of private practice medical doctors by corporations two decades earlier (Jared Skillings, APA Practice Directorate, personal communication, 10-17-2022).

When telepsychology first appeared, prior to the pandemic, guidelines suggested initial interviews be done in person to better assess the ability of the person's safety if telepsychology were to be used. Practitioners were urged to get an emergency contact person or even a nearby hospital should the patient have difficulties with uncovering difficult psychological material. Care to properly assess suicidal patients was also routine at that time. However, during the COVID-19 emergency, people were not available for any in-person interviews, as they too were in lockdown and the hospital emergency rooms to which they previously might have been sent were filled with COVID-19 patients. Thus, the crisis caused relaxation of some of these guidelines, and initial interviews were done online as well and followed up with treatment sessions. It is hoped that these relaxed guidelines remain in place as, according to data collected by DHHS, there was a 63-fold increase in traditional

Medicare telehealth visits in 2020 that are considered a direct result of the PHE waivers and new state statues permitting flexibility during the pandemic (https://www.apa.org/news/press/releases/2020/05//phone-only-telehealth-medicare). However, practitioners still strive to collect emergency data whenever possible.

Some psychological tests also became available to be administered online with computerized scoring available. This opened the way for forensic evaluations to be performed even though the courts were closed in most jurisdictions. Performing psychological assessment using telehealth methods became possible using objective personality tests and trauma tests. It was more difficult to perform neuropsychological tests or cognitive intelligence tests using digital technologies. Many neuropsychologists and forensic psychologists who performed essential services did go into their offices to work with patients there especially in the second year, once vaccines were available. Interestingly, psychologists were among the first group of essential workers eligible for vaccination even though their services were not always seen by the administration as essential. Many psychologists found themselves dealing with patients with profound grief as multiple deaths occurred in some families. During this time, a new disorder appeared in the DSM-V-TR called Profound Grief Disorder. Psychologists were also called upon to deal with those hesitant to accept the vaccine, but not until it became apparent that almost half of the USA were hesitant or refusing it. Vaccine hesitancy is an area that behavioral health might have been able to assist the government to avoid politicization and help it remain in the province of healthcare.

One of the biggest problems related to the new use of technology that was mentioned by those in our work groups during the pandemic was the inability to separate work from their personal life. Generally, practitioners set hours that they will see patients or talk with them except for emergencies. Call most doctors and you will hear on their voice mail the instruction to go to the nearest hospital if they are in an emergency. However, as we've mentioned, hospitals were overloaded, so many patients would call their psychotherapist who would answer the phone during off-hours. Further, the amount of exhaustion reported at the end of the day seeing the same number of patients was greater than if seen in their offices. Some suggested they were better able to get up and do something else between patients when in their office while others suggested they were experiencing what became known as "Zoom" fatigue. New ways of combatting accompanying eye strain from staring at boxes on the computer needed to be developed and tested. The IPV and Whole Person Group presented a roundtable featuring Erik Peper, a professor at San Francisco State University, author of a book on combatting Zoom fatigue to help develop ways to avoid it (Peper et al., 2020). Dr. Jana Martin, CEO of the Trust and Morgan Sammons and CEO of the National Register of Health Service Providers, presented a roundtable that discussed risk management strategies for psychologists they had developed for their subscribers.

Developing an appropriate informed consent document to give patients became an important issue as the laws and regulations varied from state to state. Many states changed their requirements for out-of-state practitioners to conduct psychotherapy with patients in that state. Legally, informed consent consists of three elements: (1)

sufficiency of information, (2) competence, and (3) voluntariness. Sufficiency of information generally includes an understanding of the role of the practitioner, the nature of the service, or intervention being provided, with whom a report or consultation will be shared and for what purpose and any limitations on confidentiality that might apply. One of the differences in informed consent in telepsychology patients is the need to specify a specific plan to deal with emergencies and crisis situations that might arise during treatment. This became difficult during COVID-19 since neither patients nor support persons were supposed to leave their home and many local hospitals were unable to deal with emergencies due to coping with huge numbers of critically ill COVID-19 patients. Nonetheless, practitioners were encouraged to try to put together whatever plan they and the patient could do. During a roundtable presented by Jana Martin, CEO of the Trust and Morgan Stanley and CEO of the National Register, it was suggested that the following be included in an informed consent for telepsychology form:

- Risks to confidentiality
- Issues related to technology
- Crisis management and intervention
- Technology to be used
- Communication between sessions
- Effectiveness of telepsychology
- Fees and billing
- Records

The use of digital therapeutics or apps also increased during COVID-19. Most digital therapeutics are typical behavioral interventions using CBT in digital formats and are totally automated, so they don't need a practitioner to use them. Those in underserved communities are often prescribed these apps that are readily available for use on smartphones. Relaxation tapes for anxiety or sleep disturbances were popular during this period. The US Department of Veterans Affairs has designed several important apps for use with people who have experienced different traumatic events causing trauma reactions. These include PTSD, sexual assault, sex harassment, anxiety, and depression, for example. They can be used as an independent behavioral intervention or as an adjunct to psychotherapy. Sometimes they are used in a therapy session, too.

The number of these apps has proliferated by commercial companies, also, during the 2 years of COVID-19, and it became difficult for therapists to learn which ones are useful for which patients. Our IPV working group suggested the therapist practice using an app prior to suggesting it to a patient. We provided practice sessions during our weekly roundtables. In one roundtable session, psychologist Skip Rizzo demonstrated the use of virtual reality (VR) for treatment of severe PTSD or anxiety, especially being used with veterans. It was obvious that training is needed to use VR, but it has great promise as a new form of digital treatment. Other interventions using biological approaches are also available for those specially trained in their use. However, when any of these newer digital methods are integrated into treatment by a psychotherapist, the same guidelines and ethical standards need to be followed.

Issues for Researchers

Although most of our working group members were practitioners, there were some who were concerned with continuing their research programs or beginning new ones. The pandemic gave the opportunity to conduct research at home for many professors whose classes were also being taught online. As one suggested, she had no idea how much time and energy the daily commute took until she was able to stay at home. Of course, those who had small children who required home schooling or others who shared their home were less rather than more productive. Nonetheless, the use of social media, such as *LinkedIn*, *Twitter*, *Facebook*, *Instagram*, and other channels to collect data, became possible for those who wanted to capture personal data readily available for some but not all groups. The data collected are usually in survey data format as having back and forth in-depth conversations like could occur during in-person data collection is not usual.

Some of the video-based media like *TikTok* and *Snapchat* may be useful for certain types of questions especially if wanting to research a younger audience. Many of these social media platforms have significant privacy and data protection concerns. But for people with lower reading levels, video-based media may provide more accurate data. Much of this research uses qualitative methods, but some have had good psychometric development. Carell and MacRae (2020) in *The Myths of Social Media* discuss how to use social media for research.

One of the limitations of doing research using social media is the lack of Institutional Review Boards (IRB) to check that the research is ethical. This allows for the entrance of "trolls" and "bots" who can attempt to influence the research. Trolls tend to lure professionals to give unethical responses online in order to normalize pathology. However, if you are clear about what you are setting out to do online and what your personal and professional boundaries are, you will recognize those attempts to draw you off topic. Bots are people who intentionally complete a phony response to the questions asked. Bots are more likely to try to use your research to sell their own products or introduce their own agenda. These are interesting issues that do not often come up in institution-based research but are manageable by putting some security controls in place when using social media to collect data.

Guidelines for Telepsychology

In 2013, the American Psychological Association (APA) put forward guidelines for using telehealth in the practice of telepsychology. They outlined eight areas that are important, most of which are familiar to psychologists as they apply in other areas. Guidelines are not mandatory to be followed, although they are encouraged unless there are sufficient reasons not to follow them. These guidelines remained helpful in telepsychology practice during COVID-19. They are (1) Competence of the Psychologist, (2) Standards of Care, (3) Informed Consent, (4) Confidentiality of Data and Information, (5) Security and Transmission of Data and Information, (6) Disposal of Data and Information and Technologies, (7) Testing and Assessment, and (8) Interjurisdictional Practice.

1. *Competence of the Psychologist. Psychologists who provide telepsychology services strive to take reasonable steps to ensure their competence with both the technologies used and the potential impact of the technologies on clients/patients, supervisees, or other professionals.*

This guideline is consistent with the Ethical Standard in the APA Code of Ethics in which psychologists are expected to monitor their own competence. This means they only practice within the boundaries of their competence based on their education, training, supervised experience, consultation, study, or professional experience. It is noted that this is a new and emerging area and therefore recognized standards for preparatory training do not yet exist. Nonetheless, psychologists are responsible for assessing and continuously evaluating their own competencies, training, consultation, experience, and risk management practices for competent practice.

2. *Standards of Care in the Delivery of Telepsychology Services. Psychologists make every effort to ensure that ethical and professional standards of care and practice are met at the outset and throughout the duration of the telepsychology they provide.*

This guideline suggested that psychologists practicing telepsychology use the same ethical and professional standards of care they would use if it were in-person practice. They do suggest that given the newness of using technology to deliver services, it would be prudent to evaluate for themselves the usefulness of technologies they use before engaging in providing services to a particular client/patient. This also includes assessing patient preferences for technologies used as well as the environment in which the patient will be for privacy concerns.

3. *Informed Consent. Psychologists strive to obtain and document informed consent that specifically addresses the unique concerns related to telepsychology services they provide. When doing so, psychologists are cognizant of the applicable laws and regulations, as well as organizational requirements that govern informed consent in this area.*

This guideline reminds psychologists that the process of informed consent is one way to develop the relationship between the patient and the psychologist by setting out the services to be performed and seeking consent of the patient. This is similarly stated in APA Ethics Code Standard 3.0. Details of how this can be developed are presented earlier in this document on page __.

4. *Confidentiality of Data and Information: Psychologists who provide telepsychology services make reasonable effort to protect and maintain the confidentiality of the data and information relating to their clients/patients and inform them of the potentially increased risks to loss of confidentiality inherent in the use of the telecommunication technologies, if any.*

   The guideline to protect confidentiality of data and information is similar to what is required of psychologists, but it is more difficult given the nature of technologies, especially those that are broadcast. Some of the additional risks include the use of social media and search engines on those sites. It is also difficult to anticipate breaches of data as the practitioner does not have control over the electronics as is possible with office files. However, this is also true with electronic medical records, so security measures are constantly being developed.

5. *Security and Transmission of Data and Information. Psychologists who provide telepsychology services take reasonable steps to ensure that security measures are in place to protect data and information related to their clients/patients from unintended access or disclosure.*

   This guideline suggests that the psychologist be mindful of unintended breaches of security such as computer viruses, hackers, theft of technology devices, damage to hard drives or portable drives, failure of security systems, flawed software, and ease of accessibility to unsecured electronic files which are all possibilities that must be prepared. Outdated software or unscrupulous vendors also are potential threats. Preparation of reasonable security measures and awareness of relevant jurisdictional and federal laws and regulations governing electronic storage are necessary.

6. *Disposal of Data and Information and Technologies. Psychologists who provide telepsychology services make reasonable efforts to dispose of data and information and the technologies used in a manner that facilitates protection from unauthorized access and accounts for safe and appropriate disposal.*

   This guideline encourages psychologists to create their own policies and procedures for destruction of data and the technologies used when obtaining the data such as computers. There are new guidelines for recordkeeping that specifically address electronic medical records that are now being required by some third-party payors.

7. *Testing and Assessment. Psychologists are encouraged to consider the unique issues that may arise with test instruments and assessment approaches designed for in-person implementation when providing telepsychology services.*

   This guideline reminds psychologists that they are uniquely trained in test administration and interpretation usually administered in person settings, although some screening tests were already being administered online. Special cautions for working with diverse populations and making appropriate accommodations are included. Interpretation of tests and written reports include the limitations, if any, when administered online. If there are norms based on telehealth assessment, psychologists strive to use them. Psychologists are encouraged to be consistent with the most recent edition of *Standards for Educational and Psychological Testing*.

8. *Interjurisdictional Practice. Psychologists are encouraged to be familiar with and comply with all relevant laws and regulations when providing telepsychology services to clients/patients across jurisdictional borders.*

The practice of psychology, like other licensed practices, is regulated in each individual state of country. Telepsychology exists in cyberspace, not real borders, which poses challenges for state regulatory boards, practitioners, and patients. In some cases, patients go out of their state temporarily while in others they permanently reside in another jurisdiction. In either case offering services across these borders using technologies has posed numerous issues for psychologists. Being familiar with the laws in both your own and your patient's jurisdictions is important, and psychologists are encouraged to make reasonable attempts to do so. We include an entire section in this chapter outlining some of the concerns that psychologists have raised and responses from both a risk management and a legal regulation perspective.

Interjurisdictional Practice

Interjurisdictional practice became a big issue during the pandemic as telehealth permitted psychotherapists to treat people anywhere where there was an internet connection without concern for travel. It became especially important when many businesses closed and psychotherapy patients moved out of small urban apartments to larger homes across state lines. Young people left colleges and workplaces and went to their parents' homes for shelter, also crossing state lines. Suddenly, practitioners were faced with immediate decisions about licensure and ethical practice as well as prioritizing continuity of care, therapeutic alliance, and safety over confusion over interstate practice. As was mentioned earlier, the practice of psychology is usually regulated by state licensing boards according to their own laws, rules, and regulations. Crossing state lines to practice, as occurs when providing remote services on electronic platforms, poses difficulties in regulating providers and protecting consumers. Many of the questions that have arisen have not yet been satisfactorily addressed due to the individuality of the different state laws and the boards charged with their regulations. This is especially true when working across two states where the laws are different and the provider must choose how to follow one or both. Several common examples are as follows:

1. When a provider licensed in state A was counseling a person in state B where they were not licensed, when did they need to apply for temporary licensure?
2. If state A specified that remote testing was permissible but state B was silent on that rule.

3. If a provider left their home state to shelter in place in another state, could they continue to provide services from their home to their patients in their original state where they held a license?

Since many state licensing board employees were working remotely themselves, psychologists had difficulty finding out if they needed a temporary license to continue to treat their patients and, if so, how to apply. It is clear that both states cannot have regulatory authority at the same time. If families who live in different states are in treatment, the issue of who has regulatory authority becomes even more complex. The question that our working groups now pose is whether states really need to adopt their own credentials? Perhaps instead, all states should permit those with the highest level of qualifications in the model licensing act provided by APA to practice interjurisdictionally for a period of time, perhaps 30 days, without having to become licensed in that state.

The Association of State & Provincial Psychology Boards (ASPPB) developed an interstate compact, PSYPACT, that if adopted by each state permitted eligible psychologists to practice in another PSYPACT state. While the idea seemed like a positive solution to the interstate jurisdictional problem, in fact, PSYPACT has created other problems. First, only 28 states have signed on to PSYPACT. Second, there are onerous restrictions on which psychologists are eligible to apply. For example, only psychologists who have graduated from an APA-approved program are eligible, and anyone who has had a board complaint filed, even if satisfactorily resolved, may not be eligible. Third, a psychologist who is practicing in a state where there are legal restrictions on what they can do or say to patients must follow them. Currently, some states do not permit discussing abortion with a patient even if it has implications for healthcare. It is possible for a psychologist from another state that does not have such a law to be criminally prosecuted for practicing competently and ethically (Younggren et al., 2022).

The providers we worked with during COVID-19 were continually questioning the complexity of these issues. Not surprisingly, the answers to many of the questions raised were different depending upon who was asked. State licensing boards insist the letter of the law must be followed but often leave it to the individual psychotherapist to decide how to follow it. Insurance risk management teams often give conservative responses in how to follow the issue in question but leave it up to the provider to decide how much risk to take. APA developed webinars to help figure out some of the issues but again made it clear that without guidance from the specific state, providers must make their own decisions. Given the fact that the rules were both rapidly changing and confusing, it is not surprising that many providers were unsure of how to proceed. Nonetheless, to date, our working groups have not reported any problems either in the USA or with global practices.

Psychologists need to be aware of the specific laws regarding the provision of remote services. Generally, the psychologist must be licensed, even if only temporarily, in the state where the patient resides as well as in the state where they practice. Problems arose when the length of treatment extended beyond the time specified by state law for temporary practice. But it wasn't clear if this meant that the practitioner needed to apply for a full license in the other state in order to maintain continuity of care, or refer to another local practitioner when the temporary license expired. During COVID-19 many states suspended the need for temporary licensure if the provider was licensed in another state. In general, this occurred for as long as the US government declared we were in a public health emergency or PHE. However, it was often unclear when the PHE was extended beyond the original dates. Those providers who accepted third-party payment for their services, such as insurance companies, were also confused by the various rules different providers had for payment in different jurisdictions.

These issues were not new to the complex field of licensing and reimbursement for services by psychologists. However, as Younggren et al. (2022) have commented, "The rapid development of electronic media and the increased mobility of both patients and psychologists have led to unintended barriers and potentially adverse consequences for both practitioners and consumers." They concur that the lessons learned during COVID-19 suggest that unified credentials in all states would better serve the public, especially by reducing barriers. We agree with their conclusion that "ASPPB should recognize that all states take high-quality care seriously and encourage the adoption of a 30-day temporary practice exemption for all member boards. This would clearly increase the availability of professional services, lower health-care costs, arguably allow sufficient time to achieve most clinical goals, and reduce the confusion that currently exists in the regulatory landscape" (p. 3).

Is Telepsychology Working?

There has not been a lot of time to fully evaluate whether telepsychology is able to provide equivalent services to in-person treatment during the pandemic. However, there are a number of areas that have been investigated, previously. First, the Treatment and Preventive Intervention Research Branch at the National Institute of Mental Health (NIMH) has suggested telepsychology has changed the paradigm of psychotherapy from one that was delivered by a patient sitting in a room for 45 minutes with a psychotherapist. Second, more people are being reached through telepsychology, which is important given recent research showing that healthcare equity has not been available for large sectors of the population, both due to cost and availability of services. Third, it is suggested that attending sessions in your own home may reduce stigma of mental health services for some people.

There has been research on populations that do well with telepsychology, such as the US Department of Veterans Affairs trials with PTSD interventions (Turgoose et al., 2018) even before COVID-19. They found that in-person and videoconferencing treatments were equally effective in the majority of cases studied. The VA also is using apps they've developed both as a separate and an adjunct to treatment effectively. There have been reviews of effective treatment via telepsychology for depression, anxiety, and adjustment disorders (Varker et al., 2019) and substance abuse, eating disorders, and other problems for children and adolescents (Slone et al., 2012). There have been studies of treatment methods used with telepsychology that found it effective, such as Mohr's (2012) study of cognitive behavioral therapy (CBT) delivered in person or over the telephone to 325 persons with major depressive disorder. Interestingly, although in-person treatment had slightly more lasting effects, those in that in-person treatment group were also more likely to drop out of therapy. Patient satisfaction surveys have shown high levels of patient satisfaction with telepsychology (Glueckauf et al., 2018) although transition periods when switching from in-person to remote sessions can cause some temporary anxiety (Jenkins-Guarnieri, 2015).

Although there have been concerns that telepsychology may not be as useful in reaching lower-income populations as they might not have access to digital equipment, COVID-19 has shown that almost all households have access to smartphones or even tablets, especially since they were essential for school children to use for learning during the pandemic. In some areas, schools actually provided tablets or computers to each child that parents could use at a different time. Access to privacy is an important issue in homes where there are crowded conditions, although there have been reports of consumers finding spaces in closets, bathrooms, cars, or other creative solutions when necessary. Some therapists responded by changing the session duration, frequency, and payment rates as well, generating what has been positively called "creative self-efficacy" or "creative adaptability" (Brahnam, 2017, Orkibi, 2021).

Maheu,[4] one of the earliest proponents for telepsychology, warned that distractions can easily occur during telehealth treatment and cautioned providers to be aware of temptations to read emails, text messages, or other ways to multitask for both them and their patients. She also cautions that platforms used are not always sufficient in making sure patient's surroundings are conducive to a productive session, especially if other people are also present in the patient's home. There hasn't been a lot of research comparing platforms, although one study found only 46% of patients experienced effective interventions (Hull & Mahan, 2017). Again, this was not during the pandemic, but it raises the caution that it is critical to be sure that the patient is in a safe and private space before beginning a telehealth session. It is also important to make sure that the provider has worked out a procedure for intervention should suicide or other emergency arise.

Conclusion

The need to change from in-person psychotherapy to delivering services remotely, using technology, probably sped up a transition that was happening anyhow. Some of the major ethical issues had already been determined, and guidelines were put

[4] https://telehealth.org/

forward for best practices by APA. This undoubtedly made the transition easier for clinicians as well as consumers, as the choice often was using technology or not obtaining treatment. Medical doctors were also transitioning to telehealth visits at the same time, and technology products were adapting to the new world we found ourselves in globally. New ways of practicing ethically were essential to keeping themselves and their patients safe. Informed consent and confidentiality issues were paramount as practitioners switched to remote practice.

It was interesting to see how quickly the resistance to telepsychology began to disappear in our own COVID-19 task force psychologists. Providers often used trial and error to find their preferred platforms, but once their new routines were established, they felt they functioned well with most of their patients. Many began to talk about new ways of experiencing their patients, such as listening to tone of voice, cadence of words used, and even how they breathe. Others had to learn new ways of detecting if a patient was high on alcohol or other substances, since the usual methods such as odor or even their gait were not always visible. Learning to interpret different nonverbal cues was another skill they had to develop. They also had to adjust their workflow, master the technology they chose to use, and maybe even change their office setting to accommodate better lighting and different seating and sometimes purchase a new computer. Nonetheless, many of the therapists appreciated the ability to stay at home and not drive distances to offices. Many who gave up their office space will not go back, while others are still not sure if they will remain at home. Others are happy to go to their offices, separating their home and professional lives. The choice will probably continue to be determined by personal preference for a while longer as COVID-19 is still with us as the virus continues to mutate into other variants.

The future for telepsychology seems to be clear. It is here to stay. Many more practitioners and patients will prefer this mode of service delivery, while others will go back to in-person practice. Although insurers have not yet committed to continuing payment once the pandemic is over, there is no guarantee that this or another pandemic is not going to keep the USA in a protective mode for some time, yet. New variants of the virus keep being reported, many people still wear protective masks despite the mandate being removed, and some at high risk still have not come out of their homes. Many people have had five doses of the vaccine. The need for psychotherapy has never been greater; children are suffering as their development has been interrupted by schools closing, friendships disrupted, and death of close family members. Parents are dealing with their inability to substitute for schoolteachers. Families have been destroyed by serious sickness, death, and the pain of not being able to support members who lived at a distance or were at too high risk to interact together. New research will help provide pathways to expand telepsychology to help people deal with all these new problems as well as others that have always been amenable to psychotherapy.

References

American Psychological Association. (2013). *Guidelines for the practice of telepsychology*. https://www.apa.org/practice/guidelines/telepsychology

Brahnam, S. (2017). Comparison of in-person and screen-based analysis using communication models: A first step toward the psychoanalysis of telecommunications and its noise. *Psychoanalytic Perspectives, 14*(2), 138–158. https://doi.org/10.1080/1551806X.2017.1304112

Brooks, S. K., Webster, R. K., Smith, L. R., Woodland, L., Wesseley, S., Greenberg, N., & Rubin, G. J. (2020). The psychological impact of quarantine and how to reduce it: Rapid review of the evidence. *The Lancet*, 912–920. https://doi.org/10.1016/S0140-6736(20)30460-8

Carrell, M., & McRae, I. (2020). *The myths of social media*. Kogan Page, Lld.

Etzelmuller, A., Radkovsky, A., Hannig, W., Berking, M., & Ebert, D. D. (2018). Patient's experience with blended video-and-internet based cognitive behavioural therapy service in routine care. *Internet Interventions, 12*, 165–175. https://doi.org/10.1016/j.invent.2018.01.003

Feniger-Schaal, R., Orkibi, H., Keisari, S., Sajnani, N., & Butler, J. (2020). Shifting to tele-creative arts therapies during the COVID-19 pandemic: An international study on helpful and challenging factors. In *The arts in psychotherapy*. Elsevier. https://doi.org/10.1016/j.aip.2022.101898

Glueckauf, R. L., Maheu, M. M., Drude, K. P., Wells, B. A., Wang, Y., Gustafson, D. J., & Nelson, E. L. (2018). Survey of psychologists' telebehavioral health practices: Technology use, ethical issues, and training needs. *Professional Psychology: Research and Practice, 49*(3), 205–219. https://doi.org/10.1037/pro0000188

Hacker, K., Briss, P., Richardson, L., Wright, J., & Petersen, R. (2021). COVID-19 and chronic disease: The impact now and in the future. *Preventing Chronic Disease, 18*. https://doi.org/10.5888/pcd18.210086

Hull, T. D., & Mahan, K. (2017). A study of asynchronous mobile-enabled SMS text psychotherapy. *Telemedicine and e-health., 23*(3). https://doi.org/10.1089/tmj.2016.0114

Jenkins- Guarnieri, M. A., Pruett, L., Luxton, D., D.D, & Johnson, K. (2015). Patient perceptions of telehealth: Review of direct comparisons to in-person psychotherapeutic treatments. *Telemedicine and e-health, 21*(8) https://doi.org/10.1089/tmj.2014.0165

Mohr. (2012). Xxx. *JAMA, 307*(21) https://www.ncbi.nim.nih.ov/pmc/articles/PMC3697075.

Orkibi, H. (2021). Creative adaptability: Conceptual framework, measurement, and outcomes in times of crisis. *Frontiers in Psychology, 11*(3695). https://doi.org/10.3389/fpsyg.2020.588172

Peper, E., Harvey, R., & Faass, N. (2020). *Tech Stress: How technology is hijacking our lives, strategies for coping, and pragmatic ergonomics*. North Atlantic Books.

Poletti, B., Tagini, S., Brugnera, A., Parolin, L., Pievani, L., Ferrucci, R., & Silani, V. (2020). Telepsychotherapy: A leaflet for psychotherapists in the age of COVID-19. A review of the evidence. *Counselling Psychology Quarterly*, 1–16. https://doi.org/10.1080/09515070.2020.1769557

Shrira, A., Hoffman, Y., Bodner, E., & Palgi, Y. (2020). COVID-19 related loneliness and psychiatric symptoms among older adults: The buffering role of subjective age. *The American Journal of Geriatric Psychiatry, 28*(11), 1200–1204. https://doi.org/10.1016/j.jagp.2020.05.018

Slone, N. C., Reese, R. J., & McClellan, M. J. (2012). Telepsychology outcome research with children and adolescents: A review of the literature. *Psychological Services, 9*(3). https://doi.org/10.1037/a0027607

Turgoose, D., Ashwick, R., & Murphy, D. (2018). Systematic review of lessons learned from delivering tele-therapy to veterans with post-traumatic stress disorder. *Journal of Telemedicine and Telecare*. https://doi.org/10.1177/1357633X17730443

Tuerk, P. W., Keller, S. M., & Acierno, R. (2018). Treatment for anxiety and depression via clinical teleconferencing: Evidence base and barriers to expanded access in practice. *Focus, 16*(4), 363–369. https://doi.org/10.1176/appi.focus.20180027

Usher, K., Bhullar, N., Durkin, J., Gyamfi, N., & Jackson, D. (2020). Family violence and COVID-19. Increased vulnerability and reduced options for support. *International Journal of Mental Health Nursing, 29*(4), 549–552. https://doi.org/10.1111/inm.12735

Varker, T., Brand, R. M., Ward, J., Tehrhaag, S., & Phelps, A. (2019). Efficacy of synchronous telepsychology interventions for people with anxiety, depression, posttraumatic stress disorder and adjustment disorder: A rapid evidence assessment. *Psychological Services, 16*(4), 621–635. https://doi.org/10.1037/ser0000239

Wind, T. R., Rijkeboer, G., & Riper, H. (2020). The COVID-19 pandemic: The 'black swan' for mental health care and a turning point for e-health. *Internet Interventions*. https://doi.org/10.1016/j.invent.2020.100317

World Health Organization. (2020). *Coronavirus disease 2019 (COVID-19) situation reports*. (https://www.who.int/emergencies/diseases/novel-coronavirus-2019/situation-reports). Accessed 2020-05-13.

Younggren, J. N., Gottlieb, M. C., & Baker, E. (2022). Navigating the labyrinth of professional regulations: Surviving in a flawed regulatory system. *Professional Psychology, 53*.

Chapter 11
International Advancements on COVID-19 Scholarship Through the Research Initiatives Working Group at the APA Interdivisional Task Force on the Pandemic

Arzu Karakulak, Rita Rivera, Radosveta Dimitrova, Denise Carballea, Bin-Bin Chen, Priyoth Kittiteerasack, Carlos Miguel Rios González, Ebrar Yildirim, and Yue Yu

This chapter provides an introduction and presentation of the Research Initiatives Working Group advancing multidimensional COVID-19-related scholarship from a global international perspective. The chapter begins by outlining the mission statement (i.e., to support all group members in identifying and supporting other scholars around the world as well as produce needed scholarly research and disseminate information about research needs) supplemented by a brief history and current profile of the group. Noteworthy contribution of this chapter regards the main products

A. Karakulak (✉)
Department of Psychology, Bahçeşehir University, Istanbul, Turkey
e-mail: arzu.karakulak@eas.bau.edu.tr

R. Rivera · D. Carballea
Department of Psychology, Albizu University, San Juan, Puerto Rico

R. Dimitrova
Department of Psychology, Stockholm University, Stockholm, Sweden

B.-B. Chen
Department of Psychology, Fudan University, Shanghai, China

P. Kittiteerasack
Department of Mental Health and Psychiatric Nursing, Thammasat University, Bangkok, Thailand

C. M. R. González
Facultad de Ciencias Médicas, Universidad Nacional de Caaguazu, Coronel Oviedo, Paraguay

E. Yildirim
Department of Psychology, Yeditepe University, Istanbul, Turkey

Y. Yu
Centre for Research in Child Development, National Institute of Education, Nanyang Technological University, Singapore, Singapore

C. R. Figley et al. (eds.), *Pandemic Providers*,
https://doi.org/10.1007/978-3-031-27580-7_11

(e.g., global scholarship on COVID-19 research initiatives), deliverables (e.g., published papers, reports, and current projects of the group) for the advancement of theoretical and empirical knowledge base on COVID-19 in global contexts, refinement of methodological issues and measurement, and integration of relevant scholarship with research, policy, and practice. The most prominent resources of the group regard the creation of a COVID-19 research map and an international project on the multidimensional impact, experience, and perceptions of COVID-19 around the globe. The chapter concludes with relevant accomplishments of the group in the midst of challenges faced and lessons learned while providing practical tips and outlook for the current field.

The Research Initiatives Working Group Mission Statement

The Research Initiatives Working Group (RIWG) is committed to compiling a collection of the currently available knowledge base on the psychological impact of COVID-19 from a multidisciplinary and international perspective. The goal is to inform students, researchers, policymakers, practitioners, stakeholders, professionals, and relevant scholarship on the multidimensional impact of COVID-19 and related psychological treatment, prevention, and intervention resources. To this end, RIWG advances the knowledge base through a repository and dissemination of newly published materials and resources such as peer-reviewed articles, reports, calls for papers, funding opportunities, conferences, webinars, symposia, as well as a COVID-19 research map with scholars conducting relevant work in international, multidisciplinary, and global settings.

The Research Initiatives Working Group Origin and Profile

The idea for a group focusing on research came out of the initial brainstorm that emerged as an area of interest for a number of the members of the APA COVID-19 Interdisciplinary Task Force. This was also a natural professional need for most members engaged in a variety of disciplines and positions at universities, hospitals, and clinics across the world. Therefore, advancing the knowledge base on research in the global pandemic was an important addition to many mental health scholars necessary for their current work, teaching, and projects.

We did an exploratory qualitative survey with open-ended questions to all group members to give voice to the group and share narrative experiences and thoughts related to our work and various activities in the midst of the pandemic. These questions asked on reasons for joining the group and relations between group work and own work/study/interests; personal experiences during the pandemic in relation to the group activities and the TF; why this effort is important; prospects and hope to achieve; personal story based on own experience and work during this year; lessons learned from this pandemic; and opportunities to develop. Based on the responses, it was evident that all group members joined as a consequence of strong relationships and parallels with their own recent work on human development, societal and family dynamics, impact on cultural communities, and youth mental health during COVID-19.

One member mentioned that "I joined this group specifically because a lot of my current work is directly aligned most to research itself. I also, though, find research to be of greatest importance right now considering a new perspective associated with a "new" population not to mention new circumstances will require new methods and tactics, new insights about individual behaviors that have never been perpetuated by the current status of society as a whole. We have history to compare, but as history evolves, as do individuals and individual behaviors aligned to environments and nature itself."

Another relevant reason was related to the wide international network and outreach – "The group represented a nice chance to connect and network with professionals and researchers at the international level and share relevant literature and works related to the pandemic. The Task Force works to systematically compile all relevant work related to COVID-19 in the psychological field and is an important source of knowledge dissemination among its members, who in turn disseminate the same resources in their networks. The shared folder represents a rich database of empirical and theoretical articles that allows to keep up with the mounting literature on the pandemic in multiple research fields related to the broader field of psychology. Our meetings were an opportunity to keep track of the rapid evolution of the situation internationally and to draw inspiration and ideas on best ways to proceed in our research and professional activities during the pandemic."

Another member noted that the need for this group focused on research almost requires no explanation, as the word "unprecedented" has been probably the most commonly used word in relation to the COVID-19 pandemic and the circumstances it created over the recent months. "The novel challenges that individuals face during this time, and the identification of particularly vulnerable individuals and groups, as well as their specific needs, is a critical step for the timely development of public health and mental health intervention and prevention strategies."

Currently, the group has members from diverse disciplines and environmental studies and countries (the USA, Sweden, China, Canada, Italy, Japan, Malaysia, Turkey). We have compiled the group profile, including member affiliations, ethnic belonging, languages spoken, research interests, memberships in major organizations/associations, and current projects. The group is truly international, ethnically diverse, and multilingual/multicultural with a wide range of expertise and research interests across *multidisciplinary fields* (i.e., neuropsychology, psychoneuroimmunology, cross-cultural psychology, educational psychology, counselor and psychologist training, international psychology, online education and remote teaching, developmental psychology, acculturation, health communication, developmental psychopathology, human resource development, qualitative research methods, epidemiology of psychiatric disorders, psychopathology social psychology), *populations* (i.e., Hispanic/Latinx, minority (Roma) groups, college and university students, adolescents, women military family caregivers, families, children, older adults, refugee immigrant asylum seekers), and *topics* (i.e., trauma, interpersonal violence, suicidality, depressive disorders, immigration, cultural competence, trauma-informed care, positive youth development, adaptation of instruments in different cultures, violent radicalization, sociocultural diversity, self-regulated learning, interceptive sensibility, stress management, relaxation therapy, stress and coping, health behavior, religiosity, depression, mental health, trauma, intergenerational transmission, international policy and programs, disaster psychosocial resilience, traumatic brain injuries, cognitive rehabilitation, sexuality post brain trauma, Alzheimer's disease, interpersonal violence, parenting, global mental health, and culturally informed interventions, alcohol addiction and nutrition, social emotional learning, mindfulness, adolescent digital medial use, social development and well-being, school interventions for digital citizenship, emotion recognition and regulation, prosocial behavior, cooperation, volunteering, moral judgment).

The group members meet virtually when some new initiatives or discussion comes up. There is also a very intense email communication to share ideas and exchange information. Further, the group members are working on a variety of products related to the pandemic (Karakulak et al. 2023; Tepe & Karakulak, 2021; Yang et al., 2021).

Gathering Resources

In line with the mission statement, the group has been devoted to gathering resources in a digital repository within a wide range of material, including but not limited to peer-reviewed articles, reports, calls for papers, funding opportunities, conferences, webinars, and symposia related to COVID-19. While acknowledging the timeliness of some of these materials, the group is interested in documenting the scholarly research of the pandemic as well as sharing resources with other mental health professionals and scholars. Additional, relevant resources developed by the group are the COVID-19 research map with scholars conducting relevant work in international, multidisciplinary, and global settings; our COVID-19 international project and group members' publications are described in more detail below.

The COVID-19 Research Map A relevant product of the group is our COVID-19 research map. This project started as a common idea to connect with researchers in social sciences around the globe and "map" research labs, groups, and projects currently conducted on COVID-19. The map was created via our networks and colleague fellows who provided information on any ongoing COVID-19 research around the world. Additionally, we are performing an online search and adding any current projects posted on the web and relevant institutions.

Currently, the map contains over 100 projects around the globe with relevant scholarship on the multidimensional impact of COVID-19 with a special focus on well-being and mental health (see Table 11.1 and Fig. 11.1 for COVID-19 research scholarship map by country). The table and the map were limited to the first two or three projects/publications per country most representative of the local population in terms of samples, measures, mental health topics, and target groups. Given the speed of ongoing publications on the topic, much more work may be added, but for the sake of synthesis, we kept it to a limited representativeness. In addition, Table 11.2 presents a summary of global research projects involving multiple country sites and locations worldwide. The content of the map is currently allocated with all other materials on our digital repository (peer-reviewed articles, reports, calls for papers, funding opportunities, conferences, webinars, and symposia). We hope the current format and the audience of these resources, as well as how to render them accessible to various professionals.

International and Multidimensional Perspectives on the Impact of COVID-19 (IMPACT-C19) The Research Initiatives Work Group (RIWG) promoted the project entitled "International and Multidimensional Perspectives on the Impact of COVID-19 (IMPACT-C19)" with the scope to examine the impact, perceptions, and experiences of COVID-19 among young people and established adults in a multidimensional and international perspective; collect data in various countries to disseminate knowledge of such multidisciplinary expertise; as well as apply new measures on COVID-19 to provide solid psychometric and methodological evidence of measurement tools internationally. We started this project with the group members (mainly developmental, social, and cross-cultural psychologists) with academic enthusiasm to promote our science and knowledge on the pandemic. The project grew as team members suggested other colleagues interested in the topic to join and also approached authors of published papers on the pandemic. Thus, all group members were actively involved in the initiation, development, and growth of the project within a supportive research community around the world to encourage and connect with each other. Currently, the project involves over 150 members across major geographical regions in over 80 countries across all major continents. The target samples are emerging adults aged 19–29, established adults aged 30–45 (Mehta et al., 2020), and youth aged 16–18. A set of measures was adopted to reflect the group multidisciplinary expertise and recent work on COVID-19 on a wide range of topics such as international assessment, positive development, well-being, resilience, and coping (Dimitrova & Wiium, 2021a, b; Lee, 2020; Tepe & Karakulak, 2021).

On each site, data are being collected with online platforms prior ethical clearance and a committee approach largely used in cross-cultural assessment and test adaptation (van de Vijver, 2019). *The committee approach* to translation attempts to decrease the introduction of cultural bias inherent in the native language, by introducing collaborative, consensus translation efforts. The translation committee members may include three to four individuals with knowledge of the target language, society, and culture and knowledge of English. They discuss the final version and then ask a study potential participant (teacher or young person) to read the items and their appropriateness. In addition, a neighbor or person not involved in the work

Table 11.1 COVID-19 research and projects in alphabetical order by country

Country	Topic/title	PI/URL	Citation	Publication type
Afghanistan	Knowledge, attitudes, and practices of medical students; healthcare workers	Arash Nemat https://doi.org/10.4269/ajtmh.20-1367	Nemat et al. (2021)	Journal article
	Emergency Response and Health Systems Preparedness Project	The World Bank	World Bank (2021a)	Project
Albania	Emergency COVID-19 Response Project	The World Bank	World Bank (2021b)	Project
	Empowering Women against COVID-19 (EWAC)	International Labor Organization	International Labour Organization (2021)	Project
	Impact on well-being of children and families	World Vision; Enkeleint Mechili	Mechili et al. (2021) and World Vision Albania (2020)	Report; Journal article
Algeria	COVID-19 epidemic in Algeria	Mohamed Hamidouche; Mohamed Lounis	Lounis (2020)	Journal article
Angola	Sociodemographic characteristics and risk factors	Cruz S. Sebastião	Sebastião et al. (2021)	Journal article
	Physicians' perceptions, knowledge and preparedness of health facilities	Margarete Arrais	Arrais et al. (2021)	Journal article
Antigua and Barbuda	COVID Packs for Kids	Red Cross Red Crescent platform	IFRC (2020)	Internet platform
Argentina	COVID-19 Emergency Response Project	The World Bank		
	Coronavirus Unit 100 basic and translational research initiatives	Rabinovich, G.A.; Geffner, J.	Rabinovich and Geffner (2021)	Journal article
	Lockdown and domestic violence	Interamerican Bank		
	University community engagement	Daniela Perrotta	Perrotta (2021)	Journal article
Armenia	Impact study on COVID-19 on older people and caregivers	Armenia Red Cross Society	Krylova and Gevorgyan (2020a)	Report
	War in the COVID-19 era: Mental health concerns	Christopher Markosian	Markosian et al. (2021)	Journal article

Country	Topic/title	PI/URL	Citation	Publication type
Australia	COVID-19 Unmasked Survey	https://www.childrens.health.qld.gov.au/covid-19-unmasked/	De Young et al. (2021)	Survey
	The COVID-19 Pandemic Adjustment Survey (CPAS)	John Toumbourou	Westrupp et al. (2020)	Journal article
	Families in Australia Survey: Life during COVID-19	Australian Government		
	Willingness to vaccinate	Rachel Dodd	Dodd et al. (2021)	Journal article
	COVID-19 and you: mentaL heaLth in AusTralia now survey (COLLATE) project	Susan Rossell	Van Rheenen et al. (2020)	Journal article
Azerbaijan	REACT-C19 project	World Health Organization	World Health Organization (2020)	Online article
	COVID-19 Emergency Response Project	The World Bank	World Bank (2021c)	Project
	Impact study of COVID-19 on older people and caregivers	Red Cross and Crescent Societies	Krylova and Gevorgyan (2020b)	Report
Bahamas	COVID-19 Response and Recovery	The World Bank	World Bank (2021d)	Project
	Decolonial Thinking, Disasters, Development	Clara Rachel Eybalin Casseus	Clara Rachel Eybalin (2021)	Book chapter
Bahrain	Frontline healthcare workers	Haitham Jahrami	Jahrami et al. (2021)	Journal article
Bangladesh	Emergency Response and Pandemic Preparedness Project	The World Bank	World Bank (2021e)	Project
	Response to COVID-19 in Bangladesh: Strategies to Resist the Growing Trend of COVID-19	Saifur Rahman Chowdhury	Chowdhury et al. (2020)	Journal article
	Fear of COVID-19 and xenophobia, psychological consequences	Mohammed A. Mamun	Mamun et al. (2021)	Journal article
	Mental health of children	Sabina Yeasmin	Yeasmin et al. (2020)	Journal article

(continued)

Table 11.1 (continued)

Country	Topic/title	PI/URL	Citation	Publication type
	Mental health of the adult population	Hassan Al-Banna	Banna et al. (2020)	Journal article
	Depression General Population and Healthcare Professionals	Najmuj Sakib	Sakib et al. (2021)	Journal article
	Depression and anxiety among university students	Akhtarul Islam	Islam et al. (2020)	Journal article
Barbados	COVID-19 Response and Recovery	The World Bank	World Bank (2021f)	Project
	Employability Project	International Labor Organization	International Labour Organization (2020)	Project
	Barbados COVID-19 Health Resilience	European Investment Bank	European Investment Bank (2020)	Project
Belarus	Emergency COVID-19 Response Project	The World Bank	World Bank (2020a)	Project
	COVID-19 Fear	Alexander Reznik	Reznik et al. (2021)	Journal article
	Stress, Anxiety, and Substance Use among Students	Valentina Gritsenko	Gritsenko et al. (2021)	Journal article
Belgium	Large COVID SDT Project	Omer Van den Bergh; Maarten Vansteenkiste	Center for Self Determination Theory (2020)	Online article
	HELICON – Unravelling the long-term and indirect health impact of the COVID-19 crisis in Belgium	Koen Blot; Brecht Devleesschauwer; Dominique Van Beckhoven	Blot et al. (2021)	Project
	INAMI project on the telemonitoring of COVID-19 patients	National Institute for Health and Disability Insurance (2020)		Project
	Attitudes of healthcare workers towards COVID-19 vaccination	Pierre Verger	Verger et al. (2021)	Journal article
	Vulnerability to disease and attitudes towards public health measures	David De Coninck	De Coninck et al. (2020)	Journal article
Belize	Belize COVID-19 Relief Project	IFRC Disaster Response and Preparedness	IFRC (2021)	Project

Country	Topic/title	PI/URL	Citation	Publication type
	Primary education	Claire Chadwick	Chadwick et al. (2021)	Book chapter
	Containing Community Spread	Danladi Chiroma Husaini	Husaini and Abubakar (2020)	Journal article
Benin	Benin COVID-19 Preparedness and Response Project	The World Bank	World Bank (2022a)	Project
	Containment Measures	Issideen Ayinla Osseni	Osseni (2020)	Journal article
Bhutan	COVID-19 Emergency Response and Health Systems Preparedness Project	The World Bank	World Bank (2021g)	Project
	Project Gawa	UNICEF	UNICEF (n.d.)	Project
	Gross National Happiness Framework and the Health System Response to the COVID-19	Thinley Dorji	Dorji (2021)	Journal article
	Pandemic management	Nitasha Kaul	Kaul (2021)	Journal article
Bolivia	Support of healthcare workers	Stephen X. Zhang	Zhang et al. (2020)	Journal article
	Social media exposure, risk perception, preventive behaviors	Diana Reyna Zeballos Rivas	Zeballos Rivas et al. (2021)	Journal article
Bosnia and Herzegovina	Fear and depression	Armin Šljivo	Šljivo et al. (2020)	Journal article
	Emergency COVID-19 Project	The World Bank	World Bank (2021h)	Project
Botswana	Vulnerability of children	Thabile Samboma	Samboma (2020)	Journal article
	Parental Engagement in Education	Rebecca Winthrop	Winthrop et al. (2020)	Policy brief
Brazil	COVID-19 and mental health	Jeferson Ferraz Goularte	Goularte et al. (2021)	Journal article
	Mental health of healthcare professionals	Felipe Ornell	Ornell et al. (2020)	Journal article
Brunei	Norms and opportunities in higher education setting	Masitah Shahrill	Shahrill et al. (2021)	Journal article

(continued)

Table 11.1 (continued)

Country	Topic/title	PI/URL	Citation	Publication type
Bulgaria	Support United Against COVID-19 Fund	https://www.globalgiving.org/projects/united-against-covid-19-bulgaria/	Trust for Social Achievement Foundation (n.d.)	Project
Burkina Faso	Supporting Children and Their Families	International Social Service	ConnectAID (n.d.)	Outreach project
	COVID-19 Preparedness and Response Project	The World Bank	World Bank (2021i)	Project
Burundi	COVID-19 Preparedness and Response Project	The World Bank	World Bank (2021j)	Project
Côte d'Ivoire	COVID-19 Strategic Preparedness and Response Project	The World Bank	World Bank (2021m)	Project
Cabo Verde	COVID-19 Emergency Response Project	The World Bank	World Bank (2021k)	Project
Cambodia	COVID-19 Emergency Response Project	The World Bank	World Bank (2021l)	Project
	Parental and Community Participation in Education	Cambodian Education Forum		
Cameroon	COVID-19 Preparedness and Response Project	The World Bank	World Bank (2022b)	Project
	Distress among health care professionals	François Roger Nguépy Keubo	Nguépy Keubo et al. (2021)	Journal article
	Preventive Behaviours National Survey and Fear and Depression Nation-wide Observational Study	Joseph Nelson Siewe Fodjo	Siewe Fodjo et al. (2021)	Journal article
Canada	Project Pandemic: Canada Reports on COVID-19	Canadian News Organizations	Institute for Investigative Journalism (n.d.)	Project
	Maternal depressive and anxiety symptoms	Nicole Racine	Racine et al. (2021)	Journal article
	Parent-child conversations about COVID-19	Lindsay Malloy	Ontorio Tech University (2020)	Online article

Country	Topic/title	PI/URL	Citation	Publication type
	Mental health impacts of the COVID-19 nationally representative cross-sectional survey	Emily K. Jenkins	Jenkins et al. (2021)	Journal article
	COVID-19 quarantine and mental health	Zachary Daly	Daly et al. (2021)	Journal article
Central African Republic	COVID-19 Preparedness and Response Project	The World Bank	World Bank (2022c)	Project
Chad	COVID-19 Strategic Preparedness and Response Project	The World Bank	World Bank (2022d)	Project
Chile	Mental Health	Alejandra Caqueo-Urízar	Caqueo-Urízar et al. (2020)	Journal article
	Psychosocial impact of COVID-19 pandemic on LGBT people	J. Barrientos	Barrientos et al. (2021)	Journal article
	Anxiety, anhedonia and food consumption	Leslie Landaeta-Diaz	Landaeta-Díaz et al. (2021)	Journal article
China	Quarantine on mental health status among general population	Yunhe Wang	Wang et al. (2021c)	Journal article
	Mental Health Among College Students	Yuanyuan Li	Li et al. (2021b)	Journal article
	Child and adolescent mental health	Wen Li; Suqin Tang; Sifan Kang	Li et al. (2021a), Tang et al. (2021), and Kang et al. (2021)	Journal article
	Parental burnout and coping with the COVID-19	Bin-Bin Chen	Yang et al. (2021)	Journal article
Colombia	COVID-19 Crisis Response	The World Bank	World Bank (2021aw)	Website
	PSY-COVID study	Juan P. Sanabria-Mazo	Sanabria-Mazo et al. (2021)	Pre-print journal article
Comoros	Emergency DPO for COVID-19 response	The World Bank	World Bank (2020b)	Project
Congo	Lisungi Emergency COVID-19 Response project	The World Bank	World Bank (2021ao)	Project

(continued)

Table 11.1 (continued)

Country	Topic/title	PI/URL	Citation	Publication type
Costa Rica	COVID-19 Response Project	The World Bank		
Croatia	Child and adolescent mental health	Tomislav Franic	Franic and Dodig-Curkovic (2020)	Journal article
	Psychological Well-Being Adolescents and Medical Students	Ruzica Dragun	Dragun et al. (2021)	Journal article
Cuba	Anxiety, Health Self-Perception, and Worry	Yunier Broche-Pérez	Broche-Pérez et al. (2021)	Journal article
Cyprus	Impact of the pandemic on refugees, migrants and asylum seekers	Sarah Morsheimer	Morsheimer et al. (2020)	Briefing
	Public Health Interventions	Annalisa Quattrocchi	Quattrocchi et al. (2020)	Journal article
	Mental Health Disorders	Neophytos Stylianou	Stylianou et al. (2020)	Journal article
Czech Republic	Fear, anger, trauma	Radek Trnka	Trnka and Lorencova (2020)	Journal article
Congo	COVID-19 Emergency Response Project	The World Bank	World Bank (2021an)	Project
	Anxiety, depression	Jude Mary Cénat	Cénat et al. (2021)	Journal article
Denmark	Coronavirus initiatives	The Novo Nordisk Foundation	Novo Nordisk Foundation (2022)	Website
	Mental health indicators	Amy Clotworthy	Clotworthy et al. (2020)	Journal article
	Psychosocial consequences in people with diabetes	Lene Eide Joensen	Joensen et al. (2020)	Journal article
Djibouti	Djibouti COVID-19 Response	The World Bank	World Bank (2021n)	Project
Dominica	COVID-19 Response and Recovery Programmatic DPC	The World Bank	World Bank (2021o)	Project
Dominican Republic	COVID-19 Crisis Response Support	The World Bank	World Bank (2020c)	Project
	Mental health services	Eddy A. Peralta	Peralta and Taveras (2020)	Journal article
Ecuador	COVID-19 Emergency Response Project	The World Bank	World Bank (2021p)	Project

Country	Topic/title	PI/URL	Citation	Publication type
	Remote-learning, time-use, and mental health of high-school students	Igor Asanov	Asanov et al. (2021)	Journal article
	Mental health workers	Xi Chen	Chen et al. (2020)	Journal article
Egypt	COVID-19 Emergency Response	The World Bank	World Bank (2021q)	Project
	Psychological Impacts	Ahmed Arafa	Arafa et al. (2021)	Journal article
	Mental Health and Social Support	Safaa M. El-Zoghby	El-Zoghby et al. (2020)	Journal article
El Salvador	COVID-19 Emergency Response Project	The World Bank	World Bank (2021r)	Project
	Emotional Symptoms During Residential Lockdown	Carlos Iván Orellana	Orellana and Orellana (2020)	Journal article
Estonia	Mental Health Athletes	Ülle Parm	Parm et al. (2021)	Journal article
	Estonian National Mental Health Study (RVTU)	Jaan Tulviste and Kenn Konstabel https://www.tlu.ee/en/covidstudy		
Eswatini	COVID-19 Emergency Response Project	The World Bank	World Bank (2021s)	Project
Ethiopia	COVID-19 Emergency Response	The World Bank	World Bank (2022e)	Project
	Mental health of healthcare professionals	Yimenu Yitayih	Yitayih et al. (2020)	Journal article
	COVID-19-Induced Among Urban Residents	Adamu Birhanu	Birhanu et al. (2021)	Journal article
Fiji	COVID-19 Emergency Response Project	The World Bank	World Bank (2021t)	Project
Finland	The impact of the COVID-19 crisis on gender equality	Finnish Institute for Health and Welfare	Welfare State Research and Reform (2020)	Project
	Corona Consumers project	Mette Ranta	DigiConsumers (n.d.)	Research project
	Psychological and Situational Risks Workers	Iina Savolainen	Savolainen et al. (2021)	Journal article

(continued)

Table 11.1 (continued)

Country	Topic/title	PI/URL	Citation	Publication type
France	Mental health before and during COVID-19 lockdown	Leila Ramiz	Ramiz et al. (2021)	Journal article
	Mental health immigrants	Anne Gosselin	Gosselin et al. (2021)	Journal article
	Mental health university students	Marielle Wathelet; Mathilde Husky	Wathelet et al. (2020) and Husky et al. (2020)	Journal article
	Coping with COVID-19: Social Distancing, Cohesion, and Inequality	Ettore Recchi	Sciences Po (2020)	Project
Gabon	COVID-19 Strategic Preparedness and Response Project (SPRP)	The World Bank	World Bank (2021u)	Project
Gambia	COVID-19 Preparedness and Response Project	The World Bank	World Bank (2021v)	Project
Georgia	Emergency COVID-19 Response Project	The World Bank	World Bank (2021w)	Project
Germany	COVID-19 related studies and tools	National Research Data Infrastructure for Personal Health Data	Fairdom Hub (2020)	Project
	GESIS Panel Special Survey on the Coronavirus SARS-CoV-2 Outbreak in Germany	GESIS	GESIS (2021)	Survey
	Quality of life and mental health in children and adolescents	Ulrike Ravens-Sieberer	Ravens-Sieberer et al. (2021)	Journal article
	Longitudinal changes of anxiety and depressive symptoms	Antonia Bendau	Bendau et al. (2021)	Journal article
	Risk, resilience, psychological distress, and anxiety	Moritz Bruno Petzold	Petzold et al. (2020)	Journal article
Ghana	COVID-19 Emergency Preparedness and Response Project	The World Bank	World Bank (2022f)	Project

Country	Topic/title	PI/URL	Citation	Publication type
	Fear and Internal Conflict among Older Adults	Razak M Gyasi	Gyasi (2020)	Journal article
	Mental health	Nestor Asiamah	Asiamah et al. (2021)	Journal article
	Psychological impact of COVID-19 on health workers	Anthony Amanfo Ofori	Ofori et al. (2021)	Journal article
Greece	Senior high school students' mental health	Ioanna Giannopoulou	Giannopoulou et al. (2021)	Journal article
	Anxiety, depression and suicidality	Konstantinos N Fountoulakis	Fountoulakis et al. (2021)	Journal article
	University students' mental health	Chrysi K. Kaparounaki	Kaparounaki et al. (2020)	Journal article
Grenada	COVID-19 Crisis Response and Fiscal Management	The World Bank	World Bank (2021x)	Project
Guatemala	COVID-19 Response	The World Bank	World Bank (2021y)	Project
	Indigenous communities, and public health	Martha Few	Few (2020)	Journal article
Guinea	COVID-19 Preparedness and Response Project	The World Bank	World Bank (2022g)	Project
	Psychosocial impacts of COVID-19	Almamy Amara Touré	Touré et al. (2021)	Journal article
Haiti	COVID-19 Response	The World Bank	World Bank (2021z)	Project
Honduras	COVID-19 Emergency Response Project	The World Bank	World Bank (2022h)	Project
	Confinement stress, and mental health	Miguel Landa-Blanco	Landa-Blanco et al. (2021)	Journal article
Hungary	Psychological well-being and coping strategies of elderly	Beatrix Lábadi	Lábadi et al. (2021)	Journal article
	Mental well-being of university students	Andrea Lukács	Lukács (2021)	Journal article
Iceland	COVID-19 projects	University of Iceland	University of Iceland (n.d.)	Website
India	COVID-19 Emergency Response and Health Systems Preparedness Project	The World Bank	World Bank (2020e)	Project

(continued)

Table 11.1 (continued)

Country	Topic/title	PI/URL	Citation	Publication type
	Impact on education, social life and mental health of students	Kunal Chaturvedi	Chaturvedi et al. (2021)	Journal article
	Mental health of the health-care professionals; migrant workers	Dhanasekhar Kesavelu; Naveen Raghavendra	Kesavelu et al. (2021) and Raghavendra et al. (2021)	Journal article
	Mental health during COVID-19 lockdown; Women	Priya Alat; Mirai Chatterjee; Usama Rehman	Alat et al. (2021), Chatterjee (2021), and Rehman et al. (2021)	Journal article
	COVID-19: Psychological Impact and Response in the Corporate Sector	Richa Rajendra Khanna		
Indonesia	Indonesia Project on COVID-19	Australian National University	Australian National University (2022)	Project
	Emergency Response to COVID19	The World Bank	World Bank (2021aa)	Project
	Adolescent Mental Well-Being; Health care professionals; Mental Health Workers; Anxiety	Tjhin Wiguna; Deni Kurniadi Sunjaya; Heni Dwi Windarwati; Yunias Setiawati; Gina Anindyajati	Wiguna et al. (2020), Sunjaya et al. (2021), Windarwati et al. (2021), Setiawati et al. (2021), and Anindyajati et al. (2021)	Journal article
Iran	Emergency Response Project	The World Bank	World Bank (2022i)	Project
	Mental health impact	Reza Shahriarirad; Ata Farajzadeh; Fatemeh Khademian; Cuiyan Wang	Shahriarirad et al. (2021), Farajzadeh et al. (2021), Khademian et al. (2021), and Wang et al. (2021a)	Journal article
Iraq	Depression, Anxiety, and Stress	Niaz Kamal	Kamal and Othman (2020)	Journal article
Ireland	Child and Adolescent Mental Health; Mental health	Katriona O'Sullivan; Ruth Neill	O'Sullivan et al. (2021) and Neill et al. (2021)	Journal article Journal article
Israel	Mental Health, Resilience, and Quality of Life	Lena Lipskaya-Velikovsky; Mary Jo Coiro; Anat Amit Aharon; Adi Mana; Mor Yehudai; Danny Horesh	Lipskaya-Velikovsky (2021), Coiro et al. (2021), Amit Aharon et al. (2021), Mana et al. (2021), Yehudai et al. (2020), and Horesh et al. (2020)	Journal article
	Hope and Resilience	Orna Braun-Lewensohn	Braun-Lewensohn et al. (2021)	Journal article

Country	Topic/title	PI/URL	Citation	Publication type
Italy	Mental health; mental health workers	Nicola Meda; Francesco Chirico; Gabriele Prati; Maria Rosaria Gualano; Claudia Carmassi; Rodolfo Rossi; Marialaura Di Tella; Felice Iasevoli	Meda et al. (2021), Chirico et al. (2021), Prati (2021), Gualano et al. (2021), Carmassi et al. (2021), Rossi et al. (2020), Di Tella et al. (2020), and Iasevoli et al. (2021)	Journal article
	Pasquale Musso	Civic engagement		
	Italian Association of Psychologists Projects and Papers	Italian Association of Psychologists	Associazione Italiana di Psicologia (2022)	Website
Jamaica	COVID-19 Response and Recovery Development Policy	The World Bank	World Bank (2021ab)	Project
Japan	Trend in suicide	Shuhei Nomura; Takanao Tanaka	Nomura et al. (2021) Tanaka and Okamoto (2021)	Journal article Journal article
	Mental health medical workers; older adults; students	Yasuhiro Kotera; Kosuke Fujita; Ryo Horita; Yoshito Nishimura; Haruhiko Midorikawa	Kotera et al. (2021), Fujita et al. (2021), Horita et al. (2021), Nishimura et al. (2021), and Midorikawa et al. (2021)	Journal article
Jordan	COVID-19 Emergency Response	The World Bank	World Bank (2021ac)	Project
	Mental Health mothers; Students	Somaya H. Malkawi; Ensaf Y. Almomani	Malkawi et al. (2021) and Almomani and Almomany (2021)	Journal article
	Psychological Impact General Population; Mental health workers	Moawiah Khatatbeh; Abdallah Y. Naser	Khatatbeh et al. (2021) and Naser et al. (2020)	Journal article
Kazakhstan	Stress, health doctors; mental health students	Dana Bazarkulova; Aidos K. Bolatov	Bazarkulova and Compton (2021) and Bolatov et al. (2021)	Journal article
Kenya	COVID-19 Health Emergency Response Project	The World Bank	World Bank (2021ad)	
	Youth mental health; mental health response	S.O. Ogweno; Jessie Pinchoff; Florence Jaguga	Ogweno et al. (2021), Pinchoff et al. (2021), and Jaguga and Kwobah (2020)	Journal article

(continued)

Table 11.1 (continued)

Country	Topic/title	PI/URL	Citation	Publication type
Kiribati	COVID-19 Emergency Response Project	The World Bank	World Bank (2021ae)	Project
Kuwait	Mental Health of Healthcare Professionals and Students	Zahra Alsairafi	Alsairafi et al. (2021)	Journal article
Kyrgyzstan	Emergency COVID-19 Project	The World Bank	World Bank (2022j)	Project
	Maternal and newborn health	Bernd Rechel	Rechel and Moldoisaeva (2021)	Journal article
Laos	COVID-19 Response Project	The World Bank	World Bank (2021af)	Project
Latvia	Life with COVID-19	Rīga Stradiņš University	Rīga Stradiņš University (2020)	Project
	Family Health-Related Quality of Life	Inese Stars	Stars et al. (2021)	Journal article
Lebanon	Mental healthcare of older adults; Mental health; Health care professionals; University students	Rita Khoury; Radwan El Othman; Fatima Msheik El Khoury; Zaid Ayad; Ghida Kassir	Khoury and Karam (2020), El Othman et al. (2021), Msheik El Khoury et al. (2021), Ayad et al. (2021), and Kassir et al. (2021)	Journal article
Lesotho	COVID-19 Emergency Preparedness and Response Project	The World Bank	World Bank (2022k)	Project
Liberia	COVID-19 Emergency Response Project	The World Bank	World Bank (2020f)	Project
Libya	Socio-Economic Framework for the Response to COVID-19	United Nations	United Nations Country Team (2020)	Press release
	COVID-19 and its impact on vulnerable populations	International Centre for Migration Policy Development	International Centre for Migration Policy Development (2022)	Online briefing
	Mental Health and Quality of Life; Health care workers	Ayesha S. Al Dhaheri; Muhammed Elhadi; Hashem A. Kilani	Al Dhaheri et al. (2021), Elhadi et al. (2020), and Kilani et al. (2020)	Journal article
Liechtenstein	Mental health of children and adolescents	Stefanie J. Schmidt	Schmidt et al. (2021)	Journal article
Lithuania	COVIDiet Study	Vilma Kriaucioniene	Kriaucioniene et al. (2020)	Journal article
Luxembourg	COVID-19 Projects	COVID-19 Task Force	Research Luxembourg (n.d.)	Website
	Health, well-being and life satisfaction of young people	Caroline Residori	Residori et al. (2020)	Conference proceeding

Country	Topic/title	PI/URL	Citation	Publication type
	Aging and well-being	Anna Elena Kornadt	Kornadt et al. (2020)	Journal article
Madagascar	COVID-19 Response	The World Bank	World Bank (2021ag)	Project
Malawi	COVID-19 Emergency Response and Health Systems Preparedness Project	The World Bank	World Bank (2021ah)	Project
Malaysia	Adults' Mental health	Huiyang Dai	Dai et al. (2020)	Journal article
	Psychological impact university students	Sheela Sundarasen	Sundarasen et al. (2020)	Journal article
Maldives	COVID-19 Emergency Response and Health Systems Preparedness Project	The World Bank	World Bank (2022l)	Project
Mali	COVID-19 Emergency Response Project	The World Bank	World Bank (2022m)	Project
	Mental Health Outcomes	Luis Sagaon-Teyssier	Sagaon-Teyssier et al. (2020)	Journal article
Malta	Mental Health Impact	Paulann Grech and Reuben Grech	Grech and Grech (2020)	Journal article
Mauritania	COVID-19 Strategic Preparedness and Response Project	The World Bank	World Bank (2020g)	Project
Mauritius	Mental Health Older Adults	Sambaladevi Chemen	Chemen and Gopalla (2021)	Journal article
Mexico	Psychological Impact Older Adults	Alejandro González-González	González-González et al. (2020)	Journal article
	Mental Health Women; Mental Health Disturbances; Health Care Workers	Adan Silverio-Murillo; Guadalupe Terán-Pérez; Mario H. Flores-Torres; Rebeca Robles	Silverio-Murillo et al. (2021), Terán-Pérez et al. (2021), Flores et al. (2021), and Robles et al. (2021)	Journal article
Moldova	Emergency COVID-19 Response Project	The World Bank	World Bank (2021ai)	Project
Mongolia	COVID-19 Emergency Response and Health System Preparedness Project	The World Bank	World Bank (2021aj)	Project
Morocco	Mental Health	Abdelkrim Janati Idrissi; Hajar Essangri	Janati Idrissi et al. (2020) and Essangri et al. (2021)	Journal article
Mozambique	Mental health; Health Care Workers; Fear of COVID-19	Mila NuNu Htay; Rubia Carla Formighieri Giordan	Htay et al. (2021) and Giordani et al. (2021)	Journal article

(continued)

Table 11.1 (continued)

Country	Topic/title	PI/URL	Citation	Publication type
Myanmar	COVID-19 Emergency Response Project	The World Bank	World Bank (2021ak)	Project
Namibia	Mental Health and Psychosocial Support	Rachel J. Freeman	Rachel et al. (2021)	Journal article
Nepal	COVID-19 Emergency Response and Health Systems Preparedness Project	The World Bank	World Bank (2021al)	Project
	Socioeconomic and mental health aspects	Kritika Paudel	Poudel and Subedi (2020)	Journal article
	Anxiety and depression among the healthcare workers	Anoop Krishna Gupta; Khagendra Kafle; Hridaya Raj Devkota; Pratik Khanal	Gupta et al. (2020), Kafle et al. (2021), Devkota et al. (2021), and Khanal et al. (2020)	Journal article
	Adolescent and Young Adult Mental Health	Vinita Sharma	Sharma et al. (2020)	Journal article
Netherlands	Research on COVID-19 in the Netherlands	National Institute for Public Health and the Environment	National Institute for Public Health and the Environment (n.d.)	Website
	COVID-19 Programme	ZonMw	ZonMw (2022)	Program
	Mental Health Older Adults; Students Well-Being	Theo G van Tilburg; Debby L. Gerritsen; Kuan-Yu Pan; Llewellyn Ellardus van Zyl	van Tilburg et al. (2020) and Gerritsen and Oude Voshaar (2020)	Journal article
	Mental Well-Being of Chinese Immigrants	Xin Ming	Ming and De Jong (2021)	Journal article
New Zealand	COVID-19 research database	Ministry of Business, Innovation and Employment	Ministry of Busines (n.d.)	Website
	Mental Well-Being	Norina Gasteiger; Susanna Every-Palmer	Gasteiger et al. (2021) and Every-Palmer et al. (2020)	Journal article
Nicaragua	COVID-19 Education Sector Response Project	The World Bank	World Bank (2022n)	Project
Niger	COVID-19 Emergency Response Project	The World Bank	World Bank (2022o)	Project
Nigeria	Psychological distress	Chisom Adaobi Nri-Ezedi	Nri-Ezedi et al. (2020)	Journal article

Country	Topic/title	PI/URL	Citation	Publication type
	Mental and Social Health-Related Complaints among Children and Adolescents	Datonye Christopher Briggs	Briggs and Kattey (2020)	Journal article
	COVID-19 Preparedness and Response Project	The World Bank	World Bank (2022p)	Project
North Macedonia	Emergency COVID-19 Response Project	The World Bank	World Bank (2022q)	Project
	Mental health of healthcare workers and police/army forces	G. Ristevska-Dimitrovska and D. Batic	Ristevska-Dimitrovska and Batic (2020)	Journal article
Norway	Collaborative and Knowledge-building Projects for the Fight Against Coronavirus Disease	The Research Council of Norway	The Research Council of Norway (2021)	Website
	Loneliness; Mental health and sleep disturbances	Thomas Hansen; Linda Ernstsen	Hansen et al. (2021) and Ernstsen and Havnen (2021)	Journal article
	Mental disorders, suicidal ideation and suicides in the general population	Ann Kristin Skrindo Knudsen	Knudsen et al. (2021)	Journal article
	Resilience and mental health	Frederick Anyan; Amy Østertun Geirdal	Anyan et al. (2020) and Geirdal et al. (2021)	Journal article
	Face masks as layers of meaning in times of COVID-19; The social perception of risk and diffusion of COVID-19; Life at the time of COVID-19 diary study	Luca Tateo		
	Disability and Disease during the 1918 Influenza Pandemic: Implications for Preparedness Policies (#DIS2)	Jessica Dimka	Dimka (2020)	Project
Oman	Mental health of health care workers	Abdallah Badahdah; Muna Alshekaili; Abdallah M. Badahdah	Badahdah et al. (2021), Alshekaili et al. (2020), and Badahdah et al. (2020)	Journal article

(continued)

Table 11.1 (continued)

Country	Topic/title	PI/URL	Citation	Publication type
Pakistan	COVID-19 Pandemic Response Effectiveness Project	The World Bank	World Bank (2020d)	Project
	Mental health of medical workers; general population	Waleed Rana; Khezar Hayat; Ahmad Ali Tooba Lateef; Ayesha Mumtaz; Abraish Ali; Sonia Mukhtar; Sajid Rahman Khattak; Ram Sandesh	Rana et al. (2020), Hayat et al. (2022), Ali et al. (2021b), Lateef et al. (2021), Mumtaz et al. (2021), Ali et al. (2021a), Mukhtar (2020), Khattak et al. (2021), and Sandesh et al. (2020)	Journal article
Palestine	Coping, stress, mental health	Fayez Azez Mahamid; Maria Helbich	Mahamid and Bdier (2021) and Helbich and Jabr (2021)	Journal article
Panama	COVID-19 Emergency Response	The World Bank	World Bank (2022r)	Project
	Mental health outcomes among interns and residents physicians	Edward A. Espinosa-Guerra		
Papua New Guinea	COVID-19 Emergency Response Project	The World Bank	World Bank (2022s)	Project
Paraguay	COVID-19 Emergency Response Project	The World Bank	World Bank (2021am)	Project
	Stress; Mental health	Julio Torales; Carlos Miguel Rios-González; Jorge Villalba-Arias	Torales et al. (2020), Rios-González and Palacios (2020), and Villalba-Arias et al. (2020)	Journal article; pre-print journal article
Peru	Fear of COVID-19, Mental health, depression	Tomás Caycho-Rodríguez; Hever Krüger-Malpartida; Daniel Antiporta	Caycho-Rodríguez et al. (2021a, b), Krüger-Malpartida et al. (2020), and Antiporta et al. (2021)	Journal article
Philippines	COVID-19 Emergency Response Project	The World Bank	World Bank (2022t)	Project
	Mental health older adults	Robert Buenaventura; Michael Tee; Cuiyan Wang	Buenaventura et al. (2020), Tee et al. (2021), and Wang et al. (2021b)	Journal article
Poland	The Coronavirus Response Investment Initiative	European Commission	European Comission (n.d.-a)	Report

Country	Topic/title	PI/URL	Citation	Publication type
	Coping styles and mental health; student mental health	Agata Kołodziejczyk; Tomasz Wieczorek; Piotr Długosz; Adrian Bartoszek	Kołodziejczyk et al. (2021), Wieczorek et al. (2021), Długosz (2021), and Bartoszek et al. (2020)	Journal article
Portugal	Psychological impact on general population; mental health	Mauro Paulino; Margarita Jarego; Pedro Silva Moreira; Ligia Passos; Lara Pinho	Paulino et al. (2021), Jarego et al. (2021), Silva Moreira et al. (2021), Passos et al. (2020), and Pinho et al. (2021)	Journal article
Qatar	The COVID Project	Georgetown University in Qatar	Georgetown University Qatar (n.d.)	Website
	Mental health, parent and children, front care workers	Ovais Wadoo; Sami Ouanes; Mohamed Abdelrahman; Ovais Wadoo	Wadoo et al. (2020), Ouanes et al. (2021), Abdelrahman et al. (2021), and Wadoo et al. (2021)	Journal article
Romania	The Coronavirus Response Investment Initiative	European Commission	European Comission (n.d.-b)	Report
	Fear of COVID; psychological impact pregnant women	Elena Stănculescu; Ruxandra-Gabriela Cigăran	Stănculescu (2021) and Cigăran et al. (2021)	Journal article
Russia	The Coronavirus Response	The World Bank		Project
	Mental health	Julia Brailovskaia; Mor Yehudai; Valentina Gritsenko; Alexander Reznik	Brailovskaia et al. (2021), Yehudai et al. (2020), Gritsenko et al. (2021), and Reznik et al. (2021)	Journal article
Rwanda	COVID-19 Emergency Response Project	The World Bank	World Bank (2022v)	Project
	Mental health students	Hawa Iye Obaje	Obaje et al. (2021)	Journal article
Samoa	COVID-19 Emergency Response Project	The World Bank	World Bank (2021ap)	Project
Saudi Arabia	Mental health trends in various populations	Nasser F. BinDhim; Youssef Althiabi; Sultana A. Alhurishi; Maha Al Ammari	BinDhim et al. (2021), Althiabi (2021), Alhurishi et al. (2021), and Al Ammari et al. (2021)	Journal article
Senegal	COVID-19 Response Project	The World Bank	World Bank (2021aq)	Project

(continued)

Table 11.1 (continued)

Country	Topic/title	PI/URL	Citation	Publication type
Serbia	Emergency COVID-19 Response Project	The World Bank	World Bank (2021ar)	Project
	Mental health	Isidora Vujčić; Dragana Ristic; Jelena Jovičić-Bata	Vujčić et al. (2021), Ignjatović Ristić et al. (2020), and Jovičić-Bata et al. (2021)	Journal article
Seychelles	COVID-19 Crisis Response Budget Support Program	African Development Bank	African Development Bank Group (2020a)	Project
Sierra Leone	COVID-19 Emergency Preparedness and Response Project	The World Bank	World Bank (2021as)	Project
	Social consequences in a low resource setting	Danilo Buonsenso	Buonsenso et al. (2020)	Journal article
	Mental health for disabled and disadvantaged children and young people	Darren Sharpe	Sharpe et al. (2021)	Journal article
Singapore	COVID-19 Research Projects	National Medical Research Council	National Medical Research Council (2021)	Website
	Mental health, psychological well-being	Kele Ding; Benjamin Tan; Max Denning	Ding et al. (2021), Wang et al. (2021b), Tan (2020), and Denning et al. (2021)	Journal article
	Well-being of families with under aged children	Yue Yu; Yang Yang; Jallene Jia En Chua	Yu et al. (2021) and Yang et al. (2020)	Pre-print journal article
Slovakia	Mental health	Gianluca Lo Coco; Marcela Matos	Lo Coco et al. (2021) and Matos et al. (2021)	Journal article
Slovenia	Mental health, psychological functioning	Gianluca Lo Coco; Tina Kavčič	Lo Coco et al. (2021) and Kavčič et al. (2021)	Journal article
Solomon Islands	COVID-19 Emergency Response Project	The World Bank	World Bank (2022w)	Project
South Africa	COVID-19 Response Development Policy Operation	The World Bank	World Bank (2021at)	Project

Country	Topic/title	PI/URL	Citation	Publication type
	Mental health	Dorrit Posel; Andrew Kim; Anita Padmanabhanunni; Tyrone Pretorius	Posel et al. (2021), Kim et al. (2020), Padmanabhanunni and Pretorius (2021), and Pretorius and Padmanabhanunni (2021)	Journal article
South Korea	Mental health, well-being	Jung Sj; Seung Won Lee; Joo Hyun Kim	Jung and Jun (2020), Lee et al. (2020), and Kim et al. (2022)	Journal article
South Sudan	COVID-19 Emergency Response and Health Systems Preparedness Project	UNICEF	UNICEF (2021)	Report
Spain	Emotional well-being, mental health	Pastora Martínez-Castilla; Montse Ruiz; Carmen Valiente; Gonzalez-Sanguino; Ma. Inmaculada López-Núñez; Enrique G. Fernández-Abascal	Martínez-Castilla et al. (2021), Ruiz et al. (2021), Valiente et al. (2021), González-Sanguino et al. (2021), López-Núñez et al. (2021), and Fernández-Abascal and Martín-Díaz (2021)	Journal article
	Aging and health	Edad con Salud	Edad con Salud (n.d.)	Website
	Will We See a Wave of Mental Health Problems After the COVID-19 Pandemic?	Barcelona Institute for Global Health (ISGlobal)	Barcelona Institute for Global Health (2021)	Website
Sri Lanka	COVID-19 Emergency Response and Health Systems Preparedness Project	The World Bank	World Bank (2021au)	Project
	Mental health, psychological experiences	Bilesha Perera	Perera et al. (2021)	Journal article
Sudan	COVID-19 Emergency Response Project	The World Bank	World Bank (2021av)	Project
	Psychological Impact on Health Professionals, students	Muna Mohamed Elamin; Mohamed Magzob Korashi	Muna Mohamed et al. (2020) and Korashi (2021)	Journal article
Suriname	Suriname COVID-19 Survey	Inter-American Development Bank	Beuermann et al. (2021)	Survey
	Health, Risk Behavior, Mental Health and Protective Factors	Supa Pengpid and Karl Peltzer	Pengpid and Peltzer (2020)	Journal article

(continued)

Table 11.1 (continued)

Country	Topic/title	PI/URL	Citation	Publication type
Sweden	Research projects on COVID-19	COVID-19 Data Portal	COVID-19 Data Portal Sweden (n.d.)	Website
	Mental health	Victoria Blom; Yun Chen; Elisabet Rondung; Johanna Gustavsson; Ingmar Skoog	Blom et al. (2021), Chen et al. (2021), Rondung et al. (2021), Gustavsson and Beckman (2020), and Skoog (2020)	Journal article
	COVIDung – Youth mental health in a time of crisis	Sabina Kapetanovic		
Switzerland	MOBIS: COVID-19	Swiss National Science Foundation	MOBIS-COVID-19 (2022)	Project
	Mental health in various populations	Paulo Puccinelli; Meichun Mohler-Kuo; Sonja Weilenmann; Simone Amendola; Timon Elmer	Puccinelli et al. (2021), Mohler-Kuo et al. (2021), Weilenmann et al. (2021), Amendola et al. (2021), and Elmer et al. (2020)	Journal article
	Corona Immunitas Ticino study	Giovanni Piumatti	Corona Immunitas (n.d.)	Website
Syria	Mental distress and psychological disorders	Ameer Kakaje; Fatema Mohsen	Kakaje et al. (2020) and Mohsen et al. (2021)	Pre-print journal article; journal article
Tajikistan	Emergency COVID-19 Project	The World Bank	World Bank (2021ax)	Project
	Mental health	Jensolin Ebenezer	Ebenezer (2020)	Journal article
Tanzania	Tackling COVID-19	The Borgen Project	The Borgen Project (2021)	Online article
	Mental health and psychological support	Keneilwe Molebatsi	Molebatsi et al. (2021)	Journal article
Thailand	Mental health problems, resilience, well-being	Surapon Nochaiwong; Rangsiman Soonthornchaiya; Suwicha Kaewsiri Isaradisaikul	Mongkhon et al. (2021), Soonthornchaiya (2020), Nochaiwong et al. (2020), and Isaradisaikul et al. (2021)	Journal article
Timor-Leste	COVID-19 Emergency Support Project	The World Bank	World Bank (2021ay)	Project
Togo	Emergency COVID-19 DPO 2021	The World Bank	World Bank (2022x)	Project
	Mental health medical professionals	Kossi Blewussi Kounou	Kounou et al. (2020)	Journal article
Trinidad and Tobago	COVID-19 Emergency Response Project	The World Bank	World Bank (2022u)	Project

Country	Topic/title	PI/URL	Citation	Publication type
	Health, Risk Behavior, Mental Health and Protective Factors	Supa Pengpid and Karl Peltzer	Pengpid and Peltzer (2020)	Journal article
	Depression, anxiety and stress among healthcare workers	Shivananda Nayak	Nayak et al. (2021)	Journal article
Tunisia	COVID-19 Response project	The World Bank	World Bank (2022y)	Project
	Psychological impact of the Pandemic COVID-19 Outbreak among Medical Residents	Feten Fekih-Romdhane	Fekih-Romdhane et al. (2020)	Journal article
	Mental health, well-being	Noomen Guelmami; Hela Slama; Khanchel Hanen	Guelmami et al. (2021), Slama et al. (2021), and Khanchel (2021)	Journal article
Turkey	Emergency COVID-19 Health Project	The World Bank	World Bank (2022z)	Project
	Mental health, well-being	Murat Yıldırım; Oznur Korukcu; Ibrahim Kira; Hassan Huseyin; Rifat Kayis; Veysi Ceri	Yıldırım and Güler (2020), Korukcu et al. (2021), Kira et al. (2021), Cam et al. (2021), Kayis et al. (2021), and Ceri and Cicek (2021)	Journal article
	Moral judgments of COVID-19 behaviors	Beyza Tepe and Arzu Karakulak		Journal article
Uganda	COVID-19 Response and Emergency Preparedness Project	The World Bank	World Bank (2022aa)	Project
	Mental health, awareness, well-being	Joseph Matovu; Abisha Meji; Anyolitho Maxson Kenneth; Clarissa Giebel; Paul Bukuluki	Matovu et al. (2021), Abisha Meji and Dennison (2020), Anyolitho et al. (2021), Giebel et al. (2022), and Bukuluki et al. (2021)	Journal article
Ukraine	Mental health, well-being	Alexandra Rogowska	Rogowska et al. (2020)	Journal article
United Arab Emirates	Psychological impact, mental health	Basema Saddik; Leila Cheikh Ismail; Salwa Majali; Mariapaola Barbato	Saddik et al. (2021), Cheikh Ismail et al. (2021), Al Majali and Alghazo (2021), and Barbato and Thomas (2021)	Journal article
UK	COVID-19 projects	Health Data Research	Health Data Research UK (2022)	Website

(continued)

Table 11.1 (continued)

Country	Topic/title	PI/URL	Citation	Publication type
	You-COPE: Youth COVID Response Personal Experience: Tracking health and wellbeing amongst 16-24 year olds in the UK during and after the COVID-19 pandemic	UCL	Crosby et al. (2020) and Pascual-Sanchez et al. (2020)	Report
	Impact of statelessness on the right to health in relation to COVID-19	Marie Claire Van Hout		Journal article
	CO-SPACE study	Oxford University	Co-SPACE Study (2022)	Website
	Mental health	Christoph Pieh; Sanja Budimir; Meg Fluharty; Ming Bo-Liu; Yang Hu	Pieh et al. (2021), Budimir et al. (2021), Fluharty et al. (2021), Liu et al. (2021), and Hu and Qian (2021)	Journal article
USA	The COVID Tracking Project	The COVID Tracking Project	The Atlantic (2021)	Website
	Mental health, well-being	Phillip Cheng; Costas Karageorghis; Julie A. Niziurski; Lindsay C. Kobayashi	Cheng et al. (2021), Karageorghis et al. (2021), Niziurski and Schaper (2021), and Kobayashi et al. (2021)	Journal article
	Experience of therapists during the transition to online therapy	Katie Aafjes-van Doorn; Vera Békés; J. Christopher Perry		
	Coping during the COVID-19 pandemic	Annie-Lori Joseph https://www.frontiersin.org/articles/10.3389/frvir.2020.576421/full		
	COVID-19 in prisons, jails, and immigration detention centers, as well as pandemic-related prison and jail releases, legal filings and court orders, and grassroots and community organizing efforts	UCLA Law COVID Behind Bars Data Project	UCLA Law (2021)	Project

Country	Topic/title	PI/URL	Citation	Publication type
	Pandemic Journaling Project	Sarah Willen and Kate Mason	University of Connecticut (n.d.)	Website
	Life during the COVID-19 pandemic	The Emotion and Social Interaction (ESI) Lab in the Department of Psychology at UC Berkeley	Department of Psychology (n.d.)	Website
Uruguay	COVID-19 Emergency Response Project	The World Bank	World Bank (2021az)	Project
Uzbekistan	Emergency COVID-19 Response Project	The World Bank	World Bank (2021ba)	Project
	Mental health, health promotion	Vasila K. Abdullaeva; Dalal Koustuv	Abdullaeva et al. (2021) and Koustuv et al. (2021)	Journal article
Venezuela	Knowledge, attitudes, and practices	Benjamin Bates	Bates et al. (2021)	Journal article
Vietnam	Project Vietnam	Project Vietnam Foundation	Project Vietnam Foundation (n.d.)	Website
	COVID-19 Emergency Response Project	The World Bank	World Bank (2021bb)	Project
	Mental health and well-being	Phuong Thi Lan Nguyen; Nguyen Tuan; Hung Manh Than; Bach Xuan Tran; Tuyen Dinh Hoang; Nguyen, Thanh Minh; Tuyen Dinh Hoang	Nguyen et al. (2021), Tuan et al. (2021), Manh Than et al. (2020), Tran et al. (2020), Hoang et al. (2021a, b), and Nguyen and Le (2021)	Journal article; pre-print journal article
Yemen	COVID-19 Response Project	The World Bank		
	Psychological effects, mental health	Nagd Mohammed Ahmed Mahmood; Gamil Ghaleb Alrubaiee	Alrubaiee et al. (2020)	Journal article
Zambia	COVID-19 Emergency Response and Health Systems Preparedness Project	The World Bank	World Bank (2022ab)	Project
	Mental health, well-being	Steward Mudenda; Darren Sharpe	Mudenda et al. (2021) and Sharpe et al. (2021)	Journal article
Zimbabwe	COVID-19 Response Project (CRP)	Government of Zimbabwe	African Development Bank Group (2020b)	Project
	Mental Health and Psychosocial Support	Keneilwe Molebatsi; Tonderayi Mathew Matsungo	Molebatsi et al. (2021) and Matsungo and Chopera (2020)	Journal article

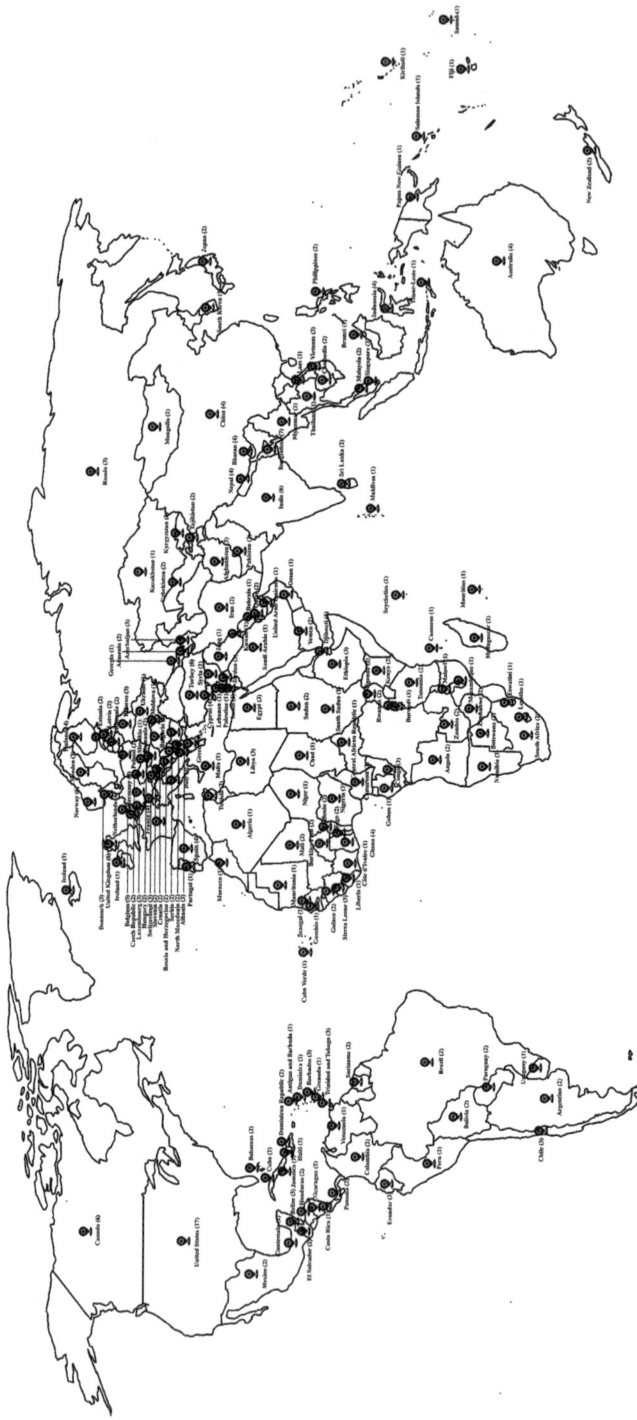

Fig. 11.1 Global research map on the COVID-19 pandemic

Table 11.2 Multinational and multisite research projects on the pandemic

Title project	Topic	PI/research team/URL	Citation
International and Multidimensional Perspectives on the Impact of COVID-19 (IMPACT-C19)	70 country study	APA Task Force Research Initiatives Group; R. Dimitrova; R. Rivera; A. Karakulak	Rivera (2021)
COVID-Minds Network	Research network with over 150 longitudinal studies on mental health and wellbeing	Daisy Fancourt https://www.covidminds.org/	COVID-Minds Network (2020)
Euro Youth Mental Health	A survey to document young people's experiences during the COVID-19 pandemic	Nicholas Morgan https://eymh.org/	Morgan (2022)
The Mental Health Million Project	Mental health and wellbeing across geographies and demographics around the world	Jennifer Newson https://sapienlabs.org/mental-health-million-post/	Newson (2020)
The COVID Tracking Project	Data from 56 US states and territories in three main areas: testing, hospitalization, and patient outcomes, racial and ethnic demographic information via the COVID Racial Data Tracker, and long-term-care facilities via the Long-Term-Care tracker	https://covidtracking.com/	The COVID Tracking Project (2021)
COVID Circle	Research in low- and middle-income countries	https://covidcircle.org/	COVID Circle (2021)
SITUATE Project	Mental health and wellbeing at transitions to and within university	Olga Chelidoni	University of Sussex (2022)
COVID-19 Unmasked Study	How young children and their parents are managing during the pandemic	Marthe Egberts	COVID-19 Unmasked Study (2022)
Time Social Distancing study	Effects of physical and social distancing on our relationship to time by using experimental psychology methods	Virginie van Wassenhove	Cognition and Brain Dynamics (n.d.)

Title project	Topic	PI/research team/URL	Citation
The HEBECO study	Health behaviors, including psychological wellbeing and participants' experience of social isolation before and during the pandemic	Lion Shahab and Aleksandra Herbec https://www.ucl-covid19research.co.uk/	The UCL Tobacco and Research Group (n.d.)
Global COVID Study	Short- and long-term effects of COVID-19 on you and your family's physical and mental health	A group of experts in psychology, neuroscience, education, and criminology https://globalcovidstudy.com/about/	Global COVID Study (2022)
Global COVID-19-related traumatic stress activities	The traumatic stress societies that are united in the Global Collaboration on Traumatic Stress (GC-TS) have collected relevant information (listed below) on the COVID-19 virus and measures we can take, the consequences, and how to respond to those who suffer from the consequences and how we support our health professionals	Sara Freedman and Tatiana Davidson https://www.global-psychotrauma.net/corona	Global Collaboration on Traumatic Stress (n.d.)
COVID and Cognition	The Impact of COVID-19 on Memory and Cognition	https://www.camblab.psychol.cam.ac.uk/participate-in-research	University of Cambridge (2022)
Alone Together Study	How factors like housing, social relationships, and resilience impact mental health and wellbeing	https://www.sydney.edu.au/matilda-centre/news-and-events/2020/12/16/alone-together-study.html	The University of Sydney (2020)
Co-Space study	Supporting Parents, Adolescents and Children during Epidemics	https://cospaceoxford.org/	Co-SPACE Study (2022)
COVID-19 Social Study	Psychological and social impact of the pandemic	https://www.covidsocialstudy.org/	UCL COVID-19 Social Study (2022)
COVID-19 Family Life Study	Effects of the coronavirus pandemic on family life across cultures	Anis Ben Brik https://www.covidfamilystudy.org/	Brik (2020)

(continued)

Table 11.2 (continued)

Title project	Topic	PI/research team/URL	Citation
COVIDiSTRESS Global Survey	Psychological stress, compliance with behavioral guidelines to slow the spread of coronavirus, and trust in governmental institutions and their preventive measures	https://covidistress.france-bioinformatique.fr/	COVIDiSTRESS Global Survey (2022)
COVID-19 Data Repository	Social, behavioral, public health, and economic impact of the novel coronavirus global pandemic	https://www.openicpsr.org/openicpsr/covid19	OPENICPSR (2022)
The Understanding Society COVID-19 study	Data on health, education, employment, income, housing, family relationships, civic engagement	Annette Jäckle, Professor Michaela Benzeval, Jonathan Burton, Institute for Social and Economic Research, University of Essex; and Professor Thomas Crossley, Department of Economics, European University Institute https://www.understandingsociety.ac.uk/topic/covid-19	The UK Household Longitudinal Study (2022)
Nordic Health Data Research Projects on COVID-19	Research projects to study COVID-19 in relation to pregnancy progression to smoking to mental health vulnerability	https://www.nordforsk.org/calls/nordic-health-data-research-projects-covid-19	NordForsk (2022)
COVID-19 Response	Revolutionary guided-practice model that reduces health disparities in under-served and remote areas of the state, nation, and world	https://hsc.unm.edu/echo/institute-programs/covid-19-response/	UNM Health Sciences (2022)
The Pandemic Stress Index (PSI)	Measure of behavior changes and stress experienced during COVID	University of Miami	University of Miami (2021)
The COVID-19 International Student Well-Being Study	Cross-sectional multi-country study that collected data on higher education students during the COVID-19 outbreak	University of Antwerp	Van de Velde et al. (2021)

Title project	Topic	PI/research team/URL	Citation
Compassion, social connectedness and trauma resilience during the COVID-19 pandemic: A multi-national study	Compassion, social connectedness and trauma resilience	Marcela Matos and Daniel Rijo https://www.fpce.uc.pt/covid19study/	Matos et al. (2020)
COVID-19 Stress and Well-Being	31-nation study on stress related to COVID-19 and well-being for individuals in a romantic relationship	Ashley K. Randall	Arizona State University (2021)
Impacts of the COVID-19 Pandemic on Life of Higher Education Students	100 country study	Aleksander Aristovnik	Aristovnik et al. (2020)
Children and Adolescents in Global Contexts: COVID-19 as a Life Course Event	SRA and societies involved in child and adolescent research seek global collaboration to document how major life events, in this instance, COVID-19, impact development	Society for Research on Adolescence	Children and Adolescents in Global Contexts: COVID-19 as a Life Course Event (2022)
Impact of COVID-19 lockdown on education in several nations		Sherry Dingman	
THEMIS: Protecting Human Rights and Public Health in Global Pandemics	Vital reference for policymaking at national, regional, and global levels for fair pandemic preparedness to cross-border health threats	Patrycja Dąbrowska-Kłosińska	European Comission (2022c)
Epidemiological mathematical model on the spread of COVID-19	Epidemiological mathematical model that infers the status of the epidemic, thereby monitoring and estimating the impact of interventions on the spread of COVID-19	European Union Research Groups	European Comission (2022a)
Projects researching COVID-19, SARS-CoV-2 and related topics	Europe	European Union	European Comission (2022b)

(continued)

Table 11.2 (continued)

Title project	Topic	PI/research team/URL	Citation
Attitudes toward COVID-19	Representations, attitudes, and reactions among the general public in the context of the COVID-19 pandemic in a number of countries	Sylvain Brouard, Michael Becher, Martial Foucault, and Pavlos Vasilopoulos	Sciences Po (2022)
Where to land after the pandemic?	Survey, groups, discussions	Sciences Po Media Lab	Sciences Po Media Lab (2022)
COVID-19 Study	How COVID-19 pandemic influences political and social aspects and the psychological perceptions of people in different societies	Keele University and the University of the Basque Country UPV/EHU, C.C.E. Research Group	Cakal and Páez (n.d.)
COH-FIT Study	Collaborative outcomes study on health and functioning during infection times (COH-FIT) in 155 countries	Christoph U. Correll and Dr. Marco Solmi, together with over 200 international scientists from around the globe	Collaborative Outcomes study on Health and Functioning during Infection Times (COH-FIT) (2019)
Moral Values under the Imprint of the Corona Pandemic	30 + country study	Christian Welzel, Klaus Boehnke, Jan Delhey, Franziska Deutsch, Jan Eichhorn, Ulrich Kühnen	Welzel et al. (2020)
COVID-19, personality and quality of life: Self-enhancement in the time of pandemic	The role of dark personality in predicting quality of life during COVID-19 pandemic across cultures	Magdalena Żemojtel-Piotrowska	CSWU Cross-Cultural Psychology Centre (2021)
Coping Responses during COVID-19 Pandemic	A cross-cultural comparison in Russia, Kyrgyzstan, and Peru coping strategies, metacognition, and in Peru and other Latin American countries	Denisse Manrique-Millones	Voronin et al. (2020)
Global Behaviors and Perceptions in the COVID-19 Pandemic	Large-scale online survey about COVID-related behaviors, beliefs, perceptions, mental health, and more, covering respondents from more than 170 countries	IPA	Innovations for Poverty Action's (IPA) (2020)

may be approached for an opinion. Then the team leader goes back to the committee and decides a final version for dissemination and data collection.

A general agreement for collaboration and data use was adopted among all partners to establish data holders, data sharing, storage, rights, obligations, authorship, and types of collaboration. Data are shared with any interested colleagues to write a paper or make cross-country comparisons or methodological papers on the measures used (upon a completion of the agreement for data use outlining main goals, data, measures, samples requested). The project members joined with data collection in their countries, with other relevant data previously collected and/or writing or helping in the publication/dissemination process. The long-term prospects see a range of products such as special issues in major journals, short reports in various newsletters, edited book/s with major publishers, and grant applications.

COVID-19 Research by Group Members Other relevant future products are ongoing research and dissemination plans. Group members are developing various ideas and topics such as the grief process amidst the coronavirus pandemic; COVID-19 as a trigger for survivor's guilt; the reactions of older adults who are children of survivors of the Holocaust to COVID-19; qualitative, in-depth interview questionnaire to examine the perceptions of professionals in various agencies offering services for older adults; insecurity about coronavirus disease on the association between childhood attachment and greed; Chinese adolescents' stereotypes about teens and health behavior during COVID-19 pandemic; and policy report with instructions and standard for online courses during the pandemic. One of our Chinese team members is working on a policy report to the local government for norms and guidelines for "homeschooling" during COVID-19 in addition to a longitudinal study on the relations between parental behaviors and youth mental health during COVID-19. We have a team member gathering data on health changes aligned to behavioral health and life-altering decisions. Finally, we collaborated in an article at the American Psychological Association released in November 2020 (De Angelis, 2020).

The Research Initiatives Working Group Key Areas

Another major area that the Research Initiatives Working Group is working on is to collect and disseminate as much research done by others outside the group members. The key areas of this work include a broad range of populations (children, youth, emerging adults, parents, older and aging adults, LGBTQ young people, ethnic minorities and ethno-cultural groups across the globe, immigrants, refugees, children and patients with disabilities, healthcare workers, at-risk populations, practitioners, caregivers, social workers, therapists). These key areas grouped by relevant literature (e.g., articles, reports, and documents on COVID-19) call for papers and special issues in relevant journals on the pandemic (see Table 11.3), local and international meetings, conferences, symposiums, and webinars related to

Table 11.3 Summary of call for papers and special issues on the COVID-19 pandemic

	Outlet	Deadline	Topic/website
1	Journal of Migration and Health	Published – still accepting	Special Articles on Migration and COVID-19 https://www.sciencedirect.com/journal/journal-of-migration-and-health/special-issue/1042295F1WB
2	Journal of Science Communication	Published	COVID-19 and Science Communication https://jcom.sissa.it/archive/19/05 https://jcom.sissa.it/archive/19/07
3	Journal of Clinical Virology	Published	Coronavirus Disease Outbreak-2019 (COVID-19) https://www.sciencedirect.com/journal/journal-of-clinical-virology/special-issue/102C3LMPFMC
4	International Journal of Psychology	Published	Psychological implications of COVID-19 https://onlinelibrary.wiley.com/toc/1464066x/2022/57/1
5	International Journal of Intercultural Relations	Published	Studying the effects of the coronavirus pandemic on Intercultural relations https://www.ncbi.nlm.nih.gov/pmc/articles/PMC7151455/
6	European Educational Research Journal	Published	Education in Europe and the COVID-19 https://journals.sagepub.com/toc/eera/20/5 https://journals.sagepub.com/toc/eera/20/4
7	Journal of Public Health in Africa	Published	Coronavirus Disease (COVID-19) in Africa https://www.publichealthinafrica.org/index.php/jphia/issue/view/24
8	Sexual and Reproductive Health Matters Journal	Published	Sexual and reproductive health and rights in the era of COVID-19 http://www.srhm.org/sexual-and-reproductive-health-and-rights-in-the-era-of-covid-19/
9	Families, Systems, & Health	Published	COVID-19 and Racial Injustice https://psycnet.apa.org/PsycARTICLES/journal/fsh/38/S1
10	Nature	Closed	Corona Discourse(s) Remaking the World: Experts, Politics, Media and Everyday Life https://www.nature.com/palcomms/calls-for-papers#Corona
11	Nature	No submission deadline	Calls for Papers: COVID-19 https://www.nature.com/srep/guestedited#covid-19

Table 11.3 (continued)

	Outlet	Deadline	Topic/website
12	Journal of Rural Mental Health	No submission deadline	Call for papers: COVID-19 and rural mental health challenges and opportunities: The Journal of Rural Mental Health is accepting submissions that focus on the impact of COVID-19 on the delivery of tele-mental health (tele-MH) services for rural persons https://www.apa.org/pubs/journals/rmh/call-for-papers-covid-19-rural-mental-health
13	Psychology of Sexual Orientation and Gender Diversity	No submission deadline	The Psychology of Sexual Orientation and Gender Diversity invites quantitative and qualitative papers related to COVID-19 that fit the larger scope and vision of the journal https://www.apa.org/pubs/journals/sgd
14	Stigma and Health	Published	Stigma and Health welcomes qualitative or quantitative papers looking at stigma associated with COVID-19 https://psycnet.apa.org/PsycARTICLES/journal/sah/7/1
15	Training and Education in Professional Psychology	Published – still accepting	All aspects of the COVID-19 pandemic relevant to health service psychology training and education at the doctoral, internship, and postdoctoral training levels. https://www.apa.org/pubs/journals/tep/call-for-papers-covid-19-pandemic
16	Translational Issues in Psychological Science	Closed	The purpose of this special issue is to bring awareness to, and promote understanding of, complex personal and societal issues arising from pandemics. The special issue will feature theoretical and empirical research, as well as scientific commentary, related to pandemics https://www.apa.org/pubs/journals/tps
17	Families, Systems, & Health	Published – still accepting	Families, Systems, & Health invites high-quality papers focusing on clinical research, training, and theoretical contributions in the areas of families and health. The journal publishes research on the systemic approach to healthcare that integrates mind and body; individual and family; and communities, clinicians, and health systems while considering cost-effectiveness and ethics. https://www.apa.org/pubs/journals/fsh/call-for-papers-general
18	Journal of Pediatric Psychology	Unspecified	Original papers should address pediatric psychology-related topics of importance to the pandemic such as child and family coping, psychological distress and trauma, diversity and/or health disparities, development and evaluation of measures or methods to capture the impact of the pandemic on children and families, behavior change interventions to improve adherence with preventive guidance, community and school efforts to promote health and wellness, remote and virtual interventions to deliver psychosocial interventions to children and families, etc. https://academic.oup.com/jpepsy/pages/covid-cfp
19	Psychological Studies	Published	Special Issue on Psychology of Uncertainty and Vulnerabilities COVID-19 Pandemic Related https://link.springer.com/journal/12646/volumes-and-issues/66-3

	Outlet	Deadline	Topic/website
20	Journal of Research on Personality	Published	Psychology and Life with COVID-19 https://www.readersinsight.net/jrp/issue/view/139
21	International Perspectives in Psychology	Published	Global Changes in the "World of Work" and "Personal Lives" in the Wake of the COVID-19 Pandemic https://psycnet.apa.org/PsycARTICLES/journal/ipp/10/4
22	Current Research in Ecological and Social Psychology	Published	This special issue will highlight research examining issues related to the COVID-19 pandemic from an ecological and social psychological perspective https://www.sciencedirect.com/journal/current-research-in-ecological-and-social-psychology/vol/3/suppl/C#article-0
23	Psychology	Published	Mental Health and Coping During COVID-19 https://www.scirp.org/genericerrorpage.htm
24	Psychologica Belgica	Published	Special Collection: Psychology and COVID-19 https://www.psychologicabelgica.com/127/volume/62/issue/1/
25	Frontiers in Psychology Journal of Applied Psychology	Published	Consumer Psychology and Corporate Social Responsibility in the post COVID-19 Era https://www.frontiersin.org/research-topics/15718/consumer-psychology-and-corporate-social-responsibility-in-the-post-covid-19-era#articleshttps://www.siop.org/Research-Publications/Items-of-Interest/ArtMID/19366/ArticleID/4661/Journal-of-Applied-Psychology-Call-for-Papers-COVID-19-Pandemic
26	Psychology	Published	Consumer Psychology and Corporate Social Responsibility in the post COVID-19 Era https://www.frontiersin.org/research-topics/15718/consumer-psychology-and-corporate-social-responsibility-in-the-post-covid-19-era#articles
27	Journal of Clinical Medicine	Closed	The paper must aim seeking the overlap among PMAD and women's health before and during the pandemic https://www.mdpi.com/journal/jcm/special_issues/Women_Health_Perinatal_Mood_Anxiety_Disorders
28	Journal of Clinical Medicine	Published	Special Issue "The Impact of the COVID-19 Emergency on the Quality of Life of the General Population" https://www.mdpi.com/journal/jcm/special_issues/COVID-19_psychology
29	Psychological Studies	Published	Special Issue on Psychology of Uncertainty and Vulnerabilities COVID-19 Pandemic Related https://link.springer.com/journal/12646/volumes-and-issues/66-3

(continued)

Table 11.3 (continued)

	Outlet	Deadline	Topic/website
30	Psychological Trauma	Published	COVID-19: Insights on the Pandemic's Traumatic Effects and Global Implications https://psycnet.apa.org/PsycARTICLES/journal/tra/12/S1
31	Psychology in Russia	Published	COVID-19: psychological challenges http://psychologyinrussia.com/volumes/13_4_2020.php
32	International Journal of Psychology	Published	Psychological implications of COVID-19 https://onlinelibrary.wiley.com/toc/1464066x/2022/57/1
33	Journal of Contextual Behavioral Science	Published	Introduction to the special issue on COVID-19 https://www.sciencedirect.com/science/article/pii/S2212144721000946
34	Training and Education in Professional Psychology	Published No submission deadline	Education and Training Through COVID-19 https://psycnet.apa.org/PsycARTICLES/journal/tep/15/4 Call for papers: COVID-19 pandemic and health service psychology education and training: it seeks manuscripts focusing on all aspects of the COVID-19 pandemic relevant to health service psychology training and education at the doctoral, internship, and postdoctoral training levels https://www.apa.org/pubs/journals/tep/call-for-papers-covid-19-pandemic
35	School Psychology	Published	Perspectives on COVID-19: Impacts on Children, Youth, Families, and Educators and the Roles of Human Services Professionals Addressing Diverse Needs https://psycnet.apa.org/PsycARTICLES/journal/spq/36/5
36	Journal of Family Communication	Published	Special Issue on Family Communication in the COVID-19 Pandemic https://www.tandfonline.com/toc/hjfc20/21/3
37	Journal of Hospitality & Tourism Education	Published	Special Issue of Journal of Hospitality, Leisure, Sport & Tourism Education https://www.sciencedirect.com/journal/journal-of-hospitality-leisure-sport-and-tourism-education/vol/30/suppl/C
38	Journal of Homosexuality	Published	Impacts of the COVID-19 Pandemic on LGBTQ+ Health and Well-Being https://www.tandfonline.com/toc/wjhm20/68/4?nav=tocList

	Outlet	Deadline	Topic/website
39	European Journal of Personality	Unspecified	Call for papers at EJP on personality and the COVID-19 pandemic: Papers that are relevant to personality and covid-19 relationship as well as personality and other mass crisis https://www.ejp-blog.com/blog/2020/3/26/call-for-papers-personality-and-covid-19-pandemic
40	Journal of Communication	Unspecified	Communication in Times of Crisis: Research Related to Coronavirus (COVID-19) https://academic.oup.com/joc/pages/coronavirus-vi
41	The Journal of Science Communication	Published	COVID-19 and science communication https://jcom.sissa.it/archive/19/05
42	Sexual and Reproductive Health Matters	Published	Sexual and reproductive health and rights in the era of COVID-19 http://www.srhm.org/sexual-and-reproductive-health-and-rights-in-the-era-of-covid-19/
43	Health Psychology Bulletin	Published	COVID-19-related behaviors https://www.healthpsychologybulletin.com/collections/special/covid-19-related-behaviours/
44	Group Dynamics: Theory, Research, and Practice	Published	Groups in a dangerous time: Virtual work and therapy in the COVID-19 era https://www.apa.org/pubs/journals/special/gdn-groups-dangerous-time-pdf
45	Developmental Psychology	Published	Parenting and Family Dynamics in Times of the COVID-19 Pandemic https://psycnet.apa.org/PsycARTICLES/journal/dev/57/10
46	International Journal of Environmental Research and Public Health	Published	The Psychological Impact of COVID-19 on Vulnerable, Marginalized or At-Risk Groups https://www.mdpi.com/journal/ijerph/special_issues/psychological_impact
47	Behavioral Sciences	Published	Psychological Impact of COVID-19 Worldwide Pandemic on Pregnancy and the Offspring https://www.mdpi.com/journal/behavsci/special_issues/COVID-19_Pregnancy
48	Child Development	Published	Special Section: The Impact of COVID-19 on Child Development around the World https://srcd.onlinelibrary.wiley.com/toc/14678624/2021/92/5
49	Child Abuse and Neglect	Published	Protecting children from maltreatment during COVID-19: First volume https://www.sciencedirect.com/journal/child-abuse-and-neglect/vol/110/part/P2
50	Journal of Research on Adolescence	Published	The impact of the COVID-19 pandemic on adolescents emotional, social, and academic adjustment https://onlinelibrary.wiley.com/toc/15327795/2021/31/3
51	Journal of Social and Personal Relationships	Published	Relationships in the time of COVID-19 https://journals.sagepub.com/toc/spra/38/6

(continued)

Table 11.3 (continued)

	Outlet	Deadline	Topic/website
52	American Psychologist	Published	COVID-19 pandemic https://psycnet.apa.org/PsycARTICLES/journal/amp/75/7
53	Creative Arts in Education and Therapy	Published	COVID-19 Special Edition https://caet.inspirees.com/caetojsjournals/index.php/caet/issue/view/15
54	Journal of Public Health in Africa	Published	2022: Focus on COVID-19 https://www.publichealthinafrica.org/index.php/jphia/issue/view/24
55	Journal of Social Issues	Closed	Ageism toward older adults during the COVID-19 pandemic and beyond https://www.spssi.org/index.cfm?fuseaction=document.viewdocument&ID=3F28EB86AE4CA3BB2EE025BE0093BF0432D8962350D367CECEBAF0E1F3DDFC798A419D9A5BFC2C3737450814D3839CB6
56	Psicología Iberoamericana	Published	El impacto psicosocial de COVID-19 https://psicologiaiberoamericana.ibero.mx/index.php/psicologia
57	Journal of Migration and Health	June 30, 2022 February	Critical Perspectives on Migrants, Migration, and COVID-19 Vaccination https://www.journals.elsevier.com/journal-of-migration-and-health/call-for-papers/critical-perspectives-on-migrants-migration-and-covid-19-vaccination
58	Journal of Clinical Virology	Published	Coronavirus Disease Outbreak-2019 (COVID-19) https://www.sciencedirect.com/journal/journal-of-clinical-virology/special-issue/102C3LMPFMC
59	Canada's Journal on Refugees	Closed	Refuge in the time of pandemic https://carleton.ca/lerrn/2020/refuge-call-for-papers-pandemic/
60	International Perspectives in Psychology	Published	Psychology and the COVID-19 pandemic: A global perspective https://econtent.hogrefe.com/toc/ipp/11/2
61	International Perspectives in Psychology	Published	Women During COVID-19 https://econtent.hogrefe.com/toc/ipp/10/3

	Outlet	Deadline	Topic/website
62	International Perspectives in Psychology	Published	Global Changes in the “World of Work” and “Personal Lives” in the Wake of the COVID-19 Pandemic https://econtent.hogrefe.com/toc/ipp/10/4
63	European Psychologist	Published	Psychology, Global Threats, Social Challenge, and the COVID-19 Pandemic: European Perspectives https://econtent.hogrefe.com/toc/epp/26/4
64	European Educational Research Journal	Published	Education in Europe and the COVID-19 Pandemic https://journals.sagepub.com/toc/eera/20/4 https://journals.sagepub.com/toc/eera/20/5
65	Healthcare	Published	Mental Health and Coping During COVID-19 https://www.mdpi.com/journal/healthcare/special_issues/Mental_Health_COVID-19
66	Emerging Adulthood	Published	The Impact of the COVID-19 Pandemic on the Lives of Emerging Adults https://journals.sagepub.com/toc/eaxa/9/5
67	Scientific American	Published	How COVID Changed the World https://www.scientificamerican.com/article/introducing-a-special-issue-on-how-covid-changed-the-world/
68	Social Psychology Quarterly	1–31 August, 2022	Organizational Behavior and Human Resource Management Perspectives on Entrepreneurship https://onlinelibrary.wiley.com/pb-assets/assets/17446570/PPsychCallforpapers_Entrepreneurship_July2_2021-1626107915633.pdf
69	Cyberpsychology, Behavior, and Social Networking	July 31, 2022	Psychosocial Impacts of Digital Travel https://home.liebertpub.com/cfp/psychosocial-impacts-of-digital-travel/385/
70	International Journal of Psychology	Closed	Psychology and Human Rights https://onlinelibrary.wiley.com/pb-assets/assets/1464066X/Psychology%20and%20Human%20Special%20Issue%20Call%20for%20Papers-1646309364483.pdf
71	Philosophical Psychology	October 31, 2022	Trustworthiness: Individual and Institutional Dimensions Although it is not a special issue directly related to the pandemic, it is planned that it will be a special issue arising from the need for trustworthiness created by the uncertainties in the pandemic https://think.taylorandfrancis.com/special_issues/trustworthiness-individual-institutional-dimensions/?utm_source=TFO&utm_medium=cms&utm_campaign=JPG15743&_gl=1*au4dqd*_ga*MTA3MzYwMTU1MS4xNjQ3Mjg1OTY3*_ga_0HYE8YG0M6*MTY0OTIzMjA5Ny41LjEuMTY0OTIzMjkyNC4w

(continued)

Table 11.3 (continued)

	Outlet	Deadline	Topic/website
72	Psychological Assessment	September 30, 2022	Clinical assessment in the time of COVID https://www.apa.org/pubs/journals/pas/clinical-assessment-covid
73	Journal of Science & Popular Culture	Closed	Vaccine Hesitancy https://www.intellectbooks.com/asset/63826/1/JSPC_CfP_Jan22.pdf
74	BMC Public Health	31 December, 2022	The COVID-19 pandemic and intimate partner violence https://www.biomedcentral.com/collections/CovIPV?sap-outbound-id=CCA139D3F81F47DA31609490C4C5071E26620C25&utm_source=hybris-campaign&utm_medium=email&utm_campaign=000_SGQ2936_0000021362_CONR_JRNLS_DEC01_GL_PMLS_COLLE_OAX422-B_JRNLS_DEC01_GL_PMLS_COLLE_OAX422-B&utm_content=EN_internal_39156_20220411&mkt-key=42010A0553051EEC8FA0F00EEA68DB5A
75	Death Studies	Published	Psychological Impacts of COVID-19: International Perspectives https://www.tandfonline.com/toc/udst20/46/5

COVID-19. Due to the time-sensitive nature of these materials, we have been disseminating them via email lists of major organizations represented by the group members as well as the APA Interdivisional Task Force network. We are also compiling a database for the Task Force members and interested scholars to be able to use well after the pandemic is over.

Books, Measurement Tools, and COVID-19 Indexes

Several texts and books were produced, used, and distributed by the membership of the RIWG. For instance, Cockerham and Cockerham (2020) developed a manuscript tailored for teachers and trainees that compiled findings regarding social implications of the pandemic. Cooper (2020) edited a series of expert testimonies on the impact of COVID-19 on issues related to work; similarly, Haslam (2020) assembled research and perspectives of international professionals on the societal changes brought by the pandemic, which included politics, social exclusion, and leadership. McMahon (2020) gathered expert testimonies on the pandemic's impact on individuals' relationship with media and technology, with topics such as fake news and conspiracy theories. In addition, Sanderman and Kwasnicka (2020) edited a volume with expert testimonies on topics of health, well-being, stress, and coping, whereas Bornstein (2020) focused their manuscript on pandemic-related issues and challenges that particularly impacted families, parents, and children. Furthermore, Ali and Davis-Floyd (2022) centered their book on cultural, national, and individual constructions of the pandemic. Other texts, such as Tosone (2020), centered on the ongoing efforts of social workers at the frontlines of the pandemic. Wallace and Wallace (2020) delivered a manuscript based on the first social epidemiological study of the COVID-19 spread in New York City, the primary epicenter of the USA. Some works, such as Kupfer and Stutz (2022), centered their research on specific lenses, such as gender perspectives and feminism and their relation to the pandemic.

The RIWG's membership researched, used, collected, and shared a diverse array of measurement tools that were assessed for their effectiveness, validity, and reliability during the pandemic. Talaee et al. (2022) examined the validity of a questionnaire for stress and burnout in healthcare workers during COVID-19. Similarly, Klok et al. (2020) measured the psychometric properties of the "Post-COVID-19 Functional Status Scale," Lotzin et al. (2022) surveyed the validity and reliability of "The Pandemic Stressor Scale," and Caycho-Rodríguez et al. (2021a, b) assessed the cross-cultural measurement invariance of the "Fear of COVID-19 Scale" across multiple Latin American countries. Moreover, many other articles examined the psychometric properties of COVID-19 scales across international and diverse samples and populations, including those in Pakistan (Ashraf et al., 2022), East Africa (Giordani et al., 2021), Arabic-speaking nations (Aljemaiah et al., 2021), Japan (Midorikawa et al., 2021), Ecuador (Moreta-Herrera et al., 2021), Ethiopia (Elemo et al., 2020), England (Freeman et al., 2022), Colombia (Vinaccia et al., 2021), and Korea (Bilgiç et al., 2022).

The RIWG also compiled and distributed multiple research products that assessed and reported findings on COVID-19 indexes. For instance, Acharya and Porwal (2020) studied a vulnerability index for the management of and response to the pandemic in India. Zhu et al. (2020) used the Stringency Index to assess social distancing in Latin America, Qin et al. (2020) employed the Social Media Search Index to predict the number of COVID-19 cases, Chang and McAleer (2020) studied alternative Global Health Security Indexes for risk analysis of COVID-19, and Belleli et al. (2020) reported the Frailty Index predicted poor outcomes for coronavirus patients. Furthermore, some studies focused on constructing and revising new indexes for the pandemic (Constantini & Mazzotti, 2020; DeCaprio et al., 2020; Haimovich et al., 2020; Salisu et al., 2020; Stephany et al., 2022).

Special Issues, Conferences, and Webinars on the COVID-19 Pandemic

With regard to special issues, we were able to retrieve a total of 75 call for papers across major disciplines in social sciences. Table 11.3 provides a summary of all special issues, and paper collections call for papers and special issues on the pandemic in relevant journals. Additionally, with regard to conferences, meetings, seminars, and webinars, we used website search within the mainstream psychological association websites. For example, APA has a section that records COVID-19-related resources. We were able to detect over 100 meetings since the beginning of the pandemic focused mainly on the impact of COVID-19 from adolescence to adulthood across different ethnic groups and nations, behavioral changes, parent-child relationships, mental health, isolation, and close relationships. The main target groups included scholars, psychological counselors, frontline workers, and students.

Use of Technology, Deliverables, and Outreach

The members of the group are setting up various actions for outreach and global impact and disseminating resources through APA listserv, social media, publications, and interviews. We have been disseminating any relevant products among our networks, our COVID-19 database, and the Task Force listserv. Further, we have been reaching out to other divisions and international organizations (local associations of psychology) to present our group and ask about COVID-19-related research projects and initiatives in various APA divisions and countries around the world. We are in contact with the chairs of the Research Group at APA Division 52-International Psychology, who are doing similar work. We are exploring ways of collaborating with their group and share common experiences, as well as exchange ideas and plan future collaboration.

Challenges Faced, Lessons Learned, and Outlook

Based on the qualitative interviews with the group members, we could clearly note that international cooperation is seen as an extremely important asset to combat the crisis. Some group members reported that data collection across countries would help learn lessons about whether human development and societal dynamics during COVID-19 vary across countries or cultures. This relates to another insight to improve understanding of human behavior during a crisis, with subsequent crisis intervention and research that can be used at any time – not only during a crisis. This is the vision with which we all started and then found it to be a critical factor in how we are different from other research networks, as having so many international and global research networks is a strong factor in the group's success.

Another group member shared the need to develop novel delivery systems of intervention and prevention service that are suited to the unprecedented limitations of social distancing. All of these can only be appropriately achieved based on solid empirical data. Preliminary findings from across the globe have already indicated that there are negative mental health effects of the pandemic on individuals who have not previously had any mental health diagnosis and that social distancing and isolation exacerbate difficulties in those who had mental health issues prior to the pandemic. In addition, there is a large population of those who suffered the untimely losses of loved ones, which was established previously by research to be the number one traumatic event reported by people across the globe. We, as psychologists, must be diligent about research into these phenomena and lead early developments in this field, to shorten the time between the trauma and the availability of adequate treatment for those who need it, or public health measures for the society at large. The interval between our profession recognizing the impact of trauma on various groups has historically been far too long (see Holocaust survivors, Vietnam veterans, victims of domestic and sexual abuse, and others). We must take steps not to repeat this tragic lapse.

The work done so far with rich global collaborations and networks within this group has been highly engaging, outlining meaningful avenues and prospects. We end this chapter from the perspective of our group members who shared insights on lessons learned from this pandemic and opportunities we may develop.

> I have learned patience, but above all else, I have learned resilience and that when necessary, we are able, and want to, work together for the greater good. I have seen inclusion. I have felt welcomed. I have seen people and individuals care more and more about one another. I see that as a sign that as professionals we have a role to play… to help create the safe space for people to be caring, understanding, more informed and involved citizens.

> The pandemic has certainly changed the research and academic environment and the possibility to collect and share experiences and reflect on best practices, risks and benefits of these rapid changes we are witnessing, and living is crucial to ensure that we learn from this experience and reduce as much as possible its harmful consequences on society. Joining forces internationally makes sense when what you are facing is an epidemic on a global scale. This initiative contributed to creating solidarity and support among professionals and researchers, a way to fight isolation, and keep an eye on the rapid evolution of our societies.

In the future, I hope this initiative can contribute to develop a better understanding and systematic analysis of the consequences of this pandemic, as to inform guidelines and best practices for our profession so that we can learn from our experiences.

This effort contributed to develop and strengthen international collaborations and was key to the implementation of an international research project on the effects of the pandemic on well-being across multiple countries. I hope this fruitful collaboration can continue and help to provide insights on how to support people's well-being during these challenging times as well as in the aftermath of this pandemic.

Author Note The Research Initiatives Working Group at the APA Interdivisional Task Force on the Pandemic is represented by Ann Rachel Wamser, Arzu Karakulak, Bin-Bin Chen, Breeda McGrath, Carlos Miguel Rios González, Danhua Lin, Denise Carballea, Diana Miconi, Irit Felsen, Judy Kuriansky, Lawrence Gerstein, Lillian Moya, Lucia Magis-Weinberg, Marta de la C. Martín Carbonell, Monica Indart, Nor Abdul Kadir, Priyoth Kittiteerasack, Rita Rivera, Roxanna Rosen, Rubia Carla Formighieri Giordani, Russell Kabir, Sadia Malik, Samson Mhizha, Sherrie Wilcox, Steven Krauss, Tina Lo Proto, Vaishali Raval, Yinka Onayemi, Yiqun Gan, Yue Yu, and Yunier Broche-Pérez. Further details or information on the chapter content (e.g., tables, work by members, conferences, research, and specific products of the project) are available from the first author upon request.

The authors would like to thank all group members and Irit Felsen for their contribution to the Task Force and sharing their experience and insightful interviews included in the chapter as well as Melis Yetkin, Emren Burak Ömür, Sure Kosulgan, and Jallene Jia En Chua for the precious editorial assistance.

References

Abdelrahman, M., Al-Adwan, D., & Hasan, Y. (2021). Impact of social distancing on the mental health of parents and children in Qatar. *International Journal of Mental Health and Addiction*. https://doi.org/10.1007/s11469-021-00555-6

Abdullaeva, V. K., Suleymanov, S. R., Rustamova, J. T., Ganikhanov, A. A., & Sattarov, T. F. (2021). Mental health of children and adolescents during the COVID-19 pandemic. *Annals of the Romanian Society for Cell Biology, 25*, 3781–3786.

Abisha Meji, M., & Dennison, M. S. (2020). Survey on general awareness, mental state and academic difficulties among students due to COVID-19 outbreak in the western regions of Uganda. *Heliyon, 6*(11), e05454. https://doi.org/10.1016/j.heliyon.2020.e05454

Acharya, R., & Porwal, A. (2020). A vulnerability index for the management of and response to the COVID-19 epidemic in India: An ecological study. *Lancet Global Health, 8*, e1142–e1151. https://doi.org/10.1016/S2214-109X(20)30300-4

African Development Bank Group. (2020a). *Seychelles – COVID-19 crisis response budget support program*. https://projectsportal.afdb.org/dataportal/VProject/show/P-SC-K00-015

African Development Bank Group. (2020b). *Zimbabwe – COVID-19 response project (CRP)*. https://projectsportal.afdb.org/dataportal/VProject/show/P-ZW-IB0-004

Al Ammari, M., Sultana, K., Thomas, A., Al Swaidan, L., & Al Harthi, N. (2021). Mental health outcomes amongst health care workers during COVID 19 pandemic in Saudi Arabia. *Frontiers in Psychiatry, 11*, 619540–619540. https://doi.org/10.3389/fpsyt.2020.619540

Al Dhaheri, A. S., Bataineh, M. A. F., Mohamad, M. N., Ajab, A., Al Marzouqi, A., Jarrar, A. H., Habib-Mourad, C., Abu Jamous, D. O., Ali, H. I., Al Sabbah, H., Hasan, H., Stojanovska, L., Hashim, M., Abd Elhameed, O. A., Shaker Obaid, R. R., ElFeky, S., Saleh, S. T., Osaili, T. M., & Cheikh Ismail, L. (2021). Impact of COVID-19 on mental health and quality of life: Is there any effect? A cross-sectional study of the MENA region. *PLoS One, 16*(3), e0249107. https://doi.org/10.1371/journal.pone.0249107

Al Majali, S. A., & Alghazo, E. M. (2021). Mental health of individuals who are deaf during COVID-19: Depression, anxiety, aggression, and fear. *Journal of Community Psychology, 49*(6), 2134–2143. https://doi.org/10.1002/jcop.22539

Alat, P., Das, S. S., Arora, A., & Jha, A. K. (2021). Mental health during COVID-19 lockdown in India: Role of psychological capital and internal locus of control. *Current Psychology*. https://doi.org/10.1007/s12144-021-01516-x

Alhurishi, S. A., Almutairi, K. M., Vinluan, J. M., Aboshaiqah, A. E., & Marie, M. A. (2021). Mental health outcomes of healthcare providers during COVID-19 pandemic in Saudi Arabia: A cross-sectional study [Original Research]. *Frontiers in Public Health, 9*, 625523. https://doi.org/10.3389/fpubh.2021.625523

Ali, I., & Davis-Floyd, R. (Eds.). (2022). *Negotiating the pandemic: Cultural, national, and individual constructions of COVID-19*. Routledge.

Ali, A., Siddiqui, A. A., Arshad, M. S., Iqbal, F., & Arif, T. B. (2021a). Effects of COVID-19 pandemic and lockdown on lifestyle and mental health of students: A retrospective study from Karachi, Pakistan. *Annales Médico-Psychologiques, Revue Psychiatrique*. https://doi.org/10.1016/j.amp.2021.02.004

Ali, A., Sohaib, M., Iqbal, S., Hayat, K., Khan, A. U., & Rasool, M. F. (2021b). Evaluation of COVID-19 disease awareness and its relation to mental health, dietary habits, and physical activity: A cross-sectional study from Pakistan. *The American Journal of Tropical Medicine and Hygiene, 104*(5), 1687–1693. https://doi.org/10.4269/ajtmh.20-1451

Aljemaiah, A. I., Osman, M., Alharbi, S., Alshehri, R., Aldggag, E. M., Aljoudi, A. T., Abdulsomad, D. S., Abdulghani, M., & Alotaibi, F. (2021). Fear at the time of the COVID-19 pandemic: Validation of the Arabic version of the Four-Dimensional Symptom Questionnaire among Saudi-based respondents. *British Journal of Psychology Open, 7*(1), e33. https://doi.org/10.1192/bjo.2020.166

Almomani, E. Y., & Almomany, A. M. (2021). The impact of COVID-19 curfew restrictions on the university students' academic learning and mental health: A study from Jordan. *Journal of Loss and Trauma, 26*(5), 501–503. https://doi.org/10.1080/15325024.2021.1886801

Alrubaiee, G. G., Al-Qalah, T. A. H., & Al-Aawar, M. S. A. (2020). Knowledge, attitudes, anxiety, and preventive behaviours towards COVID-19 among health care providers in Yemen: An online cross-sectional survey. *BMC Public Health, 20*(1), 1541. https://doi.org/10.1186/s12889-020-09644-y

Alsairafi, Z., Naser, A. Y., Alsaleh, F. M., Awad, A., & Jalal, Z. (2021). Mental health status of healthcare professionals and students of health sciences faculties in Kuwait during the COVID-19 pandemic. *International Journal of Environmental Research and Public Health, 18*(4), 2203. https://www.mdpi.com/1660-4601/18/4/2203

Alshekaili, M., Hassan, W., Al Said, N., Al Sulaimani, F., Jayapal, S. K., Al-Mawali, A., Chan, M. F., Mahadevan, S., & Al-Adawi, S. (2020). Factors associated with mental health outcomes across healthcare settings in Oman during COVID-19: Frontline versus non-frontline healthcare workers. *BMJ Open, 10*(10), e042030. https://doi.org/10.1136/bmjopen-2020-042030

Althiabi, Y. (2021). Attitude, anxiety and perceived mental health care needs among parents of children with autism spectrum disorder (ASD) in Saudi Arabia during COVID-19 pandemic. *Research in Developmental Disabilities, 111*, 103873. https://doi.org/10.1016/j.ridd.2021.103873

Amendola, S., von Wyl, A., Volken, T., Zysset, A., Huber, M., & Dratva, J. (2021). A longitudinal study on generalized anxiety among university students during the first wave of the COVID-19 pandemic in Switzerland. *Frontiers in Psychology, 12*, 643171. https://doi.org/10.3389/fpsyg.2021.643171

Amit Aharon, A., Dubovi, I., & Ruban, A. (2021). Differences in mental health and health-related quality of life between the Israeli and Italian population during a COVID-19 quarantine. *Quality of Life Research, 30*(6), 1675–1684. https://doi.org/10.1007/s11136-020-02746-5

Anindyajati, G., Wiguna, T., Murtani, B. J., Christian, H., Wigantara, N. A., Putra, A. A., Hanafi, E., Minayati, K., Ismail, R. I., Kaligis, F., Savitri, A. I., Uiterwaal, C. S. P. M., & Diatri, H. (2021). Anxiety and its associated factors during the initial phase of the COVID-19 pandemic in Indonesia. *Frontiers in Psychiatry, 12*. https://doi.org/10.3389/fpsyt.2021.634585

Antiporta, D. A., Cutipé, Y. L., Mendoza, M., Celentano, D. D., Stuart, E. A., & Bruni, A. (2021). Depressive symptoms among Peruvian adult residents amidst a national lockdown during the COVID-19 pandemic. *BMC Psychiatry, 21*(1), 111. https://doi.org/10.1186/s12888-021-03107-3

Anyan, F., Hjemdal, O., Ernstsen, L., & Havnen, A. (2020). Change in physical activity during the coronavirus disease 2019 lockdown in Norway: The buffering effect of resilience on mental health. *Frontiers in Psychology, 11*, 598481. https://doi.org/10.3389/fpsyg.2020.598481

Anyolitho, M. K., Kabunga, A., Anyayo, L. G., & Nakaziba, R. (2021). Mental health during COVID-19 pandemic: Does social support count? A cross-sectional survey among Lira University students, Northern Uganda. *CPQ Neurology and Psychology, 3*, 1–11.

Arafa, A., Mohamed, A., Saleh, L., & Senosy, S. (2021). Psychological impacts of the COVID-19 pandemic on the public in Egypt. *Community Mental Health Journal, 57*(1), 64–69. https://doi.org/10.1007/s10597-020-00701-9

Aristovnik, A., Keržič, D., Ravšelj, D., Tomaževič, N., & Umek, L. (2020). Impacts of the COVID-19 pandemic on life of higher education students: A global perspective. *Sustainability, 12*, 8438. https://doi.org/10.3390/su12208438

Arizona State University. (2021). *COVID-19 stress and well-being*. https://asu.pure.elsevier.com/en/persons/ashley-randall

Arrais, M., Dias, W., Gama, J. M. R., & Brito, M. (2021). Physicians' perceptions of their knowledge and the preparedness of health facilities in Angola to diagnose and manage COVID-19. *International Health*. https://doi.org/10.1093/inthealth/ihab017

Asanov, I., Flores, F., McKenzie, D., Mensmann, M., & Schulte, M. (2021). Remote-learning, time-use, and mental health of Ecuadorian high-school students during the COVID-19 quarantine. *World Development, 138*, 105225. https://doi.org/10.1016/j.worlddev.2020.105225

Ashraf, F., Lee, S. A., Jobe, M. C., Mathis, A. A., & Kanwal, T. (2022). Bereavement in Pakistan during the COVID-19 pandemic: Psychometric analysis of the Pandemic Grief Scale-Urdu Version (PGS-UV). *Death Studies*. https://doi.org/10.1080/07481187.2022.2048197

Asiamah, N., Opuni, F. F., Mends-Brew, E., Mensah, S. W., Mensah, H. K., & Quansah, F. (2021). Short-term changes in behaviors resulting from COVID-19-related social isolation and their influences on mental health in Ghana. *Community Mental Health Journal, 57*(1), 79–92. https://doi.org/10.1007/s10597-020-00722-4

Associazione Italiana di Psicologia. (2022). *Ricerche su aspetti psicologici COVID-19*. https://aipass.org/ricerche-su-aspetti-psicologici-covid-19

Australian National University. (2022). *The ANU Indonesia project*. https://indonesia.crawford.anu.edu.au/

Ayad, Z., Al Tabbah, S., Hazimeh, B., & Sinno, L. (2021). Depression, anxiety, and stress associated with coronavirus disease (COVID-19) pandemic among health-care professionals in Lebanon and Iraq [Original Article]. *World Social Psychiatry, 3*(1), 36–44. https://doi.org/10.4103/wsp.wsp_74_20

Badahdah, A. M., Khamis, F., & Mahyijari, N. A. (2020). The psychological well-being of physicians during COVID-19 outbreak in Oman. *Psychiatry Research, 289*, 113053. https://doi.org/10.1016/j.psychres.2020.113053

Badahdah, A., Khamis, F., Al Mahyijari, N., Al Balushi, M., Al Hatmi, H., Al Salmi, I., Albulushi, Z., & Al Noomani, J. (2021). The mental health of health care workers in Oman during the COVID-19 pandemic. *International Journal of Social Psychiatry, 67*(1), 90–95. https://doi.org/10.1177/0020764020939596

Banna, M. H. A., Sayeed, A., Kundu, S., Christopher, E., Hasan, M. T., Begum, M. R., Kormoker, T., Dola, S. T. I., Hassan, M. M., Chowdhury, S., & Khan, M. S. I. (2020). The impact of the COVID-19 pandemic on the mental health of the adult population in Bangladesh: a nationwide cross-sectional study. *International Journal of Environmental Health Research*, 1–12. https://doi.org/10.1080/09603123.2020.1802409

Barbato, M., & Thomas, J. (2021). In this together: Psychological wellbeing of foreign workers in the United Arab Emirates during the COVID-19 pandemic. *International Journal of Psychology, 56*(6), 825–833. https://doi.org/10.1002/ijop.12786

Barcelona Institute for Global Health. (2021). *Will we see a wave of mental health problems after the COVID-19 pandemic?* https://www.isglobal.org/en/-/-es-la-salud-mental-la-pandemia-despues-de-la-covid-19-

Barrientos, J., Guzmán-González, M., Urzúa, A., & Ulloa, F. (2021). Psychosocial impact of COVID-19 pandemic on LGBT people in Chile. *Sexologies, 30*(1), e35–e41. https://doi.org/10.1016/j.sexol.2020.12.006

Bartoszek, A., Walkowiak, D., Bartoszek, A., & Kardas, G. (2020). Mental well-being (depression, loneliness, insomnia, daily life fatigue) during COVID-19 related home-confinement—A study from Poland. *International Journal of Environmental Research and Public Health, 17*(20), 7417. https://www.mdpi.com/1660-4601/17/20/7417

Bates, B. R., Tami, A., Carvajal, A., & Grijalva, M. J. (2021). Knowledge, attitudes, and practices towards COVID-19 among Venezuelans during the 2020 epidemic: An online cross-sectional survey. *PLoS One, 16*(4), e0249022. https://doi.org/10.1371/journal.pone.0249022

Bazarkulova, D., & Compton, J. (2021). Gender differences in self-reported stress and health behaviors of doctors in Kazakhstan during COVID-19. *Feminist Economics, 27*(1–2), 81–102. https://doi.org/10.1080/13545701.2020.1853789

Belleli, G., Rebora, P., Valsecchi, M. G., Bonfanti, P., & Citerio, G. (2020). Frailty index predicts poor outcome in COVID-19 patients. *Intensive Care Medicine, 46*(8), 1634–1636. https://doi.org/10.1007/s00134-020-06087-2

Bendau, A., Kunas, S. L., Wyka, S., Petzold, M. B., Plag, J., Asselmann, E., & Ströhle, A. (2021). Longitudinal changes of anxiety and depressive symptoms during the COVID-19 pandemic in Germany: The role of pre-existing anxiety, depressive, and other mental disorders. *Journal of Anxiety Disorders, 79*, 102377. https://doi.org/10.1016/j.janxdis.2021.102377

Beuermann, D., Bottan, N. L., Hoffmann, B., Khadan, J., & Vera-Cossio, D. A. (2021). *Suriname COVID-19 survey.*

Bilgiç, Ş., Baloğlu, M., & Tokalilar, S. (2022). Adapting and validating the coronavirus-19 phobia scale (C19P-S) in Korea. *Death Studies, 46*(3), 590–594. https://doi.org/10.1080/07481187.2021.1924897

BinDhim, N. F., Althumiri, N. A., Basyouni, M. H., Alageel, A. A., Alghnam, S., Al-Qunaibet, A. M., Almubarak, R. A., Aldhukair, S., & Ad-Dab'bagh, Y. (2021). Saudi Arabia mental health surveillance system (MHSS): Mental health trends amid COVID-19 and comparison with pre-COVID-19 trends. *European Journal of Psychotraumatology, 12*(1), 1875642. https://doi.org/10.1080/20008198.2021.1875642

Birhanu, A., Tiki, T., Mekuria, M., Yilma, D., Melese, G., & Seifu, B. (2021). COVID-19-induced anxiety and associated factors among urban residents in West Shewa Zone, Central Ethiopia, 2020. *Psychology Research and Behavior Management, 14*, 99–108. https://doi.org/10.2147/PRBM.S298781

Blom, V., Lönn, A., Ekblom, B., Kallings, L. V., Väisänen, D., Hemmingsson, E., Andersson, G., Wallin, P., Stenling, A., Ekblom, Ö., Lindwall, M., Salier Eriksson, J., Holmlund, T., & Ekblom-Bak, E. (2021). Lifestyle habits and mental health in light of the two Covid-19 pandemic waves in Sweden, 2020. *International Journal of Environmental Research and Public Health, 18*(6), 3313. https://www.mdpi.com/1660-4601/18/6/3313

Blot, K., Cavillot, L., De Pauw, R., De Smedt, D., Devleesschauwer, B., Ghattas, J., Gadeyne, S., Khan, Y., Speybroeck, N., Van den Borre, L., Vandepitte, S., Van Lancker, W., Vanroelen, C., Vanthomme, K., & Verhaeghe, N. (2021). *HELICON – Unravelling the long-term and indirect health impact of the COVID-19 crisis in Belgium.* https://www.brain-helicon.be/

Bolatov, A. K., Seisembekov, T. Z., Askarova, A. Z., Baikanova, R. K., Smailova, D. S., & Fabbro, E. (2021). Online-learning due to COVID-19 improved mental health among medical students. *Medical Science Educator, 31*(1), 183–192. https://doi.org/10.1007/s40670-020-01165-y

Bornstein, M. H. (Ed.). (2020). *Psychological insights for understanding COVID-19 and families, parents, and children*. Routledge.

Brailovskaia, J., Cosci, F., Mansueto, G., Miragall, M., Herrero, R., Baños, R. M., Krasavtseva, Y., Kochetkov, Y., & Margraf, J. (2021). The association between depression symptoms, psychological burden caused by COVID-19 and physical activity: An investigation in Germany, Italy, Russia, and Spain. *Psychiatry Research, 295*, 113596. https://doi.org/10.1016/j.psychres.2020.113596

Braun-Lewensohn, O., Abu-Kaf, S., & Kalagy, T. (2021). Hope and resilience during a pandemic among three cultural groups in Israel: The second wave of COVID-19 [Original Research]. *Frontiers in Psychology, 12*. https://doi.org/10.3389/fpsyg.2021.637349

Briggs, D. C., & Kattey, K. A. (2020). Mental and social health-related complaints among children and adolescents in Nigeria: Parents'/caregivers' perception – An online survey. *International Neuropsychiatric Disease Journal, 14*, 1–13. https://doi.org/10.9734/indj/2020/v14i430134

Brik, A. B. (2020). *COVID 19 Family Life Study/Impact of the pandemic on family life across cultures*. https://www.covidfamilystudy.org/

Broche-Pérez, Y., Fernández-Fleites, Z., Fernández-Castillo, E., Jiménez-Puig, E., Vizcaíno-Escobar, A. E., Ferrer-Lozano, D. M., Martínez-Rodríguez, L., & Martín-González, R. (2021). Anxiety, health self-perception, and worry about the resurgence of COVID-19 predict fear reactions among genders in the Cuban population [Original Research]. *Frontiers in Global Women's Health, 2*. https://doi.org/10.3389/fgwh.2021.634088

Budimir, S., Pieh, C., Dale, R., & Probst, T. (2021). Severe mental health symptoms during COVID-19: A comparison of the United Kingdom and Austria. *Healthcare, 9*(2), 191. https://www.mdpi.com/2227-9032/9/2/191

Buenaventura, R. D., Ho, J. B., & Lapid, M. I. (2020). COVID-19 and mental health of older adults in The Philippines: A perspective from a developing country. *International Psychogeriatrics, 32*(10), 1129–1133. https://doi.org/10.1017/S1041610220000757

Bukuluki, P., Frimpong-Manso, K., & Kato, F. (2021). Chapter 2 – Care leavers' experiences of COVID-19 in Uganda and Ghana: Implications for their mental health and psychosocial wellbeing. In A. A. Moustafa (Ed.), *Mental health effects of COVID-19* (pp. 19–36). Academic Press. https://doi.org/10.1016/B978-0-12-824289-6.00018-0

Buonsenso, D., Cinicola, B., Raffaelli, F., Sollena, P., & Iodice, F. (2020). Social consequences of COVID-19 in a low resource setting in Sierra Leone, West Africa. *International Journal of Infectious Diseases, 97*, 23–26. https://doi.org/10.1016/j.ijid.2020.05.104

Cakal, H., & Páez, D. (n.d.). *Socio-political effects of COVID-19*. https://keelepsych.co1.qualtrics.com/jfe/form/SV_85DOqpI7NyTk3qZ?version=ro1&Q_Language=RO&fbclid=IwAR0bVya-BfqrvFtnNbUy72VbBV3J8MRkPNSp551q_xz7a5q7FK68RMn-Wuw

Cam, H. H., Ustuner Top, F., & Kuzlu Ayyildiz, T. (2021). Impact of the COVID-19 pandemic on mental health and health-related quality of life among university students in Turkey. *Current Psychology*. https://doi.org/10.1007/s12144-021-01674-y

Caqueo-Urízar, A., Urzúa, A., Aragón-Caqueo, D., Charles, C. H., El-Khatib, Z., Otu, A., & Yaya, S. (2020). Mental health and the COVID-19 pandemic in Chile. *Psychological Trauma: Theory, Research, Practice, and Policy, 12*(5), 521–523. https://doi.org/10.1037/tra0000753

Carmassi, C., Cerveri, G., Bertelloni, C. A., Marasco, M., Dell'Oste, V., Massimetti, E., Gesi, C., & Dell'Osso, L. (2021). Mental health of frontline help-seeking healthcare workers during the COVID-19 outbreak in the first affected hospital in Lombardy, Italy. *Psychiatry Research, 298*, 113763–113763. https://doi.org/10.1016/j.psychres.2021.113763

Caycho-Rodríguez, T., Tomás, J. M., Barboza-Palomino, M., Ventura-León, J., Gallegos, M., Reyes-Bossio, M., & Vilca, L. W. (2021a). Assessment of fear of COVID-19 in older adults: Validation of the fear of COVID-19 scale. *International Journal of Mental Health and Addiction*. https://doi.org/10.1007/s11469-020-00438-2

Caycho-Rodríguez, T., Tomás, J. M., Vilca, L. W., Carbajal-León, C., Cervigni, M., Gallegos, M., Martino, P., Barés, I., Calandra, M., Anacona, C., López-Calle, C., Moreta-Herrera, R., Chacón-Andrade, E. R., Lobos-Rivera, M. E., Del Carpio, P., Quintero, Y., Robles, E., Lombardo, M. P., Recalde, O. G., Figares, A. B., et al. (2021b). Cross-cultural measurement invariance of the fear of COVID-19 scale in seven Latin American countries. *Death Studies*. https://doi.org/10.1080/07481187.2021.1879318

Cénat, J. M., Noorishad, P.-G., Kokou-Kpolou, C. K., Dalexis, R. D., Hajizadeh, S., Guerrier, M., Clorméus, L. A., Bukaka, J., Birangui, J.-P., Adansikou, K., Ndengeyingoma, A., Sezibera, V., Derivois, D., & Rousseau, C. (2021). Prevalence and correlates of depression during the COVID-19 pandemic and the major role of stigmatization in low- and middle-income countries: A multinational cross-sectional study. *Psychiatry Research, 297*, 113714. https://doi.org/10.1016/j.psychres.2021.113714

Center for Self Determination Theory. (2020). *Large Covid SDT project in Belgium*. https://selfdeterminationtheory.org/covid-19-sdt-study-how-motivated-are-belgian-citizens-to-adhere-to-the-prevention/

Ceri, V., & Cicek, I. (2021). Psychological well-being, depression and stress during COVID-19 pandemic in Turkey: A comparative study of healthcare professionals and non-healthcare professionals. *Psychology, Health & Medicine, 26*(1), 85–97. https://doi.org/10.1080/13548506.2020.1859566

Chadwick, C., Kenyon, C., & Nagel, M. (2021). Resiliency in uncertainty: Sustaining and strengthening primary education in Belize during the COVID-19 pandemic. In F. M. Reimers, U. Amaechi, A. Bamerji, & M. Wang (Eds.), *An educational calamity. Learning and teaching during the COVID-19 pandemic*.

Chang, C. L., & McAleer, M. (2020). Alternative Global Health Security Indexes for risk analysis of COVID-19. *International Journal of Environmental Research and Public Health, 17*. https://doi.org/10.3390/ijerph17093161

Chatterjee, M. (2021). Safeguarding the mental health of women of India in times of COVID 19: Challenges and ways forward [Invited Perspective]. *Indian Journal of Social Psychiatry, 37*(1), 3–6. https://doi.org/10.4103/ijsp.ijsp_37_21

Chaturvedi, K., Vishwakarma, D. K., & Singh, N. (2021). COVID-19 and its impact on education, social life and mental health of students: A survey. *Children and Youth Services Review, 121*, 105866. https://doi.org/10.1016/j.childyouth.2020.105866

Cheikh Ismail, L., Mohamad, M. N., Bataineh, M. A. F., Ajab, A., Al-Marzouqi, A. M., Jarrar, A. H., Abu Jamous, D. O., Ali, H. I., Al Sabbah, H., Hasan, H., Stojanovska, L., Hashim, M., Shaker Obaid, R. R., Saleh, S. T., Osaili, T. M., & Al Dhaheri, A. S. (2021). Impact of the coronavirus pandemic (COVID-19) lockdown on mental health and well-being in the United Arab Emirates [Original Research]. *Frontiers in Psychiatry, 12*. https://doi.org/10.3389/fpsyt.2021.633230

Chemen, S., & Gopalla, Y. N. (2021). Lived experiences of older adults living in the community during the COVID-19 lockdown – The case of Mauritius. *Journal of Aging Studies, 57*, 100932. https://doi.org/10.1016/j.jaging.2021.100932

Chen, X., Zhang, S. X., Jahanshahi, A. A., Alvarez-Risco, A., Dai, H., Li, J., & Ibarra, V. G. (2020). Belief in a COVID-19 conspiracy theory as a predictor of mental health and well-being of health care workers in Ecuador: Cross-sectional survey study. *JMIR Public Health and Surveillance, 6*(3), e20737. https://doi.org/10.2196/20737

Chen, Y., Osika, W., Henriksson, G., Dahlstrand, J., & Friberg, P. (2021). Impact of COVID-19 pandemic on mental health and health behaviors in Swedish adolescents. *Scandinavian Journal of Public Health*, 14034948211021724. https://doi.org/10.1177/14034948211021724

Cheng, P., Park, H. R. P., & Gatt, J. M. (2021). Approach coping mitigates distress of COVID-19 isolation for young men with low well-being in a sample of 1,749 youth from Australia and the USA [Original Research]. *Frontiers in Psychiatry, 12*. https://doi.org/10.3389/fpsyt.2021.634925

Children and Adolescents in Global Contexts: COVID-19 as a Life Course Event. (2022). *Children and adolescents in global contexts: COVID-19 as a life course event.*

Chirico, F., Nucera, G., & Magnavita, N. (2021). Protecting the mental health of healthcare workers during the COVID-19 emergency. *BJPsych International, 18*(1), E1. https://doi.org/10.1192/bji.2020.39

Chowdhury, S. R., Sunna, T. C., & Sanjoy, S. (2020). Response to COVID-19 in Bangladesh: Strategies to resist the growing trend of COVID-19 in a less restricted situation. *Asia Pacific Journal of Public Health, 32*(8), 471–472. https://doi.org/10.1177/1010539520951689

Cigăran, R.-G., Botezatu, R., Mînecan, E.-M., Gică, C., Panaitescu, A. M., Peltecu, G., & Gică, N. (2021). The psychological impact of the COVID-19 pandemic on pregnant women. *Healthcare, 9*(6), 725. https://www.mdpi.com/2227-9032/9/6/725

Clara Rachel Eybalin, C. (2021). Facing the three Ds: Decolonial thinking, disasters, development – The case of The Bahamas. In C. C. R. Eybalin, O. S. Aguto, & A. A. Adel (Eds.), *Memory, conflicts, disasters, and the geopolitics of the displaced* (pp. 25–41). IGI Global. https://doi.org/10.4018/978-1-7998-4438-9.ch002

Clotworthy, A., Dissing, A. S., Nguyen, T.-L., Jensen, A. K., Andersen, T. O., Bilsteen, J. F., Elsenburg, L. K., Keller, A., Kusumastuti, S., Mathisen, J., Mehta, A., Pinot de Moira, A., Rod, M. H., Skovdal, M., Strandberg-Larsen, K., Tapager, I. W., Varga, T. V., Vinther, J. L., Xu, T., Hoeyer, K., & Hulvej Rod, N. (2020). 'Standing together – At a distance': Documenting changes in mental-health indicators in Denmark during the COVID-19 pandemic. *Scandinavian Journal of Public Health, 49*(1), 79–87. https://doi.org/10.1177/1403494820956445

Cockerham, W. C., & Cockerham, G. B. (Eds.). (2020). *The COVID-19 reader: The science and what it says about the social.* Routledge.

Cognition and Brain Dynamics. (n.d.). *Does the confinement situation change our relationship to time?* https://brainthemind.com/temps-distanciation-sociale/

Coiro, M. J., Asraf, K., Tzischinsky, O., Hadar-Shoval, D., Tannous-Haddad, L., & Wolfson, A. R. (2021). Sleep quality and COVID-19-related stress in relation to mental health symptoms among Israeli and U.S. adults. *Sleep Health, 7*(2), 127–133. https://doi.org/10.1016/j.sleh.2021.02.006

Collaborative Outcomes study on Health and Functioning during Infection Times (COH-FIT). (2019). *How the COVID-19 pandemic affects physical and mental well-being in the general population.* https://www.coh-fit.com/

ConnectAID. (n.d.). *Supporting children and their families in the face of COVID-19.* https://connectaid.com/en/project/covidburkina

Constantini, A., & Mazzotti, E. (2020). Italian validation of CoViD-19 Peritraumatic Distress Index and preliminary data in a sample of general population. *Rivista Psichiatrica, 55*(3), 145–151.

Cooper, C. L. (Ed.). (2020). *Psychological insights for understanding COVID-19 and work.* Routledge.

Corona Immunitas. (n.d.). *F1 corona iImmunitas ticino.* https://www.corona-immunitas.ch/en/program/studies/f1-corona-immunitas-ticino/

Co-SPACE Study. (2022). *COVID-19: Supporting parents, adolescents and children during epidemics.* https://cospaceoxford.org/

Covid Circle. (2021). *Supporting delivery of a more effective and coherent global research response to the COVID-19 pandemic.* https://covidcircle.org/

COVID-19 Data Portal Sweden. (n.d.). *Research projects on COVID-19 in Sweden.* https://covid19dataportal.se/projects/

COVID-19 Unmasked Study. (2022). *How young children and their parents are managing during the pandemic.* https://www.uu.nl/onderzoek/covid-19-en-het-jonge-gezin-aandacht-voor-de-allerkleinsten

COVIDiSTRESS Global Survey. (2022). *Psychological stress, compliance with behavioral guidelines to slow the spread of coronavirus, and trust in governmental institutions and their preventive measures.* https://covidistress.france-bioinformatique.fr/

Covid-Minds Network. (2020). *Global mental health in the COVID-19 pandemic*. https://www.covidminds.org/

Crosby, L., McCloud, T., Hudson, L., Nicholls, D., De Stavola, B., Fowler, D., Viner, R., & Patalay, P. (2020). *You-COPE: Disruptions experienced by young people aged 16-24 during first months of the COVID-19 lockdown*. https://www.ucl.ac.uk/child-health/sites/child_health/files/ppp-youcope-briefing-disruptions_2020-06-23.pdf

CSWU Cross-Cultural Psychology Centre. (2021). *COVID-19, personality and quality of life: Self-enhancement in the time of pandemic*. https://www.crossculturalpsychlab.com/covid-19

Dai, H., Zhang, S. X., Looi, K. H., Su, R., & Li, J. (2020). Perception of health conditions and test availability as predictors of adults' mental health during the COVID-19 pandemic: A survey study of adults in Malaysia. *International Journal of Environmental Research and Public Health, 17*(15), 5498. https://www.mdpi.com/1660-4601/17/15/5498

Daly, Z., Slemon, A., Richardson, C. G., Salway, T., McAuliffe, C., Gadermann, A. M., Thomson, K. C., Hirani, S., & Jenkins, E. K. (2021). Associations between periods of COVID-19 quarantine and mental health in Canada. *Psychiatry Research, 295*, 113631. https://doi.org/10.1016/j.psychres.2020.113631

De Coninck, D., d'Haenens, L., & Matthijs, K. (2020). Perceived vulnerability to disease and attitudes towards public health measures: COVID-19 in Flanders, Belgium. *Personality and Individual Differences, 166*, 110220. https://doi.org/10.1016/j.paid.2020.110220

De Young, A., Hoehn, E., Vasileva, M., Alisic, E., March, S., Cobham, V., Donovan, C., & Middeldorp, C. (2021). *COVID-19 unmasked survey*.

DeCaprio, D., Gartner, J., McCall, C. J., Burgess, T., Garcia, K., Kothari, S., & Sayed, S. (2020). Building a COVID-19 vulnerability index. *Journal of Medical Artificial Intelligence, 3*. https://doi.org/10.21037/jmai-20-47

Denning, M., Goh, E. T., Tan, B., Kanneganti, A., Almonte, M., Scott, A., Martin, G., Clarke, J., Sounderajah, V., Markar, S., Przybylowicz, J., Chan, Y. H., Sia, C.-H., Chua, Y. X., Sim, K., Lim, L., Tan, L., Tan, M., Sharma, V., Ooi, S., Winter Beatty, J., Flott, K., Mason, S., Chidambaram, S., Yalamanchili, S., Zbikowska, G., Fedorowski, J., Dykowska, G., Wells, M., Purkayastha, S., & Kinross, J. (2021). Determinants of burnout and other aspects of psychological well-being in healthcare workers during the COVID-19 pandemic: A multinational cross-sectional study. *PLoS One, 16*(4), e0238666. https://doi.org/10.1371/journal.pone.0238666

Department of Psychology. (n.d.). *Emotion and social interaction laboratory*. https://esilab.berkeley.edu/research/

Devkota, H. R., Sijali, T. R., Bogati, R., Ahmad, M., Shakya, K. L., & Adhikary, P. (2021). The impact of COVID-19 on mental health outcomes among hospital fever clinic attendants across Nepal: A cross-sectional study. *PLoS One, 16*(3), e0248684. https://doi.org/10.1371/journal.pone.0248684

De Angelis, T. (2020). How APA is helping COVID's overlooked populations. Consider joining one of the 10 working groups tasked with culling resources to aid clinicians in working with underserved groups during the pandemic. *American Psychological Association*. https://www.apaservices.org/practice/news/covid-19-overlookedpopulations

Di Tella, M., Romeo, A., Benfante, A., & Castelli, L. (2020). Mental health of healthcare workers during the COVID-19 pandemic in Italy. *Journal of Evaluation in Clinical Practice, 26*(6), 1583–1587. https://doi.org/10.1111/jep.13444

DigiConsumers. (n.d.). *Improving young people's financial skills in a digitalised consumer society*. https://digiconsumers.fi/en/home/

Dimka, J. (2020). Disability and disease during the 1918 influenza pandemic. https://uni.oslomet.no/dis2/about-the-project/

Dimitrova, R., & Wiium, N. (2021a). Handbook of positive youth development: Advancing the next generation of research, policy and practice in global contexts. In R. Dimitrova & N. Wiium (Eds.), Handbook of positive youth development. *Advancing research, policy and practice in global contexts* (pp. 3-17). Springer. https://www.springer.com/gp/book/9783030702618

Dimitrova, R., & Wiium, N. (2021b) (Eds.). Handbook of positive youth development. *Advancing research, policy and practice in global contexts*. Springer. https://www.springer.com/gp/book/9783030702618

Ding, K., Yang, J., Chin, M.-K., Sullivan, L., Demirhan, G., Violant-Holz, V., Uvinha, R. R., Dai, J., Xu, X., Popeska, B., Mladenova, Z., Khan, W., Kuan, G., Balasekaran, G., Smith, G. A., & On Behalf of Global Community Health-COVID-Collaborative Research Team. (2021). Mental health among adults during the COVID-19 pandemic lockdown: A cross-sectional multi-country comparison. *International Journal of Environmental Research and Public Health, 18*(5), 2686. https://www.mdpi.com/1660-4601/18/5/2686

Długosz, P. (2021). Predictors of mental health after the first wave of the COVID-19 pandemic in Poland. *Brain Sciences, 11*(5), 544. https://www.mdpi.com/2076-3425/11/5/544

Dodd, R. H., Cvejic, E., Bonner, C., Pickles, K., McCaffery, K. J., Ayre, J., Batcup, C., Copp, T., Cornell, S., Dakin, T., Isautier, J. M. J., & Nickel, B. (2021). Willingness to vaccinate against COVID-19 in Australia. *The Lancet Infectious Diseases, 21*(3), 318–319. https://doi.org/10.1016/S1473-3099(20)30559-4

Dorji, T. (2021). The Gross National Happiness framework and the health system response to the COVID-19 pandemic in Bhutan. *The American Journal of Tropical Medicine and Hygiene, 104*(2), 441–445. https://doi.org/10.4269/ajtmh.20-1416

Dragun, R., Veček, N. N., Marendić, M., Pribisalić, A., Đivić, G., Cena, H., Polašek, O., & Kolčić, I. (2021). Have lifestyle habits and psychological well-being changed among adolescents and medical students due to COVID-19 lockdown in Croatia? *Nutrients, 13*(1), 97. https://www.mdpi.com/2072-6643/13/1/97

Ebenezer, J. (2020). Mental health in Tajikistan and COVID pandemic. *Social Science Research Network*. https://doi.org/10.2139/ssrn.3752562

Edad con Salud. (n.d.). *What we evaluate*. http://edadconsalud.com/que-evaluamos/?lang=en

El Othman, R., Touma, E., El Othman, R., Haddad, C., Hallit, R., Obeid, S., Salameh, P., & Hallit, S. (2021). COVID-19 pandemic and mental health in Lebanon: A cross-sectional study. *International Journal of Psychiatry in Clinical Practice, 25*(2), 152–163. https://doi.org/10.1080/13651501.2021.1879159

Elemo, A. S., Satici, S. A., & Griffiths, M. D. (2020). The Fear of COVID-19 Scale: Psychometric properties of the Ethiopian Amharic Version. *International Journal of Mental Health and Addiction*, 1–12. https://doi.org/10.1007/s11469-020-00448-0

Elhadi, M., Msherghi, A., Elgzairi, M., Alhashimi, A., Bouhuwaish, A., Biala, M., Abuelmeda, S., Khel, S., Khaled, A., Alsoufi, A., Elmabrouk, A., Alshiteewi, F. B., Alhadi, B., Alhaddad, S., Gaffaz, R., Elmabrouk, O., Hamed, T. B., Alameen, H., Zaid, A., Elhadi, A., & Albakoush, A. (2020). Psychological status of healthcare workers during the civil war and COVID-19 pandemic: A cross-sectional study. *Journal of Psychosomatic Research, 137*, 110221. https://doi.org/10.1016/j.jpsychores.2020.110221

Elmer, T., Mepham, K., & Stadtfeld, C. (2020). Students under lockdown: Comparisons of students' social networks and mental health before and during the COVID-19 crisis in Switzerland. *PLoS One, 15*(7), e0236337. https://doi.org/10.1371/journal.pone.0236337

El-Zoghby, S. M., Soltan, E. M., & Salama, H. M. (2020). Impact of the COVID-19 pandemic on mental health and social support among adult Egyptians. *Journal of Community Health, 45*(4), 689–695. https://doi.org/10.1007/s10900-020-00853-5

Ernstsen, L., & Havnen, A. (2021). Mental health and sleep disturbances in physically active adults during the COVID-19 lockdown in Norway: Does change in physical activity level matter? *Sleep Medicine, 77*, 309–312. https://doi.org/10.1016/j.sleep.2020.08.030

Essangri, H., Sabir, M., Benkabbou, A., Majbar, M. A., Amrani, L., Ghannam, A., Lekehal, B., Mohsine, R., & Souadka, A. (2021). Predictive factors for impaired mental health among medical students during the early stage of the COVID-19 pandemic in Morocco. *The American Journal of Tropical Medicine and Hygiene, 104*(1), 95–102. https://doi.org/10.4269/ajtmh.20-1302

European Comission. (2022a). *Epidemiological mathematical model on the spread of COVID-19*. https://ec.europa.eu/info/funding-tenders/opportunities/portal/screen/opportunities/horizon-results-platform/22936;campaigns=1

European Comission. (2022b). *Marie Skłodowska-Curie Actions: Projects researching COVID–19, SARS-Cov-2 and related topics*. https://ec.europa.eu/research/mariecurieactions/about-msca/covid-19-information/projects-researching-covid-19-sars-cov-2-and-related-topics

European Comission. (2022c). *THEMIS project: Protecting human rights and public health in global pandemics: A map of the standards applied by EU and US courts*. https://cordis.europa.eu/project/id/746014?fbclid=IwAR1NiLQYuGqkKLTvS1oVlaOU6NfAjjPLO9mup6nNv975MSaRfAqBnS7K_ic

European Comission. (n.d.-a). *The coronavirus response investment initiative in Poland*. https://ec.europa.eu/regional_policy/sources/newsroom/crii/coronavirus_response_poland_en.pdf

European Comission. (n.d.-b). *The coronavirus response investment initiative in Romania*. https://ec.europa.eu/regional_policy/sources/newsroom/crii/coronavirus_response_romania_en.pdf

European Investment Bank. (2020). *Barbados COVID-19 health resilience*. https://www.eib.org/en/projects/pipelines/all/20200764

Every-Palmer, S., Jenkins, M., Gendall, P., Hoek, J., Beaglehole, B., Bell, C., Williman, J., Rapsey, C., & Stanley, J. (2020). Psychological distress, anxiety, family violence, suicidality, and well-being in New Zealand during the COVID-19 lockdown: A cross-sectional study. *PLoS One, 15*(11), e0241658. https://doi.org/10.1371/journal.pone.0241658

Fairdom Hub. (2020). *COVID-19 related studies and tools in Germany*. https://fairdomhub.org/projects/191

Farajzadeh, A., Dehghanizadeh, M., Maroufizadeh, S., Amini, M., & Shamili, A. (2021). Predictors of mental health among parents of children with cerebral palsy during the COVID-19 pandemic in Iran: A web-based cross-sectional study. *Research in Developmental Disabilities, 112*, 103890. https://doi.org/10.1016/j.ridd.2021.103890

Fekih-Romdhane, F., Snene, H., Jebri, A., Ben Rhouma, M., & Cheour, M. (2020). Psychological impact of the pandemic COVID-19 outbreak among medical residents in Tunisia. *Asian Journal of Psychiatry, 53*, 102349–102349. https://doi.org/10.1016/j.ajp.2020.102349

Fernández-Abascal, E. G., & Martín-Díaz, M. D. (2021). Longitudinal study on affect, psychological well-being, depression, mental and physical health, prior to and during the COVID-19 pandemic in Spain. *Personality and Individual Differences, 172*, 110591. https://doi.org/10.1016/j.paid.2020.110591

Few, M. (2020). Epidemics, indigenous communities, and public health in the COVID-19 era: Views from smallpox inoculation campaigns in colonial Guatemala. *Journal of Global History, 15*(3), 380–393. https://doi.org/10.1017/S1740022820000297

Flores, M., Murchland, A., Espinosa-Tamez, P., Jaen, J., Brochier, M., Bautista-Arredondo, S., Lamadrid-Figueroa, H., Lajous, M., & Koenen, K. (2021). Prevalence and correlates of mental health outcomes during the SARS-Cov-2 epidemic in Mexico City and their association with non-adherence to stay-at-home directives, June 2020 [Original Article]. *International Journal of Public Health, 66*. https://doi.org/10.3389/ijph.2021.620825

Fluharty, M., Bu, F., Steptoe, A., & Fancourt, D. (2021). Coping strategies and mental health trajectories during the first 21 weeks of COVID-19 lockdown in the United Kingdom. *Social Science & Medicine, 279*, 113958. https://doi.org/10.1016/j.socscimed.2021.113958

Fountoulakis, K. N., Apostolidou, M. K., Atsiova, M. B., Filippidou, A. K., Florou, A. K., Gousiou, D. S., Katsara, A. R., Mantzari, S. N., Padouva-Markoulaki, M., Papatriantafyllou, E. I., Sacharidi, P. I., Tonia, A. I., Tsagalidou, E. G., Zymara, V. P., Prezerakos, P. E., Koupidis, S. A., Fountoulakis, N. K., & Chrousos, G. P. (2021). Self-reported changes in anxiety, depression and suicidality during the COVID-19 lockdown in Greece. *Journal of Affective Disorders, 279*, 624–629. https://doi.org/10.1016/j.jad.2020.10.061

Franic, T., & Dodig-Curkovic, K. (2020). Covid-19, child and adolescent mental health – Croatian (in)experience. *Irish Journal of Psychological Medicine, 37*(3), 214–217. https://doi.org/10.1017/ipm.2020.55

Freeman, D., Waite, F., Rosebrock, L., Petit, A., Causier, C., East, A., Jenner, L., Teale, A. L., Carr, L., Mulhall, S., Bold, E., & Lambe, S. (2022). Coronavirus conspiracy beliefs, mistrust, and compliance with government guidelines in England. *Psychological Medicine, 52*(2), 251–263. https://doi.org/10.1017/S0033291720001890

Fujita, K., Inoue, A., Kuzuya, M., Uno, C., Huang, C. H., Umegaki, H., & Onishi, J. (2021). Mental health status of the older adults in Japan during the COVID-19 pandemic. *Journal of the American Medical Directors Association, 22*(1), 220–221. https://doi.org/10.1016/j.jamda.2020.11.023

Gasteiger, N., Vedhara, K., Massey, A., Jia, R., Ayling, K., Chalder, T., Coupland, C., & Broadbent, E. (2021). Depression, anxiety and stress during the COVID-19 pandemic: Results from a New Zealand cohort study on mental well-being. *BMJ Open, 11*(5), e045325. https://doi.org/10.1136/bmjopen-2020-045325

Geirdal, A. Ø., Ruffolo, M., Leung, J., Thygesen, H., Price, D., Bonsaksen, T., & Schoultz, M. (2021). Mental health, quality of life, wellbeing, loneliness and use of social media in a time of social distancing during the COVID-19 outbreak. A cross-country comparative study. *Journal of Mental Health, 30*(2), 148–155. https://doi.org/10.1080/09638237.2021.1875413

Georgetown University Qatar. (n.d.). *The COVID project.* https://cirs.qatar.georgetown.edu/research/research-initiatives/covid-project/

Gerritsen, D. L., & Oude Voshaar, R. C. (2020). The effects of the COVID-19 virus on mental healthcare for older people in The Netherlands. *International Psychogeriatrics, 32*(11), 1353–1356. https://doi.org/10.1017/S1041610220001040

GESIS. (2021). *GESIS panel special survey on the coronavirus SARS-CoV-2 outbreak in Germany.* https://www.gesis.org/gesis-panel/coronavirus-outbreak

Giannopoulou, I., Efstathiou, V., Triantafyllou, G., Korkoliakou, P., & Douzenis, A. (2021). Adding stress to the stressed: Senior high school students' mental health amidst the COVID-19 nationwide lockdown in Greece. *Psychiatry Research, 295*, 113560. https://doi.org/10.1016/j.psychres.2020.113560

Giebel, C., Ivan, B., & Ddumba, I. (2022). COVID-19 public health restrictions and older adults' well-being in Uganda: Psychological impacts and coping mechanisms. *Clinical Gerontologist, 45*(1), 97–105. https://doi.org/10.1080/07317115.2021.1910394

Giordani, R. C. F., Giolo, S. R., Muhl, C., Estavela, A. J., & Mabuie Gove, J. I. (2021). Validation of the FCV-19 scale and assessment of fear of COVID-19 in the population of Mozambique, East Africa. *Psychology Research and Behaviour Management, 14*, 345–354. https://doi.org/10.2147/PRBM.S298948

Global Collaboration on Traumatic Stress. (n.d.). *Global crises: Global COVID-19-related traumatic stress activities.* https://www.global-psychotrauma.net/covid-19-projects

Global Covid Study. (2022). *COVID-19: Global study of social trust and mental health.* https://globalcovidstudy.com/about/

González-González, A., Toledo-Fernández, A., Romo-Parra, H., Reyes-Zamorano, E., & Betancourt-Ocampo, D. (2020). Psychological impact of sociodemographic factors and medical conditions in older adults during the COVID-19 pandemic in Mexico. *Salud Mental, 43*, 293–301. http://www.scielo.org.mx/scielo.php?script=sci_arttext&pid=S0185-33252020000600293&nrm=iso

González-Sanguino, C., Ausín, B., Castellanos, M. A., Saiz, J., & Muñoz, M. (2021). Mental health consequences of the COVID-19 outbreak in Spain. A longitudinal study of the alarm situation and return to the new normality. *Progress in Neuro-Psychopharmacology and Biological Psychiatry, 107*, 110219. https://doi.org/10.1016/j.pnpbp.2020.110219

Gosselin, A., Melchior, M., Carillon, S., Gubert, F., Ridde, V., Kohou, V., Zoumenou, I., Senne, J.-N., & Desgrées du Loû, A. (2021). Deterioration of mental health and insufficient COVID-19 information among disadvantaged immigrants in the greater Paris area. *Journal of Psychosomatic Research, 146*, 110504. https://doi.org/10.1016/j.jpsychores.2021.110504

Goularte, J. F., Serafim, S. D., Colombo, R., Hogg, B., Caldieraro, M. A., & Rosa, A. R. (2021). COVID-19 and mental health in Brazil: Psychiatric symptoms in the general population. *Journal of Psychiatric Research, 132*, 32–37. https://doi.org/10.1016/j.jpsychires.2020.09.021

Grech, P., & Grech, R. (2020). COVID-19 in Malta: The mental health impact. *Psychological Trauma: Theory, Research, Practice, and Policy, 12*(5), 534–535. https://doi.org/10.1037/tra0000925

Gritsenko, V., Skugarevsky, O., Konstantinov, V., Khamenka, N., Marinova, T., Reznik, A., & Isralowitz, R. (2021). COVID 19 fear, stress, anxiety, and substance use among Russian and Belarusian university students. *International Journal of Mental Health and Addiction, 19*(6), 2362–2368. https://doi.org/10.1007/s11469-020-00330-z

Gualano, M. R., Lo Moro, G., Voglino, G., Bert, F., & Siliquini, R. (2021). Monitoring the impact of COVID-19 pandemic on mental health: a public health challenge? Reflection on Italian data. *Social Psychiatry and Psychiatric Epidemiology, 56*(1), 165–167. https://doi.org/10.1007/s00127-020-01971-0

Guelmami, N., Ben Khalifa, M., Chalghaf, N., Kong, J. D., Amayra, T., Wu, J., Azaiez, F., & Bragazzi, N. L. (2021). Development of the 12-item social media disinformation scale and its association with social media addiction and mental health related to COVID-19 in Tunisia: Survey-based pilot case study. *JMIR Formative Research, 5*(6), e27280. https://doi.org/10.2196/27280

Gupta, A. K., Mehra, A., Niraula, A., Kafle, K., Deo, S. P., Singh, B., Sahoo, S., & Grover, S. (2020). Prevalence of anxiety and depression among the healthcare workers in Nepal during the COVID-19 pandemic. *Asian Journal of Psychiatry, 54*, 102260–102260. https://doi.org/10.1016/j.ajp.2020.102260

Gustavsson, J., & Beckman, L. (2020). Compliance to recommendations and mental health consequences among elderly in Sweden during the initial phase of the COVID-19 pandemic—A cross sectional online survey. *International Journal of Environmental Research and Public Health, 17*(15), 5380. https://www.mdpi.com/1660-4601/17/15/5380

Gyasi, R. M. (2020). Fighting COVID-19: Fear and internal conflict among older adults in Ghana. *Journal of Gerontological Social Work, 63*(6–7), 688–690. https://doi.org/10.1080/01634372.2020.1766630

Haimovich, A., Ravindra, N. G., Stoytchev, S., Young, H. P., Wilson, F. P., Dijk, D., Schulz, W. L., & Taylor, A. R. (2020). Development and validation of the COVID-19 severity index (CSI): A prognostic tool for early respiratory decompensation. *Annals of Emergency Medicine, 76*(4), 442–453. https://doi.org/10.1016/j.annemergmed.2020.07.022

Hansen, T., Nilsen, T. S., Yu, B., Knapstad, M., Skogen, J. C., Vedaa, Ø., & Nes, R. B. (2021). Locked and lonely? A longitudinal assessment of loneliness before and during the COVID-19 pandemic in Norway. *Scandinavian Journal of Public Health, 49*(7), 766–773. https://doi.org/10.1177/1403494821993711

Haslam, S. A. (Ed.). (2020). *Psychological insights for understanding COVID-19 and society*. Routledge.

Hayat, K., Haq, M. I. U., Wang, W., Khan, F. U., Rehman, A. U., Rasool, M. F., Kadirhaz, M., Omer, S., Rasheed, U., & Fang, Y. (2022). Impact of the COVID-19 outbreak on mental health status and associated factors among general population: A cross-sectional study from Pakistan. *Psychology, Health & Medicine, 27*(1), 54–68. https://doi.org/10.1080/13548506.2021.1884274

Health Data Research UK. (2022). *COVID-19 projects*. https://www.hdruk.ac.uk/covid-19/covid-19-projects/

Helbich, M., & Jabr, S. (2021). Analysis of the mental health response to COVID-19 and human rights concerns in the occupied Palestinian territories. *International Journal of Human Rights in Healthcare, 14*(3), 255–269. https://doi.org/10.1108/IJHRH-06-2020-0039

Hoang, T. D., Colebunders, R., Fodjo, J. N. S., Nguyen, N. P. T., Tran, T. D., & Vo, T. V. (2021a). Vietnamese people's well-being during the COVID-19 pandemic: An online survey.

International Journal of Environmental Research and Public Health, 18, 4737. https://doi.org/10.3390/ijerph18094737

Hoang, T. D., Colebunders, R., Fodjo, J. N. S., Nguyen, N. P. T., Tran, T. D., & Vo, T. V. (2021b). Well-being of healthcare workers and the general public during the COVID-19 pandemic in Vietnam: An online survey. *International Journal of Environmental Research and Public Health, 18*(9), 4737. https://www.mdpi.com/1660-4601/18/9/4737

Horesh, D., Kapel Lev-Ari, R., & Hasson-Ohayon, I. (2020). Risk factors for psychological distress during the COVID-19 pandemic in Israel: Loneliness, age, gender, and health status play an important role. *British Journal of Health Psychology, 25*(4), 925–933. https://doi.org/10.1111/bjhp.12455

Horita, R., Nishio, A., & Yamamoto, M. (2021). The effect of remote learning on the mental health of first year university students in Japan. *Psychiatry Research, 295*, 113561. https://doi.org/10.1016/j.psychres.2020.113561

Htay, M. N. N., Marzo, R. R., Bahari, R., AlRifai, A., Kamberi, F., El-Abasiri, R. A., Nyamache, J. M., Hlaing, H. A., Hassanein, M., Moe, S., Abas, A. L., & Su, T. T. (2021). How healthcare workers are coping with mental health challenges during COVID-19 pandemic? – A cross-sectional multi-countries study. *Clinical Epidemiology and Global Health, 11*, 100759. https://doi.org/10.1016/j.cegh.2021.100759

Hu, Y., & Qian, Y. (2021). COVID-19 and adolescent mental health in the United Kingdom. *Journal of Adolescent Health, 69*(1), 26–32. https://doi.org/10.1016/j.jadohealth.2021.04.005

Husaini, D. C., & Abubakar, Y. I. (2020). COVID-19: Belize's success story in containing community spread has suffered a setback! *Asia Pacific Journal of Public Health, 32*(8), 536–538. https://doi.org/10.1177/1010539520962604

Husky, M. M., Kovess-Masfety, V., & Swendsen, J. D. (2020). Stress and anxiety among university students in France during COVID-19 mandatory confinement. *Comprehensive Psychiatry, 102*, 152191. https://doi.org/10.1016/j.comppsych.2020.152191

Iasevoli, F., Fornaro, M., D'Urso, G., Galletta, D., Casella, C., Paternoster, M., Buccelli, C., & de Bartolomeis, A. (2021). Psychological distress in patients with serious mental illness during the COVID-19 outbreak and one-month mass quarantine in Italy. *Psychological Medicine, 51*(6), 1054–1056. https://doi.org/10.1017/S0033291720001841

IFRC. (2020). *Antigua and Barbuda: COVID-19*. https://go.ifrc.org/emergencies/4222#details

IFRC. (2021). *Belize COVID 19 relief project*. https://go.ifrc.org/reports/14088

Ignjatović Ristić, D., Hinić, D., Banković, D., Kočović, A., Ristić, I., Rosić, G., Ristić, B., Milovanović, D., Janjić, V., Jovanović, M., Selaković, D., Jovičić, M., Stevanović, N., Milanović, P., Milenković, N., Paunović, M., Stašević Karličić, I., Novaković, I., Aleksić, J., Drašković, M., Ranđelović, N., Đorđić, M., & Gavrilović, J. (2020). Levels of stress and resilience related to the COVID-19 pandemic among academic medical staff in Serbia. *Psychiatry and Clinical Neurosciences, 74*(11), 604–605. https://doi.org/10.1111/pcn.13124

Innovations for Poverty Action's (IPA). (2020). *Global behaviors and perceptions in the COVID-19 pandemic*. https://www.poverty-action.org/recovr-study/global-behaviors-and-perceptions-covid-19-pandemic

Institute for Investigative Journalism. (n.d.). *Project pandemic: Canada reports on COVID-19*. https://projectpandemic.concordia.ca/

International Centre for Migration Policy Development. (2022). *The role of information (technology) in the context of irregular migration: The private sector perspective*. Virtual briefing for ICMPD Member States. https://www.icmpd.org/news/the-role-of-information-technology-in-the-context-of-irregular-migration-the-private-sector-perspective.-virtual-briefing-for-icmpd-member-states

International Labour Organization. (2020). *Employability project (Barbados)*. https://www.ilo.org/caribbean/projects/WCMS_751092/lang%2D%2Den/index.htm

International Labour Organization. (2021). *Empowering women against COVID-19 (EWAC) in Albania*. https://www.ilo.org/budapest/what-we-do/projects/WCMS_764072/lang%2D%2Den/index.htm

Isaradisaikul, S. K., Thansuwonnont, P., & Sangthongluan, P. (2021). Impact of COVID-19 pandemic on happiness and stress: Comparison of preclinical and clinical medical students. *Korean Journal of Medical Education, 33*(2), 75–85. https://doi.org/10.3946/kjme.2021.189

Islam, M. A., Barna, S. D., Raihan, H., Khan, M. N. A., & Hossain, M. T. (2020). Depression and anxiety among university students during the COVID-19 pandemic in Bangladesh: A web-based cross-sectional survey. *PLoS One, 15*(8), e0238162. https://doi.org/10.1371/journal.pone.0238162

Jaguga, F., & Kwobah, E. (2020). Mental health response to the COVID-19 pandemic in Kenya: A review. *International Journal of Mental Health Systems, 14*(1), 68. https://doi.org/10.1186/s13033-020-00400-8

Jahrami, H., BaHammam, A. S., AlGahtani, H., Ebrahim, A., Faris, M., AlEid, K., Saif, Z., Haji, E., Dhahi, A., Marzooq, H., Hubail, S., & Hasan, Z. (2021). The examination of sleep quality for frontline healthcare workers during the outbreak of COVID-19. *Sleep and Breathing, 25*(1), 503–511. https://doi.org/10.1007/s11325-020-02135-9

Janati Idrissi, A., Lamkaddem, A., Benouajjit, A., Ben El Bouaazzaoui, M., El Houari, F., Alami, M., Labyad, S., Chahidi, A., Benjelloun, M., Rabhi, S., Kissani, N., Zarhbouch, B., Ouazzani, R., Kadiri, F., Alouane, R., Elbiaze, M., Boujraf, S., El Fakir, S., & Souirti, Z. (2020). Sleep quality and mental health in the context of COVID-19 pandemic and lockdown in Morocco. *Sleep Medicine, 74*, 248–253. https://doi.org/10.1016/j.sleep.2020.07.045

Jarego, M., Pimenta, F., Pais-Ribeiro, J., Costa, R. M., Patrão, I., Coelho, L., & Ferreira-Valente, A. (2021). Do coping responses predict better/poorer mental health in Portuguese adults during Portugal's national lockdown associated with the COVID-19? *Personality and Individual Differences, 175*, 110698. https://doi.org/10.1016/j.paid.2021.110698

Jenkins, E. K., McAuliffe, C., Hirani, S., Richardson, C., Thomson, K. C., McGuinness, L., Morris, J., Kousoulis, A., & Gadermann, A. (2021). A portrait of the early and differential mental health impacts of the COVID-19 pandemic in Canada: Findings from the first wave of a nationally representative cross-sectional survey. *Preventive Medicine, 145*, 106333. https://doi.org/10.1016/j.ypmed.2020.106333

Joensen, L. E., Madsen, K. P., Holm, L., Nielsen, K. A., Rod, M. H., Petersen, A. A., Rod, N. H., & Willaing, I. (2020). Diabetes and COVID-19: Psychosocial consequences of the COVID-19 pandemic in people with diabetes in Denmark—What characterizes people with high levels of COVID-19-related worries? *Diabetic Medicine, 37*(7), 1146–1154. https://doi.org/10.1111/dme.14319

Jovičić-Bata, J., Pavlović, N., Milošević, N., Gavarić, N., Goločorbin-Kon, S., Todorović, N., & Lalić-Popović, M. (2021). Coping with the burden of the COVID-19 pandemic: A cross-sectional study of community pharmacists from Serbia. *BMC Health Services Research, 21*(1), 304. https://doi.org/10.1186/s12913-021-06327-1

Jung, S. J., & Jun, J. Y. (2020). Mental health and psychological intervention amid COVID-19 outbreak: Perspectives from South Korea. *Yonsei Medical Journal, 61*(4), 271–272. https://doi.org/10.3349/ymj.2020.61.4.271

Kafle, K., Shrestha, D. B., Baniya, A., Lamichhane, S., Shahi, M., Gurung, B., Tandan, P., Ghimire, A., & Budhathoki, P. (2021). Psychological distress among health service providers during COVID-19 pandemic in Nepal. *PLoS One, 16*(2), e0246784. https://doi.org/10.1371/journal.pone.0246784

Kakaje, A., Fadel, A., & Ghareeb, A. (2020). Mental distress and psychological disorders of Syrians in fragile Syria and multiple countries related to COVID-19. *Social Science Research Network*. https://doi.org/10.2139/ssrn.3631240

Kamal, N. M., & Othman, N. (2020). Depression, anxiety, and stress in the time of COVID-19 pandemic in Kurdistan Region, Iraq. *Kurdistan Journal of Applied Research*, 37–44. https://doi.org/10.24017/covid.5

Kang, S., Sun, Y., Zhang, X., Sun, F., Wang, B., & Zhu, W. (2021). Is physical activity associated with mental health among Chinese adolescents during isolation in COVID-19 pandemic? *Journal of Epidemiology and Global Health, 11*(1), 26–33. https://doi.org/10.2991/jegh.k.200908.001

Kaparounaki, C. K., Patsali, M. E., Mousa, D.-P. V., Papadopoulou, E. V. K., Papadopoulou, K. K. K., & Fountoulakis, K. N. (2020). University students' mental health amidst the COVID-19 quarantine in Greece. *Psychiatry Research, 290*, 113111. https://doi.org/10.1016/j.psychres.2020.113111

Karakulak, A., Tepe, B., Dimitrova, R., Abdelrahman, M., Akaliyski, P., Alaseel, R. R., ... & da Silva, M. Z. (2023). Empathy, Fear of Disease and Support for COVID-19 Containment Behaviors: Evidence from 34 Countries on the Moderating Role of Governmental Trust. Retrieved from https://assets.researchsquare.com/files/rs-2412449/v1/2ce45f20-1d94-4166-b550-44a7ad3d7026.pdf?c=1676916039

Karageorghis, C. I., Bird, J. M., Hutchinson, J. C., Hamer, M., Delevoye-Turrell, Y. N., Guérin, S. M. R., Mullin, E. M., Mellano, K. T., Parsons-Smith, R. L., Terry, V. R., & Terry, P. C. (2021). Physical activity and mental well-being under COVID-19 lockdown: A cross-sectional multination study. *BMC Public Health, 21*(1), 988. https://doi.org/10.1186/s12889-021-10931-5

Kassir, G., El Hayek, S., Zalzale, H., Orsolini, L., & Bizri, M. (2021). Psychological distress experienced by self-quarantined undergraduate university students in Lebanon during the COVID-19 outbreak. *International Journal of Psychiatry in Clinical Practice, 25*(2), 172–179. https://doi.org/10.1080/13651501.2021.1900872

Kaul, N. (2021). Small state, big example: Covid pandemic management in Bhutan. *Critical Studies on Security, 9*(1), 58–62. https://doi.org/10.1080/21624887.2021.1904359

Kavčič, T., Avsec, A., & Zager Kocjan, G. (2021). Psychological functioning of Slovene adults during the COVID-19 pandemic: Does resilience matter? *Psychiatric Quarterly, 92*(1), 207–216. https://doi.org/10.1007/s11126-020-09789-4

Kayis, A. R., Satici, B., Deniz, M. E., Satici, S. A., & Griffiths, M. D. (2021). Fear of COVID-19, loneliness, smartphone addiction, and mental wellbeing among the Turkish general population: A serial mediation model. *Behaviour & Information Technology*, 1–13. https://doi.org/10.1080/0144929X.2021.1933181

Kesavelu, D., Inuganti, A., & Karthikeyan, N. (2021). Evaluation of the impact of the COVID-19 pandemic on the mental health of the health-care professionals across India [Original Article]. *Apollo Medicine, 18*(1), 7–11. https://doi.org/10.4103/am.am_126_20

Khademian, F., Delavari, S., Koohjani, Z., & Khademian, Z. (2021). An investigation of depression, anxiety, and stress and its relating factors during COVID-19 pandemic in Iran. *BMC Public Health, 21*(1), 275. https://doi.org/10.1186/s12889-021-10329-3

Khanal, P., Devkota, N., Dahal, M., Paudel, K., & Joshi, D. (2020). Mental health impacts among health workers during COVID-19 in a low resource setting: A cross-sectional survey from Nepal. *Globalization and Health, 16*(1), 89. https://doi.org/10.1186/s12992-020-00621-z

Khanchel, H. (2021). Measuring innovative practices for workplace safety, health and Well-being in Tunisia during the COVID-19 pandemic. *Human Systems Management, Preprint*, 1–10. https://doi.org/10.3233/HSM-201154

Khatatbeh, M., Khasawneh, A., Hussein, H., Altahat, O., & Alhalaiqa, F. (2021). Psychological impact of COVID-19 pandemic among the general population in Jordan. *Frontiers in Psychiatry, 12*, 618993. https://doi.org/10.3389/fpsyt.2021.618993

Khattak, S. R., Saeed, I., Rehman, S. U., & Fayaz, M. (2021). Impact of fear of COVID-19 pandemic on the mental health of nurses in Pakistan. *Journal of Loss and Trauma, 26*(5), 421–435. https://doi.org/10.1080/15325024.2020.1814580

Khoury, R., & Karam, G. (2020). Impact of COVID-19 on mental healthcare of older adults: Insights from Lebanon (Middle East). *International Psychogeriatrics, 32*(10), 1177–1180. https://doi.org/10.1017/S104161022000068X

Kilani, H. A., Bataineh, M. A. F., Al-Nawayseh, A., Atiyat, K., Obeid, O., Abu-Hilal, M. M., Mansi, T., Al-Kilani, M., Al-Kitani, M., El-Saleh, M., Jaber, R. M., Sweidan, A., Himsi, M., Yousef, I., Alzeer, F., Nasrallah, M., Al Dhaheri, A. S., Al-Za'abi, A., Allala, O., Al-Kilani, L., Alhasan, A. M., Ghieda, M., Najah, Y., Alsheekhly, S., Alhaifi, A., Shukri, R., Al Adwani, J., Waly, M., Kilani, L., Kilani, L. H., al Shareef, A. S., & Kilani, A. (2020). Healthy lifestyle behaviors are major predictors of mental wellbeing during COVID-19 pandemic confinement:

A study on adult Arabs in higher educational institutions. *PLoS One, 15*(12), e0243524. https://doi.org/10.1371/journal.pone.0243524

Kim, A. W., Nyengerai, T., & Mendenhall, E. (2020). Evaluating the mental health impacts of the COVID-19 pandemic: Perceived risk of COVID-19 infection and childhood trauma predict adult depressive symptoms in urban South Africa. *Psychological Medicine*, 1–13. https://doi.org/10.1017/S0033291720003414

Kim, J. H., Shim, Y., Choi, I., & Choi, E. (2022). The role of coping strategies in maintaining well-being during the COVID-19 outbreak in South Korea. *Social Psychological and Personality Science, 13*(1), 320–332. https://doi.org/10.1177/1948550621990595

Kira, I. A., Alpay, E. H., Ayna, Y. E., Shuwiekh, H. A. M., Ashby, J. S., & Turkeli, A. (2021). The effects of COVID-19 continuous traumatic stressors on mental health and cognitive functioning: A case example from Turkey. *Current Psychology*. https://doi.org/10.1007/s12144-021-01743-2

Klok, F. A., Boon, G. J. A. M., Barco, S., Endres, M., Geelhoed, M. J. J., Knauss, S., Rezek, S. A., Spruit, M. A., Vehreschild, J., & Siegerink, B. (2020). The post-COVID-19 functional status scale: A tool to measure functional status over time after COVID-19. *European Respiratory Journal, 56*, 2001494. https://doi.org/10.1183/13993003.01494-2020

Knudsen, A. K. S., Stene-Larsen, K., Gustavson, K., Hotopf, M., Kessler, R. C., Krokstad, S., Skogen, J. C., Øverland, S., & Reneflot, A. (2021). Prevalence of mental disorders, suicidal ideation and suicides in the general population before and during the COVID-19 pandemic in Norway: A population-based repeated cross-sectional analysis. *The Lancet Regional Health – Europe, 4*, 100071. https://doi.org/10.1016/j.lanepe.2021.100071

Kobayashi, L. C., O'Shea, B. Q., Kler, J. S., Nishimura, R., Palavicino-Maggio, C. B., Eastman, M. R., Vinson, Y. R., & Finlay, J. M. (2021). Cohort profile: The COVID-19 coping study, a longitudinal mixed-methods study of middle-aged and older adults' mental health and well-being during the COVID-19 pandemic in the USA. *BMJ Open, 11*(2), e044965. https://doi.org/10.1136/bmjopen-2020-044965

Kołodziejczyk, A., Misiak, B., Szcześniak, D., Maciaszek, J., Ciułkowicz, M., Łuc, D., Wieczorek, T., Fila-Witecka, K., Chladzinska-Kiejna, S., & Rymaszewska, J. (2021). Coping styles, mental health, and the COVID-19 quarantine: A nationwide survey in Poland [Original Research]. *Frontiers in Psychiatry, 12*. https://doi.org/10.3389/fpsyt.2021.625355

Korashi, M. M. (2021). The academic and psychological impact of COVID-19 outbreak on medical students in Sudan. *Gezira Journal of Health Sciences*, (16), 1–6. http://journals.uofg.edu.sd/index.php/gjhs/article/view/1572

Kornadt, A., Hoffmann, M., Murdock, E., Nell, J., & Albert, I. (2020). Views on aging and well-being in the covid crisis – A longitudinal study in Luxembourg. *Innovation in Aging, 4*(Supplement_1), 961–961. https://doi.org/10.1093/geroni/igaa057.3513

Korukcu, O., Ozkaya, M., Faruk Boran, O., & Boran, M. (2021). The effect of the COVID-19 pandemic on community mental health: A psychometric and prevalence study in Turkey. *Health & Social Care in the Community, 29*(5), e204–e213. https://doi.org/10.1111/hsc.13270

Kotera, Y., Ozaki, A., Miyatake, H., Tsunetoshi, C., Nishikawa, Y., & Tanimoto, T. (2021). Mental health of medical workers in Japan during COVID-19: Relationships with loneliness, hope and self-compassion. *Current Psychology, 40*(12), 6271–6274. https://doi.org/10.1007/s12144-021-01514-z

Kounou, K. B., Guédénon, K. M., Dogbe Foli, A. A., & Gnassounou-Akpa, E. (2020). Mental health of medical professionals during the COVID-19 pandemic in Togo. *Psychiatry and Clinical Neurosciences, 74*(10), 559–560. https://doi.org/10.1111/pcn.13108

Koustuv, D., Vikhrov, I., Azimova, N., & Chakraborty, S. (2021). The role of social messaging in the health promotion against COVID-19 in Uzbekistan. *Interdisciplinary Approaches to Medicine, 2*. https://doi.org/10.26577/IAM.2021.v2.i1.012

Kriaucioniene, V., Bagdonaviciene, L., Rodríguez-Pérez, C., & Petkeviciene, J. (2020). Associations between changes in health behaviours and body weight during the COVID-19 quarantine in Lithuania: The Lithuanian COVIDiet study. *Nutrients, 12*(10), 3119. https://www.mdpi.com/2072-6643/12/10/3119

Krüger-Malpartida, H., Pedraz-Petrozzi, B., Arevalo-Flores, M., Samalvides-Cuba, F., Anculle-Arauco, V., & Dancuart-Mendoza, M. (2020). Effects on mental health after the COVID-19 lockdown period: Results from a population survey study in Lima, Peru. *Clinical Medicine Insights: Psychiatry, 11*, 1179557320980423. https://doi.org/10.1177/1179557320980423

Krylova, O., & Gevorgyan, L. (2020a). *Impact study of COVID-19 on older people and caregivers in Armenia*. https://reliefweb.int/sites/reliefweb.int/files/resources/Armenia-report-COVID19_V06_13012021.pdf

Krylova, O., & Gevorgyan, L. (2020b). *Impact study of COVID-19 on older people and caregivers in Azerbaijan*. https://reliefweb.int/sites/reliefweb.int/files/resources/Azerbaijan-report-COVID19_V04_13012021.pdf

Kupfer, A., & Stutz, C. (Eds.). (2022). *Covid, crisis, care, and change? International gender perspectives on re/production, state, and feminist traditions*. Verlag Barbara Budrich.

Lábadi, B., Arató, N., Budai, T., Inhóf, O., Stecina, D. T., Sík, A., & Zsidó, A. N. (2021). Psychological well-being and coping strategies of elderly people during the COVID-19 pandemic in Hungary. *Aging & Mental Health*, 1–8. https://doi.org/10.1080/13607863.2021.1902469

Landa-Blanco, M., Mejía, C. J., Landa-Blanco, A. L., Martínez-Martínez, C. A., Vásquez, D., Vásquez, G., Moraga-Vargas, P., Echenique, Y., Del Cid, G. M., & Montoya, B. D. (2021). Coronavirus awareness, confinement stress, and mental health: Evidence from Honduras, Chile, Costa Rica, Mexico and Spain. *Social Science & Medicine, 277*, 113933. https://doi.org/10.1016/j.socscimed.2021.113933

Landaeta-Díaz, L., González-Medina, G., & Agüero, S. D. (2021). Anxiety, anhedonia and food consumption during the COVID-19 quarantine in Chile. *Appetite, 164*, 105259. https://doi.org/10.1016/j.appet.2021.105259

Lateef, T., Chen, J., Tahir, M., Lateef, T. A., Chen, B. Z., Li, J., & Zhang, S. X. (2021). Typhoon eye effect versus ripple effect: The role of family size on mental health during the COVID-19 pandemic in Pakistan. *Globalization and Health, 17*(1), 32. https://doi.org/10.1186/s12992-021-00685-5

Lee, S. W., Yang, J. M., Moon, S. Y., Yoo, I. K., Ha, E. K., Kim, S. Y., Park, U. M., Choi, S., Lee, S.-H., Ahn, Y. M., Kim, J.-M., Koh, H. Y., & Yon, D. K. (2020). Association between mental illness and COVID-19 susceptibility and clinical outcomes in South Korea: A nationwide cohort study. *The Lancet Psychiatry, 7*(12), 1025–1031. https://doi.org/10.1016/S2215-0366(20)30421-1

Li, W., Wang, Z., Wang, G., Ip, P., Sun, X., Jiang, Y., & Jiang, F. (2021a). Socioeconomic inequality in child mental health during the COVID-19 pandemic: First evidence from China. *Journal of Affective Disorders, 287*, 8–14. https://doi.org/10.1016/j.jad.2021.03.009

Li, Y., Zhao, J., Ma, Z., McReynolds, L. S., Lin, D., Chen, Z., Wang, T., Wang, D., Zhang, Y., Zhang, J., Fan, F., & Liu, X. (2021b). Mental health among college students during the COVID-19 pandemic in China: A 2-wave longitudinal survey. *Journal of Affective Disorders, 281*, 597–604. https://doi.org/10.1016/j.jad.2020.11.109

Lipskaya-Velikovsky, L. (2021). COVID-19 isolation in healthy population in Israel: Challenges in daily life, mental health, resilience, and quality of life. *International Journal of Environmental Research and Public Health, 18*(3), 999. https://www.mdpi.com/1660-4601/18/3/999

Liu, M.-B., Dufour, G., Sun, Z.-E., Galante, J., Xing, C.-Q., Zhan, J.-Y., & Wu, L.-L. (2021). The impact of the COVID-19 pandemic on the mental health of young people: A comparison between China and the United Kingdom. *Chinese Journal of Traumatology, 24*(4), 231–236. https://doi.org/10.1016/j.cjtee.2021.05.005

Lo Coco, G., Gentile, A., Bosnar, K., Milovanović, I., Bianco, A., Drid, P., & Pišot, S. (2021). A cross-country examination on the fear of COVID-19 and the sense of loneliness during the first wave of COVID-19 outbreak. *International Journal of Environmental Research and Public Health, 18*(5), 2586. https://www.mdpi.com/1660-4601/18/5/2586

López-Núñez, M. I., Díaz-Morales, J. F., & Aparicio-García, M. E. (2021). Individual differences, personality, social, family and work variables on mental health during COVID-19 outbreak in Spain. *Personality and Individual Differences, 172*, 110562. https://doi.org/10.1016/j.paid.2020.110562

Lotzin, A., Ketelsen, R., Zrnic, I., Lueger-Shuster, B., Böttche, M., & Schäfer, I. (2022). The Pandemic Stressor Scale: Factorial validity and reliability of a measure of stressors during a pandemic. *BMC Psychology, 10*, 92. https://doi.org/10.1186/s40359-022-00790-z

Lounis, M. (2020). A descriptive study of the current situation of COVID-19 in Algeria. *Electronic Journal of General Medicine, 17*, em253.

Lukács, A. (2021). *Mental well-being of university students in social isolation*. Hogrefe Publishing. https://doi.org/10.1027/2512-8442/a000065

Mahamid, F. A., & Bdier, D. (2021). The association between positive religious coping, perceived stress, and depressive symptoms during the spread of coronavirus (COVID-19) among a sample of adults in Palestine: Across sectional study. *Journal of Religion and Health, 60*(1), 34–49. https://doi.org/10.1007/s10943-020-01121-5

Malkawi, S. H., Almhdawi, K., Jaber, A. F., & Alqatarneh, N. S. (2021). COVID-19 quarantine-related mental health symptoms and their correlates among mothers: A cross sectional study. *Maternal and Child Health Journal, 25*(5), 695–705. https://doi.org/10.1007/s10995-020-03034-x

Mamun, M. A., Sakib, N., Gozal, D., Bhuiyan, A. K. M. I., Hossain, S., Bodrud-Doza, M., Al Mamun, F., Hosen, I., Safiq, M. B., Abdullah, A. H., Sarker, M. A., Rayhan, I., Sikder, M. T., Muhit, M., Lin, C.-Y., Griffiths, M. D., & Pakpour, A. H. (2021). The COVID-19 pandemic and serious psychological consequences in Bangladesh: A population-based nationwide study. *Journal of Affective Disorders, 279*, 462–472. https://doi.org/10.1016/j.jad.2020.10.036

Mana, A., Super, S., Sardu, C., Juvinya Canal, D., Moran, N., & Sagy, S. (2021). Individual, social and national coping resources and their relationships with mental health and anxiety: A comparative study in Israel, Italy, Spain, and The Netherlands during the coronavirus pandemic. *Global Health Promotion, 28*(2), 17–26. https://doi.org/10.1177/1757975921992957

Manh Than, H., Minh Nong, V., Trung Nguyen, C., Phu Dong, K., Ngo, H. T., Thu Doan, T., Thu Do, N., Huyen Thi Nguyen, T., Van Do, T., Xuan Dao, C., Quang Nguyen, T., Ngoc Pham, T., & Duy Do, C. (2020). Mental health and health-related quality-of-life outcomes among frontline health workers during the peak of COVID-19 outbreak in Vietnam: A cross-sectional study. *Risk Management and Healthcare Policy, 13*, 2927–2936. https://doi.org/10.2147/RMHP.S280749

Markosian, C., Layne, C. M., Petrosyan, V., Shekherdimian, S., Kennedy, C. A., & Khachadourian, V. (2021). War in the COVID-19 era: Mental health concerns in Armenia and Nagorno-Karabakh. *International Journal of Social Psychiatry*, 00207640211003940. https://doi.org/10.1177/00207640211003940

Martínez-Castilla, P., Gutiérrez-Blasco, I. M., Spitz, D. H., & Granot, R. (2021). The efficacy of music for emotional wellbeing during the COVID-19 lockdown in Spain: An analysis of personal and context-related variables [Original Research]. *Frontiers in Psychology, 12*. https://doi.org/10.3389/fpsyg.2021.647837

Matos, M., Rijo, D., McEwan, K., Steindl, S., Linharelhos, M., Lunding-Gregersen, V., Asano, K., Cheli, S., Bortolon, C., Gregório, S., Halamová, J., Kolts, R., Brito, G., Gumiy, N., Kelly, A., Santos, P., Ferreira, N., Tholouli, E., Wahl, J., & Zhang, A. (2020). *Compassion, social connectedness and trauma resilience during the COVID-19 pandemic: A multi-national study*. https://www.fpce.uc.pt/covid19study/

Matos, M., McEwan, K., Kanovský, M., Halamová, J., Steindl, S. R., Ferreira, N., Linharelhos, M., Rijo, D., Asano, K., Gregório, S., Márquez, M. G., Vilas, S. P., Brito-Pons, G., Lucena-Santos, P., da Silva Oliveira, M., de Souza, E. L., Llobenes, L., Gumiy, N., Costa, M. I., Habib, N., Hakem, R., Khrad, H., Alzahrani, A., Cheli, S., Petrocchi, N., Tholouli, E., Issari, P., Simos, G., Lunding-Gregersen, V., Elklit, A., Kolts, R., Kelly, A. C., Bortolon, C., Delamillieure, P., Paucsik, M., Wahl, J. E., Zieba, M., Zatorski, M., Komendziński, T., Zhang, S., Basran, J., Kagialis, A., Kirby, J., & Gilbert, P. (2021). Fears of compassion magnify the harmful effects of threat of COVID-19 on mental health and social safeness across 21 countries. *Clinical Psychology & Psychotherapy, 28*(6), 1317–1333. https://doi.org/10.1002/cpp.2601

Matovu, J. K. B., Kabwama, S. N., Ssekamatte, T., Ssenkusu, J., & Wanyenze, R. K. (2021). COVID-19 awareness, adoption of COVID-19 preventive measures, and effects of COVID-19 lockdown among adolescent boys and young men in Kampala, Uganda. *Journal of Community Health, 46*(4), 842–853. https://doi.org/10.1007/s10900-021-00961-w

Matsungo, T. M., & Chopera, P. (2020). Effect of the COVID-19-induced lockdown on nutrition, health and lifestyle patterns among adults in Zimbabwe. *BMJ Nutrition, Prevention & Health, 3*(2), 205–212. https://doi.org/10.1136/bmjnph-2020-000124

McMahon, C. (2020). *Psychological insights for understanding COVID-19 and media and technology*. Routledge.

Mechili, E. A., Saliaj, A., Kamberi, F., Girvalaki, C., Peto, E., Patelarou, A. E., Bucaj, J., & Patelarou, E. (2021). Is the mental health of young students and their family members affected during the quarantine period? Evidence from the COVID-19 pandemic in Albania. *Journal of Psychiatric and Mental Health Nursing, 28*(3), 317–325. https://doi.org/10.1111/jpm.12672

Meda, N., Pardini, S., Slongo, I., Bodini, L., Zordan, M. A., Rigobello, P., Visioli, F., & Novara, C. (2021). Students' mental health problems before, during, and after COVID-19 lockdown in Italy. *Journal of Psychiatric Research, 134*, 69–77. https://doi.org/10.1016/j.jpsychires.2020.12.045

Mehta, C. M., Arnett, J. J., Palmer, C. G., & Nelson, L. J. (2020). Established adulthood: A new conception of ages 30 to 45. *American Psychologist, 75*(4), 431–444. https://doi.org/10.1037/amp0000600

Midorikawa, H., Aiba, M., Lebowitz, A., Taguchi, T., Shiratori, Y., Ogawa, T., Takahashi, A., Takahashi, S., Nemoto, K., Arai, T., & Tachikawa, H. (2021). Confirming validity of The Fear of COVID-19 Scale in Japanese with a nationwide large-scale sample. *PLoS One, 16*(2), e0246840. https://doi.org/10.1371/journal.pone.0246840

Ming, X., & De Jong, M. D. T. (2021). Mental well-being of chinese immigrants in The Netherlands during the COVID-19 pandemic: A survey investigating personal and societal antecedents. *Sustainability, 13*(8), 4198. https://www.mdpi.com/2071-1050/13/8/4198

Ministry of Business, I. a. E. (n.d.). *COVID-19 research database*. https://www.mbie.govt.nz/science-and-technology/science-and-innovation/research-and-data/nzris/covid-19-research-database/

MOBIS-COVID-19. (2022). *Mobility behaviour in Switzerland Coronavirus Study*. https://ivtmobis.ethz.ch/mobis/covid19/reports/latest

Mohler-Kuo, M., Dzemaili, S., Foster, S., Werlen, L., & Walitza, S. (2021). Stress and mental health among children/adolescents, their parents, and young adults during the first COVID-19 lockdown in Switzerland. *International Journal of Environmental Research and Public Health, 18*(9), 4668. https://www.mdpi.com/1660-4601/18/9/4668

Mohsen, F., Bakkar, B., Melhem, S., Aldakkak, S., McHantaf, D., Marrawi, M., & Latifeh, Y. (2021). Psychological health problems among Syrians during war and the COVID-19 pandemic: National survey. *British Journal of Psychology International, 18*(3), E8. https://doi.org/10.1192/bji.2021.16

Molebatsi, K., Musindo, O., Ntlantsana, V., & Wambua, G. N. (2021). Mental health and psychosocial support during COVID-19: A review of health guidelines in Sub-Saharan Africa [Policy and Practice Reviews]. *Frontiers in Psychiatry, 12*. https://doi.org/10.3389/fpsyt.2021.571342

Mongkhon, P., Ruengorn, C., Awiphan, R., Thavorn, K., Hutton, B., Wongpakaran, N., Wongpakaran, T., & Nochaiwong, S. (2021). Exposure to COVID-19-related information and its association with mental health problems in Thailand: Nationwide, cross-sectional survey study. *Journal of Medical Internet Research, 23*(2), e25363. https://doi.org/10.2196/25363

Moreta-Herrera, R., López-Calle, C., Caycho-Rodríguez, T., Guerra, C. C., Gallegos, M., Cervigni, M., Martino, P., Barés, I., & Calandra, M. (2021). Is it possible to find a bifactor structure in the Fear of COVID-19 Scale (FCV-19S)? Psychometric evidence in an Ecuadorian sample. *Death Studies*. https://doi.org/10.1080/07481187.2021.1914240

Morgan, R. N. (2022). *Euro Youth Mental Health: A survey to document young people's experiences during the COVID-19 pandemic*. https://eymh.org/

Morsheimer, S., Chatzipanagiotou, K., Mykkänen, T., & Sandilya, H. (2020). *A systemic analysis of the impact of the COVID-19 pandemic on the refugees, migrants and asylum seekers in Cyprus* (Project Phoenix, Issue). https://reliefweb.int/sites/reliefweb.int/files/resources/FESSystemic%20Analysis%20of%20the%20Impact%20of%20the%20COVID-19_30.10.pdf

Msheik El Khoury, F., Talih, F., Khatib, M. F. E., Abi Younes, N., Siddik, M., & Siddik-Sayyid, S. (2021). Factors associated with mental health outcomes: Results from a tertiary referral hospital in Lebanon during the COVID-19 pandemic. *Libyan Journal of Medicine, 16*(1), 1901438. https://doi.org/10.1080/19932820.2021.1901438

Mudenda, S., Mukosha, M., Mwila, C., Saleem, Z., Kalungia, A., Munkombwe, D., Daka, V., Witika, B., Kampamba, M., Hikaambo, C., Jaffar, M., Chileshe, M., Kasanga, M., Mufwambi, W., Mfune, R., Matafwali, S., Masebe, P., Muungo, T., Bwalya, A., & Kazonga, E. (2021). Impact of the coronavirus disease on the mental health and physical activity of pharmacy students at the university of Zambia: A cross-sectional study. *International Journal of Basic & Clinical Pharmacology, 10*, 324. https://doi.org/10.18203/2319-2003.ijbcp20211010

Mukhtar, S. (2020). Mental health and psychosocial aspects of coronavirus outbreak in Pakistan: Psychological intervention for public mental health crisis. *Asian Journal of Psychiatry, 51*, 102069. https://doi.org/10.1016/j.ajp.2020.102069

Mumtaz, A., Manzoor, F., Jiang, S., & Anisur Rahaman, M. (2021). COVID-19 and mental health: A study of stress, resilience, and depression among the older population in Pakistan. *Healthcare, 9*(4), 424. https://www.mdpi.com/2227-9032/9/4/424

Muna Mohamed, E., Salih Boushra, H., Yassin Abdelrahim, A., Ahmed Alsayed Mohammed, M., Mosab Abbas, A., Maria Adam, M., Radi Tofaha, A., & Mohamed Fathelrahman Mohammed, A. (2020). The psychological impact of the COVID-19 pandemic on health professionals in Sudan 2020. *Sudan Journal of Medical Sciences (SJMS), 15*(5). https://doi.org/10.18502/sjms.v15i5.7136

Naser, A. Y., Dahmash, E. Z., Al-Rousan, R., Alwafi, H., Alrawashdeh, H. M., Ghoul, I., Abidine, A., Bokhary, M. A., AL-Hadithi, H. T., Ali, D., Abuthawabeh, R., Abdelwahab, G. M., Alhartani, Y. J., Al Muhaisen, H., Dagash, A., & Alyami, H. S. (2020). Mental health status of the general population, healthcare professionals, and university students during 2019 coronavirus disease outbreak in Jordan: A cross-sectional study. *Brain and Behavior, 10*(8), e01730. https://doi.org/10.1002/brb3.1730

National Institute for Health and Disability Insurance. (2020). *Institut national d'assurance maladie-invalidité (INAMI) pilot project on the telemonitoring of COVID-19 patients at home in Belgium*.

National Institute for Public Health and the Environment. (n.d.). *Research on COVID-19 in the Netherlands*. https://www.rivm.nl/en/coronavirus-covid-19/research

National Medical Research Council. (2021). *COVID-19 research*. https://www.nmrc.gov.sg/grants/awarded-projects/covid-19-research-projects

Nayak, B. S., Sahu, P. K., Ramsaroop, K., Maharaj, S., Mootoo, W., Khan, S., & Extavour, R. M. (2021). Prevalence and factors associated with depression, anxiety and stress among healthcare workers of Trinidad and Tobago during COVID-19 pandemic: A cross-sectional study. *BMJ Open, 11*(4), e044397. https://doi.org/10.1136/bmjopen-2020-044397

Neill, R. D., Blair, C., Best, P., McGlinchey, E., & Armour, C. (2021). Media consumption and mental health during COVID-19 lockdown: a UK cross-sectional study across England, Wales, Scotland and Northern Ireland. *Journal of Public Health*. https://doi.org/10.1007/s10389-021-01506-0

Nemat, A., Asady, A., Raufi, N., Zaki, N., Ehsan, E., Noor, N. A. S., & Zeng, Q. (2021). A survey of the healthcare workers in Afghanistan during the COVID-19 pandemic. *The American Journal of Tropical Medicine and Hygiene, 104*(2), 537–539. https://doi.org/10.4269/ajtmh.20-1367

Newson, J. J. (2020). *The Mental Health Million Project seeks to create an evolving map of global mental wellbeing and its demographic and situational drivers*. https://sapienlabs.org/mentalog/mental-health-million-post/

Nguépy Keubo, F. R., Mboua, P. C., Djifack Tadongfack, T., Fokouong Tchoffo, E., Tasson Tatang, C., Ide Zeuna, J., Noupoue, E. M., Tsoplifack, C. B., & Folefack, G. O. (2021). Psychological distress among health care professionals of the three COVID-19 most affected regions in Cameroon: Prevalence and associated factors. *Annales Médico-Psychologiques, Revue Psychiatrique, 179*(2), 141–146. https://doi.org/10.1016/j.amp.2020.08.012

Nguyen, T. M., & Le, G. N. H. (2021). The influence of COVID-19 stress on psychological well-being among Vietnamese adults: The role of self-compassion and gratitude. *Traumatology, 27*(1), 86–97. https://doi.org/10.1037/trm0000295

Nguyen, P. T. L., Nguyen, T. B. L., Pham, A. G., Duong, K. N. C., Gloria, M. A. J., Vo, T. V., Vo, B. V., & Phung, T. L. (2021). Psychological stress risk factors, concerns and mental health support among mealth care workers in Vietnam during the coronavirus disease 2019 (COVID-19) outbreak [Original Research]. *Frontiers in Public Health, 9*. https://doi.org/10.3389/fpubh.2021.628341

Nishimura, Y., Ochi, K., Tokumasu, K., Obika, M., Hagiya, H., Kataoka, H., & Otsuka, F. (2021). Impact of the COVID-19 pandemic on the psychological distress of medical students in Japan: Cross-sectional survey study. *Journal of Medical Internet Research, 23*(2), e25232. https://doi.org/10.2196/25232

Niziurski, J. A., & Schaper, M. L. (2021). Psychological wellbeing, memories, and future thoughts during the COVID-19 pandemic. *Current Psychology*. https://doi.org/10.1007/s12144-021-01969-0

Nochaiwong, S., Ruengorn, C., Awiphan, R., Ruanta, Y., Boonchieng, W., Nanta, S., Kowatcharakul, W., Pumpaisalchai, W., Kanjanarat, P., Mongkhon, P., Thavorn, K., Hutton, B., Wongpakaran, N., Wongpakaran, T., & Health Outcomes and Mental Health Care Evaluation Survey Research Group (HOME-Survey). (2020). Mental health circumstances among health care workers and general public under the pandemic situation of COVID-19 (HOME-COVID-19). *Medicine, 99*(26), e20751–e20751. https://doi.org/10.1097/MD.0000000000020751

Nomura, S., Kawashima, T., Yoneoka, D., Tanoue, Y., Eguchi, A., Gilmour, S., Kawamura, Y., Harada, N., & Hashizume, M. (2021). Trends in suicide in Japan by gender during the COVID-19 pandemic, up to September 2020. *Psychiatry Research, 295*, 113622. https://doi.org/10.1016/j.psychres.2020.113622

NordForsk. (2022). *Nordic health data research projects on COVID-19*. https://www.nordforsk.org/calls/nordic-health-data-research-projects-covid-19

Novo Nordisk Foundation. (2022). *Coronavirus initiatives*. https://novonordiskfonden.dk/en/about-the-foundation/initiatives-covid-19/

Nri-Ezedi, C. A., Nnamani, C. P., Ezeh, N. I., Okechukwu, C., Fasesan, O., & Ulasi, T. O. (2020). Psychological distress among residents in Nigeria during the COVID-19 pandemic. *International Neuropsychiatric Disease Journal, 14*, 8–21. https://doi.org/10.9734/indj/2020/v14i330129

O'Sullivan, K., Clark, S., McGrane, A., Rock, N., Burke, L., Boyle, N., Joksimovic, N., & Marshall, K. (2021). A qualitative study of child and adolescent mental health during the COVID-19 pandemic in Ireland. *International Journal of Environmental Research and Public Health, 18*(3), 1062. https://www.mdpi.com/1660-4601/18/3/1062

Obaje, H. I., Okengwu, G. C., Kenan, J. J., Uwimana, A., Ndayambaje, A., Carey, T. A., & Wong, R. (2021). Assessing the knowledge, perceptions, and mental health impact of COVID-19 among students in Rwanda. *Journal of Public Mental Health, 20*(3), 210–220. https://doi.org/10.1108/JPMH-10-2020-0125

Ofori, A. A., Osarfo, J., Agbeno, E. K., Manu, D. O., & Amoah, E. (2021). Psychological impact of COVID-19 on health workers in Ghana: A multicentre, cross-sectional study. *SAGE Open Medicine, 9*, 20503121211000919. https://doi.org/10.1177/20503121211000919

Ogweno, S. O., Oduor, K., & Mutisya, R. (2021). Sources of information on COVID-19 among the youths and its implications on mental health. A cross-sectional study in Nairobi, Kenya. *East African Medical Journal, 98*, 3390–3400.

Ontorio Tech University. (2020). *Ontario Tech researcher exploring parent-child conversations about COVID-19.* https://news.ontariotechu.ca/archives/2020/03/ontario-tech-researcher-exploring-parent-child-conversations-about-covid-19.php

OPENICPSR. (2022). *COVID-19 Data Repository: the social, behavioral, public health, and economic impact of the novel coronavirus global pandemic*. https://www.openicpsr.org/openicpsr/search/covid19

Orellana, C. I., & Orellana, L. M. (2020). Predictores de síntomas emocionales durante la cuarentena domiciliar por pandemia de COVID-19 en El Salvador. *Actualidades en Psicología, 34*, 103–120. http://www.scielo.sa.cr/scielo.php?script=sci_arttext&pid=S2215-35352020000100103&nrm=iso

Ornell, F., Halpern, S. C., Kessler, F. H. P., & de Magalhães Narvaez, J. C. (2020). The impact of the COVID-19 pandemic on the mental health of healthcare professionals. *Cadernos De Saude Publica, 36*. https://doi.org/10.1590/0102-311X00063520

Osseni, I. A. (2020). Benin responds to COVID-19: Sanitary cordon without generalized containment or lockdown? *Tropical Medicine and Health, 48*(1), 46. https://doi.org/10.1186/s41182-020-00235-6

Ouanes, S., Kumar, R., Doleh, E. S. I., Smida, M., Al-Kaabi, A., Al-Shahrani, A. M., Mohamedsalih, G. A., Ahmed, N. E., Assar, A., Khoodoruth, M. A. S., AbuKhattab, M., Maslamani, M. A., & AlAbdulla, M. A. (2021). Mental health, resilience, and religiosity in the elderly under COVID-19 quarantine in Qatar. *Archives of Gerontology and Geriatrics, 96*, 104457. https://doi.org/10.1016/j.archger.2021.104457

Padmanabhanunni, A., & Pretorius, T. (2021). The loneliness–life satisfaction relationship: The parallel and serial mediating role of hopelessness, depression and ego-resilience among young adults in South Africa during COVID-19. *International Journal of Environmental Research and Public Health, 18*(7), 3613. https://www.mdpi.com/1660-4601/18/7/3613

Parm, Ü., Aluoja, A., Tomingas, T., & Tamm, A.-L. (2021). Impact of the COVID-19 pandemic on Estonian elite athletes: Survey on mental health characteristics, training conditions, competition possibilities, and perception of supportiveness. *International Journal of Environmental Research and Public Health, 18*(8), 4317. https://www.mdpi.com/1660-4601/18/8/4317

Pascual-Sanchez, A., Nicholls, D., Patalay, P., Crosby, L., McCloud, T., Hudson, L., De Stavola, B., Fowler, D., & Viner, R. (2020). *You-COPE: Mental health consequences experienced by young people aged 16-24 during first months of the COVID-19 lockdown*. https://www.ucl.ac.uk/child-health/sites/child_health/files/youcope_briefing_mental_health_impact_final_version.pdf

Passos, L., Prazeres, F., Teixeira, A., & Martins, C. (2020). Impact on mental health due to COVID-19 pandemic: Cross-sectional study in Portugal and Brazil. *International Journal of Environmental Research and Public Health, 17*(18), 6794. https://www.mdpi.com/1660-4601/17/18/6794

Paulino, M., Dumas-Diniz, R., Brissos, S., Brites, R., Alho, L., Simões, M. R., & Silva, C. F. (2021). COVID-19 in Portugal: Exploring the immediate psychological impact on the general population. *Psychology, Health & Medicine, 26*(1), 44–55. https://doi.org/10.1080/13548506.2020.1808236

Pengpid, S., & Peltzer, K. (2020). Hand and oral hygiene practices among adolescents in Dominican Republic, Suriname and Trinidad and Tobago: Prevalence, health, risk behavior, mental health and protective factors. *International Journal of Environmental Research and Public Health, 17*(21), 7860. https://www.mdpi.com/1660-4601/17/21/7860

Peralta, E. A., & Taveras, M. (2020). Effectiveness of teleconsultation use in access to mental health services during the coronavirus disease 2019 pandemic in the Dominican Republic. *Indian Journal of Psychiatry, 62*(Suppl 3), S492–S494. https://doi.org/10.4103/psychiatry.IndianJPsychiatry_1047_20

Perera, B., Wickramarachchi, B., Samanmalie, C., & Hettiarachchi, M. (2021). Psychological experiences of healthcare professionals in Sri Lanka during COVID-19. *BMC Psychology, 9*(1), 49. https://doi.org/10.1186/s40359-021-00526-5

Perrotta, D. (2021). Universities and Covid-19 in Argentina: From community engagement to regulation. *Studies in Higher Education, 46*(1), 30–43. https://doi.org/10.1080/03075079.2020.1859679

Petzold, M. B., Bendau, A., Plag, J., Pyrkosch, L., Mascarell Maricic, L., Betzler, F., Rogoll, J., Große, J., & Ströhle, A. (2020). Risk, resilience, psychological distress, and anxiety at the beginning of the COVID-19 pandemic in Germany. *Brain and Behavior, 10*(9), e01745. https://doi.org/10.1002/brb3.1745

Pieh, C., Budimir, S., Delgadillo, J., Barkham, M., Fontaine, J. R. J., & Probst, T. (2021). Mental health during COVID-19 lockdown in the United Kingdom. *Psychosomatic Medicine, 83*(4). https://journals.lww.com/psychosomaticmedicine/Fulltext/2021/05000/Mental_Health_During_COVID_19_Lockdown_in_the.5.aspx

Pinchoff, J., Friesen, E. L., Kangwana, B., Mbushi, F., Muluve, E., Ngo, T. D., & Austrian, K. (2021). How has COVID-19-related income loss and household stress affected adolescent mental health in Kenya? *Journal of Adolescent Health, 69*(5), 713–720. https://doi.org/10.1016/j.jadohealth.2021.07.023

Pinho, L., Correia, T., Sampaio, F., Sequeira, C., Teixeira, L., Lopes, M., & Fonseca, C. (2021). The use of mental health promotion strategies by nurses to reduce anxiety, stress, and depression during the COVID-19 outbreak: A prospective cohort study. *Environmental Research, 195*, 110828. https://doi.org/10.1016/j.envres.2021.110828

Posel, D., Oyenubi, A., & Kollamparambil, U. (2021). Job loss and mental health during the COVID-19 lockdown: Evidence from South Africa. *PLoS One, 16*(3), e0249352. https://doi.org/10.1371/journal.pone.0249352

Poudel, K., & Subedi, P. (2020). Impact of COVID-19 pandemic on socioeconomic and mental health aspects in Nepal. *International Journal of Social Psychiatry, 66*(8), 748–755. https://doi.org/10.1177/0020764020942247

Prati, G. (2021). Mental health and its psychosocial predictors during national quarantine in Italy against the coronavirus disease 2019 (COVID-19). *Anxiety, Stress, & Coping, 34*(2), 145–156. https://doi.org/10.1080/10615806.2020.1861253

Pretorius, T., & Padmanabhanunni, A. (2021). A looming mental health pandemic in the time of COVID-19? Role of fortitude in the interrelationship between loneliness, anxiety, and life satisfaction among young adults. *South Africa Journal of Psychology, 51*(2), 256–268. https://doi.org/10.1177/0081246321991030

Project Vietnam Foundation. (n.d.). *Their smile begins with you*. https://projectvietnam.org/

Puccinelli, P. J., Costa, T. S., Seffrin, A., de Lira, C. A. B., Vancini, R. L., Knechtle, B., Nikolaidis, P. T., & Andrade, M. S. (2021). Physical activity levels and mental health during the COVID-19 pandemic: Preliminary results of a comparative study between convenience samples from Brazil and Switzerland. *Medicina, 57*(1), 48. https://www.mdpi.com/1648-9144/57/1/48

Qin, L., Sun, Q., Wang, Y., Wu, K. F., Chen, M., Shia, B. C., & Wu, S. Y. (2020). Prediction of number of cases of 2019 novel coronavirus (COVID-19) using Social Media Search Index. *International Journal of Environmental Research and Public Health, 17*(7), 2365. https://doi.org/10.3390/ijerph17072365

Quattrocchi, A., Mamais, I., Tsioutis, C., Christaki, E., Constantinou, C., Koliou, M., Pana, Z.-D., Silvestros, V., Theophanous, F., Haralambous, C., Stylianou, A., Sotiriou, S., Athanasiadou, M., Kyprianou, T., Demetriou, A., Demetriou, C. A., Kolokotroni, O., Gregoriou, I., Paphitou, N., Panos, G., Kostrikis, L., Karayiannis, P., Petrikkos, G., Agathangelou, P., Mixides, G., Siakallis, G., Hadjihannas, L., Palazis, L., Vavlitou, A., Matsentidou-Timiliotou, C., Koukios, D., Adamidi, T., Frangopoulos, F., Constantinou, E., & Nikolopoulos, G. (2020). Extensive testing and public health interventions for the control of COVID-19 in the Republic of Cyprus between March and May 2020. *Journal of Clinical Medicine, 9*(11), 3598. https://www.mdpi.com/2077-0383/9/11/3598

Rabinovich, G. A., & Geffner, J. (2021). Facing up to the COVID-19 pandemic in Argentina. *Nature Immunology, 22*(3), 264–265. https://doi.org/10.1038/s41590-021-00873-w

Rachel, J. F., Simon George, T., & Eveline Ndinelao, K. (2021). Mental health and psychosocial support for persons in quarantine and isolation facilities during the COVID-19 pandemic in Namibia: A multi-sectoral response. In T. Simon George (Ed.), *Epidemiological research applications for public health measurement and intervention* (pp. 40–52). IGI Global. https://doi.org/10.4018/978-1-7998-4414-3.ch003

Racine, N., Hetherington, E., McArthur, B. A., McDonald, S., Edwards, S., Tough, S., & Madigan, S. (2021). Maternal depressive and anxiety symptoms before and during the COVID-19 pandemic in Canada: a longitudinal analysis. *The Lancet Psychiatry, 8*(5), 405–415. https://doi.org/10.1016/S2215-0366(21)00074-2

Raghavendra, N. K., Gopal, S., & Munuswamy, J. (2021). Data set on impact of COVID-19 on mental health of internal migrant workers in India: Corona Virus Anxiety Scale (CAS) approach. *Data in Brief, 36*, 107052. https://doi.org/10.1016/j.dib.2021.107052

Ramiz, L., Contrand, B., Rojas Castro, M. Y., Dupuy, M., Lu, L., Sztal-Kutas, C., & Lagarde, E. (2021). A longitudinal study of mental health before and during COVID-19 lockdown in the French population. *Globalization and Health, 17*(1), 29. https://doi.org/10.1186/s12992-021-00682-8

Rana, W., Mukhtar, S., & Mukhtar, S. (2020). Mental health of medical workers in Pakistan during the pandemic COVID-19 outbreak. *Asian Journal of Psychiatry, 51*, 102080–102080. https://doi.org/10.1016/j.ajp.2020.102080

Ravens-Sieberer, U., Kaman, A., Erhart, M., Devine, J., Schlack, R., & Otto, C. (2021). Impact of the COVID-19 pandemic on quality of life and mental health in children and adolescents in Germany. *European Child & Adolescent Psychiatry*. https://doi.org/10.1007/s00787-021-01726-5

Rechel, B., & Moldoisaeva, S. (2021). Improving maternal and newborn health in Kyrgyzstan. *The Lancet. Global Health, 9*(3), e237–e238. https://doi.org/10.1016/S2214-109X(20)30511-8

Rehman, U., Shahnawaz, M. G., Khan, N. H., Kharshiing, K. D., Khursheed, M., Gupta, K., Kashyap, D., & Uniyal, R. (2021). Depression, anxiety and stress among Indians in times of COVID-19 lockdown. *Community Mental Health Journal, 57*(1), 42–48. https://doi.org/10.1007/s10597-020-00664-x

Research Luxembourg. (n.d.). *COVID-19 task force*. https://researchluxembourg.lu/covid-19-taskforce/

Residori, C., Schomaker, L., & Samuel, R. (2020). *The health, well-being and life satisfaction of young people in Luxembourg before the COVID-19 pandemic and during deconfinement*. HBSC Autumn Meeting 2020, Online.

Reznik, A., Gritsenko, V., Konstantinov, V., Khamenka, N., & Isralowitz, R. (2021). COVID-19 fear in Eastern Europe: Validation of the Fear of COVID-19 Scale. *International Journal of Mental Health and Addiction, 19*(5), 1903–1908. https://doi.org/10.1007/s11469-020-00283-3

Rīga Stradiņš University. (2020). *Life with COVID-19: Evaluation of overcoming the coronavirus crisis in Latvia and recommendations for societal resilience in the future*. https://www.rsu.lv/en/project/life-with-covid-19#:~:text=The%20project%20is%20based%20on,and%20analysing%20socio%2Dpolitical%20processes.&text=The%20interdisciplinary%20approach%20is%20designed,COVID%2D19%20on%20Latvian%20society

Rios-González, C. M., & Palacios, J. M. (2020). Symptoms of anxiety and depression during the outbreak of COVID-19 in Paraguay. *SciELO*. https://doi.org/10.1590/SciELOPreprints.152

Ristevska-Dimitrovska, G., & Batic, D. (2020). The impact of COVID-19 on mental health of healthcare workers and police/army forces in the Republic of North Macedonia. *European Neuropsychopharmacology, 40*, S479–S479. https://doi.org/10.1016/j.euroneuro.2020.09.622

Rivera, R. (2021). The Research Initiatives Working Group at the APA Interdivisional Task Force on the Pandemic. How to advance multidimensional Covid-19 scholarship from a global international perspective. *International Psychology Bulletin, 25*. http://div52.net/ipb-2021-25-3/#collaborations

Robles, R., Rodríguez, E., Vega-Ramírez, H., Álvarez-Icaza, D., Madrigal, E., Durand, S., Morales-Chainé, S., Astudillo, C., Real-Ramírez, J., Medina-Mora, M. E., Becerra, C., Escamilla, R., Alcocer-Castillejos, N., Ascencio, L., Díaz, D., González, H., Barrón-Velázquez, E., Fresán, A., Rodríguez-Bores, L., Quijada-Gaytán, J. M., Zabicky, G., Tejadilla-Orozco, D., González-Olvera, J. J., & Reyes-Terán, G. (2021). Mental health problems among healthcare workers involved with the COVID-19 outbreak. *Brazilian Journal of Psychiatry, 43*(5), 494–503. https://doi.org/10.1590/1516-4446-2020-1346

Rogowska, A. M., Pavlova, I., Kuśnierz, C., Ochnik, D., Bodnar, I., & Petrytsa, P. (2020). Does physical activity matter for the mental health of university students during the COVID-19 pandemic? *Journal of Clinical Medicine, 9*(11), 3494. https://www.mdpi.com/2077-0383/9/11/3494

Rondung, E., Leiler, A., Meurling, J., & Bjärtå, A. (2021). Symptoms of depression and anxiety during the early phase of the COVID-19 pandemic in Sweden [Original Research]. *Frontiers in Public Health, 9*. https://doi.org/10.3389/fpubh.2021.562437

Rossi, R., Socci, V., Talevi, D., Mensi, S., Niolu, C., Pacitti, F., Di Marco, A., Rossi, A., Siracusano, A., & Di Lorenzo, G. (2020). COVID-19 pandemic and lockdown measures impact on mental health among the general population in Italy [Brief Research Report]. *Frontiers in Psychiatry, 11*. https://doi.org/10.3389/fpsyt.2020.00790

Ruiz, M. C., Devonport, T. J., Chen-Wilson, C.-H., Nicholls, W., Cagas, J. Y., Fernandez-Montalvo, J., Choi, Y., & Robazza, C. (2021). A cross-cultural exploratory study of health behaviors and wellbeing during COVID-19 [Original Research]. *Frontiers in Psychology, 11*. https://doi.org/10.3389/fpsyg.2020.608216

Saddik, B., Hussein, A., Albanna, A., Elbarazi, I., Al-Shujairi, A., Temsah, M.-H., Saheb Sharif-Askari, F., Stip, E., Hamid, Q., & Halwani, R. (2021). The psychological impact of the COVID-19 pandemic on adults and children in the United Arab Emirates: A nationwide cross-sectional study. *BMC Psychiatry, 21*(1), 224. https://doi.org/10.1186/s12888-021-03213-2

Sagaon-Teyssier, L., Kamissoko, A., Yattassaye, A., Diallo, F., Rojas Castro, D., Delabre, R., Pouradier, F., Maradan, G., Bourrelly, M., Cissé, M., Vidal, L., Keïta, B. D., & Spire, B. (2020). Assessment of mental health outcomes and associated factors among workers in community-based HIV care centers in the early stage of the COVID-19 outbreak in Mali. *Health Policy OPEN, 1*, 100017. https://doi.org/10.1016/j.hpopen.2020.100017

Sakib, N., Akter, T., Zohra, F., Bhuiyan, A. K. M. I., Mamun, M. A., & Griffiths, M. D. (2021). Fear of COVID-19 and depression: A comparative study among the general population and healthcare professionals during COVID-19 pandemic crisis in Bangladesh. *International Journal of Mental Health and Addiction*. https://doi.org/10.1007/s11469-020-00477-9

Salisu, A. A., Akanni, L., & Raheem, I. (2020). The COVID-19 global fear index and the predictability of commodity price returns. *Journal of Behavioral and Experimental Finance, 27*, 100383. https://doi.org/10.1016/j.jbef.2020.100383

Samboma, T. A. (2020). Vulnerability of children in Botswana during COVID-19. *International Social Work, 63*(6), 807–810. https://doi.org/10.1177/0020872820949904

Sanabria-Mazo, J. P., Useche-Aldana, B., Ochoa, P. P., Rojas-Gualdrón, D. F., Mateo-Canedo, C., Carmona-Cervelló, M., Crespo-Puig, N., Selva-Olid, C., Méndez-Ulrich, A. M. L., Soler, A. F., Luciano, J. V., & Sanz, A. (2021). *Social inequities in the impact of COVID-19 lockdown measures on the mental health of a large sample of the Colombian population (PSY-COVID study)*. https://doi.org/10.31219/osf.io/bt9p2

Sanderman, R., & Kwasnicka, D. (Eds.). (2020). *Psychological insights for understanding COVID-19 and health*. Routledge.

Sandesh, R., Shahid, W., Dev, K., Mandhan, N., Shankar, P., Shaikh, A., & Rizwan, A. (2020). Impact of COVID-19 on the mental health of healthcare professionals in Pakistan. *Cureus, 12*(7), e8974. https://doi.org/10.7759/cureus.8974

Savolainen, I., Oksa, R., Savela, N., Celuch, M., & Oksanen, A. (2021). COVID-19 anxiety—A longitudinal survey study of psychological and situational risks among Finnish workers.

International Journal of Environmental Research and Public Health, 18(2), 794. https://www.mdpi.com/1660-4601/18/2/794

Schmidt, S. J., Barblan, L. P., Lory, I., & Landolt, M. A. (2021). Age-related effects of the COVID-19 pandemic on mental health of children and adolescents. *European Journal of Psychotraumatology, 12*(1), 1901407. https://doi.org/10.1080/20008198.2021.1901407

Sciences Po. (2020). *Coping with COVID-19: Social distancing, cohesion and inequality in 2020.* https://www.sciencespo.fr/osc/en/node/2232.html

Sciences Po. (2022). *Attitudes toward COVID-19.* https://www.sciencespo.fr/cevipof/attitudesoncovid19/

Sciences Po Media Lab. (2022). *Where to land after the pandemic?* https://ouatterrir.medialab.sciences-po.fr/

Sebastião, C. S., Neto, Z., Martinez, P., Jandondo, D., Antonio, J., Galangue, M., de Carvalho, M., David, K., Miranda, J., Afonso, P., Inglês, L., Carrelero, R. R., de Vasconcelos, J. N., & Morais, J. (2021). Sociodemographic characteristics and risk factors related to SARS-CoV-2 infection in Luanda, Angola. *PLoS One, 16*(3), e0249249. https://doi.org/10.1371/journal.pone.0249249

Setiawati, Y., Wahyuhadi, J., Joestandari, F., Maramis, M. M., & Atika, A. (2021). Anxiety and resilience of healthcare workers during COVID-19 pandemic in Indonesia. *Journal of Multidisciplinary Healthcare, 14*, 1–8. https://doi.org/10.2147/JMDH.S276655

Shahriarirad, R., Erfani, A., Ranjbar, K., Bazrafshan, A., & Mirahmadizadeh, A. (2021). The mental health impact of COVID-19 outbreak: a Nationwide Survey in Iran. *International Journal of Mental Health Systems, 15*(1), 19. https://doi.org/10.1186/s13033-021-00445-3

Shahrill, M., Petra, M. I., Naing, L., Yacob, J., Santos, J. H., & Abdul Aziz, A. B. Z. (2021). New norms and opportunities from the COVID-19 pandemic crisis in a higher education setting: Perspectives from Universiti Brunei Darussalam. *International Journal of Educational Management, 35*(3), 700–712. https://doi.org/10.1108/IJEM-07-2020-0347

Sharma, V., Reina Ortiz, M., & Sharma, N. (2020). Risk and protective factors for adolescent and young adult mental health within the context of COVID-19: A perspective from Nepal. *The Journal of Adolescent Health, 67*(1), 135–137. https://doi.org/10.1016/j.jadohealth.2020.04.006

Sharpe, D., Rajabi, M., Chileshe, C., Joseph, S. M., Sesay, I., Williams, J., & Sait, S. (2021). Mental health and wellbeing implications of the COVID-19 quarantine for disabled and disadvantaged children and young people: Evidence from a cross-cultural study in Zambia and Sierra Leone. *BMC Psychology, 9*(1), 79. https://doi.org/10.1186/s40359-021-00583-w

Siewe Fodjo, J. N., Ngarka, L., Njamnshi, W. Y., Nfor, L. N., Mengnjo, M. K., Mendo, E. L., Angwafor, S. A., Basseguin, J. G. A., Nkouonlack, C., Njit, E. N., Ahidjo, N., Chokote, E. S., Dema, F., Fonsah, J. Y., Tatah, G. Y., Palmer, N., Seke Etet, P. F., Palmer, D., Nsagha, D. S., Etya'ale, D. E., Perrig, S., Sztajzel, R., Annoni, J.-M., Bissek, A.-C. Z.-K., Leke, R. G. F., Obama, M.-T. A. O., Nkengasong, J. N., Colebunders, R., & Njamnshi, A. K. (2021). COVID-19 preventive behaviours in Cameroon: A six-month online national survey. *International Journal of Environmental Research and Public Health, 18*(5), 2554. https://www.mdpi.com/1660-4601/18/5/2554

Silva Moreira, P., Ferreira, S., Couto, B., Machado-Sousa, M., Fernández, M., Raposo-Lima, C., Sousa, N., Picó-Pérez, M., & Morgado, P. (2021). Protective elements of mental health status during the COVID-19 outbreak in the Portuguese population. *International Journal of Environmental Research and Public Health, 18*(4), 1910. https://www.mdpi.com/1660-4601/18/4/1910

Silverio-Murillo, A., Hoehn-Velasco, L., Balmori de la Miyar, J. R., & Rodríguez, A. (2021). COVID-19 and women's health: Examining changes in mental health and fertility. *Economics Letters, 199*, 109729. https://doi.org/10.1016/j.econlet.2021.109729

Skoog, I. (2020). COVID-19 and mental health among older people in Sweden. *International Psychogeriatrics, 32*(10), 1173–1175. https://doi.org/10.1017/S104161022000143X

Slama, H., El Kefi, H., Taamallah, K., Stambouli, N., Baffoun, A., Samoud, W., Bechikh, C., Oumaya, A., Lamine, K., Hmida, M. J., Slama, H., Ferjani, M., & Gharsallah, H. (2021). Immediate psychological responses, stress factors, and coping behaviors in military health-care professionals during the COVID-19 pandemic in Tunisia [Brief Research Report]. *Frontiers in Psychiatry, 12*. https://doi.org/10.3389/fpsyt.2021.622830

Šljivo, A., Kačamaković, M., Quraishi, I., & Džubur Kulenović, A. (2020). Fear and depression among residents of Bosnia and Herzegovina during COVID-19 outbreak – Internet survey. *Psychiatria Danubina, 32*(2), 266–272. https://doi.org/10.24869/psyd.2020.266

Soonthornchaiya, R. (2020). Resilience for psychological impacts of COVID-19 pandemic on older adults in Thailand. *Gerontology and Geriatric Medicine, 6*. https://doi.org/10.24966/GGM-8662/100053

Stănculescu, E. (2021). Fear of COVID-19 in Romania: Validation of the Romanian version of the fear of COVID-19 scale using graded response model analysis. *International Journal of Mental Health and Addiction*. https://doi.org/10.1007/s11469-020-00428-4

Stars, I., Smane, L., Pucuka, Z., Roge, I., & Pavare, J. (2021). Impact of pediatric COVID-19 on family health-related quality of life: A qualitative study from Latvia. *Global Pediatric Health, 8*, 2333794X211012394. https://doi.org/10.1177/2333794x211012394

Stephany, F., Neuhäuser, L., Stoehr, N., Darius, P., Teutloff, O., & Braesemann, F. (2022). The CoRisk-Index: A data-mining approach to identify industry-specific risk perceptions related to COVID-19. *Humanities and Social Sciences Communications, 9*(41). https://doi.org/10.1057/s41599-022-01039-1

Stylianou, N., Samouti, G., & Samoutis, G. (2020). Mental health disorders during the COVID-19 outbreak in Cyprus. *Journal of Medicine and Life, 13*(3), 300–305. https://doi.org/10.25122/jml-2020-0114

Sundarasen, S., Chinna, K., Kamaludin, K., Nurunnabi, M., Baloch, G. M., Khoshaim, H. B., Hossain, S. F. A., & Sukayt, A. (2020). Psychological impact of COVID-19 and lockdown among university students in Malaysia: Implications and policy recommendations. *International Journal of Environmental Research and Public Health, 17*(17), 6206. https://www.mdpi.com/1660-4601/17/17/6206

Sunjaya, D. K., Herawati, D. M. D., & Siregar, A. Y. M. (2021). Depressive, anxiety, and burnout symptoms on health care personnel at a month after COVID-19 outbreak in Indonesia. *BMC Public Health, 21*(1), 227. https://doi.org/10.1186/s12889-021-10299-6

Talaee, N., Varahram, M., Jamaati, H., Salimi, A., Attarchi, M., Kazempour-dizaji, M., Sadr, M., Hassani, S., Farzanegan, B., Monjazebi, F., & Seyedmehdi, S. M. (2022). Stress and burnout in health care workers during COVID-19 pandemic: Validation of a questionnaire. *Journal of Public Health, 30*, 531–536. https://doi.org/10.1007/s10389-020-01313-z

Tan, B. Y. Q. (2020). Psychological impact of the COVID-19 pandemic on health care workers in Singapore. *Annals of Internal Medicine, 173*(4), 317–320. https://doi.org/10.7326/M20-1083

Tanaka, T., & Okamoto, S. (2021). Increase in suicide following an initial decline during the COVID-19 pandemic in Japan. *Nature Human Behaviour, 5*(2), 229–238. https://doi.org/10.1038/s41562-020-01042-z

Tang, S., Xiang, M., Cheung, T., & Xiang, Y.-T. (2021). Mental health and its correlates among children and adolescents during COVID-19 school closure: The importance of parent-child discussion. *Journal of Affective Disorders, 279*, 353–360. https://doi.org/10.1016/j.jad.2020.10.016

Tee, M., Wang, C., Tee, C., Pan, R., Reyes, P. W., Wan, X., Anlacan, J., Tan, Y., Xu, L., Harijanto, C., Kuruchittham, V., Ho, C., & Ho, R. (2021). Impact of the COVID-19 pandemic on physical and mental health in lower and upper middle-income asian countries: A comparison between the Philippines and China. *Frontiers in Psychiatry, 11*, 568929. https://doi.org/10.3389/fpsyt.2020.568929

Tepe, B., & Karakulak, A. (2021). Linking judging moral to acting moral: a relational motivations approach to judging and practicing Covid-19 behaviors. Psychological Reports, 00332941211061077.

Terán-Pérez, G., Portillo-Vásquez, A., Arana-Lechuga, Y., Sánchez-Escandón, O., Mercadillo-Caballero, R., González-Robles, R. O., & Velázquez-Moctezuma, J. (2021). Sleep and mental health disturbances due to social isolation during the COVID-19 pandemic in Mexico. *International Journal of Environmental Research and Public Health, 18*(6), 2804. https://www.mdpi.com/1660-4601/18/6/2804

The Atlantic. (2021). *The COVID tracking project*. https://covidtracking.com/

The Borgen Project. (2021). *Tracking COVID-19 in Tanzania*. https://borgenproject.org/covid-19-in-tanzania/

The COVID Tracking Project. (2021). *US federal COVID data*. https://covidtracking.com/

The Research Council of Norway. (2021). *COVID-19 emergency call for proposals: Collaborative and knowledge-building projects for the fight against Coronavirus Disease (COVID-19)*. https://www.forskningsradet.no/en/call-for-proposals/2020/covid-19-emergency-call-proposals-collaborative-and-knowledge-building-projects-for-the-fight-against-coronavirus-disease-covid-19/

The UCL Tobacco and Research Group. (n.d.). *Health behaviors during the COVID-19 pandemic (HEBECO STUDY)*. https://www.ucl-covid19research.co.uk/

The UK Household Longitudinal Study. (2022). *The Understanding Society COVID-19 survey about participants experiences during the COVID-19 outbreak*. https://www.understandingsociety.ac.uk/topic/covid-19

The University of Sydney. (2020). *Alone together study: How has 2020 affected you? Have your say today*. https://www.sydney.edu.au/matilda-centre/news-and-events/2020/12/16/alone-together-study.html

Torales, J., Ríos-González, C., Barrios, I., O'Higgins, M., González, I., García, O., Castaldelli-Maia, J. M., & Ventriglio, A. (2020). Self-perceived stress during the quarantine of COVID-19 pandemic in Paraguay: An exploratory survey. *Frontiers in Psychiatry, 11*, 558691. https://doi.org/10.3389/fpsyt.2020.558691

Tosone, C. (Ed.). (2020). *Shared trauma, shared resilience during a pandemic: Social work in the time of COVID-19*. Springer.

Touré, A. A., Camara, L. M., Magassouba, A. S., Doumbouya, A., Camara, G., Camara, A. Y., Loua, G., Cissé, D., Sylla, M., Bereté, A. O., & Beavogui, A. H. (2021). Psychosocial impacts of COVID-19 in the Guinean population. An online cross-sectional survey. *PLoS One, 16*(2), e0245751. https://doi.org/10.1371/journal.pone.0245751

Tran, B. X., Nguyen, H. T., Le, H. T., Latkin, C. A., Pham, H. Q., Vu, L. G., Le, X. T. T., Nguyen, T. T., Pham, Q. T., Ta, N. T. K., Nguyen, Q. T., Ho, C. S. H., & Ho, R. C. M. (2020). Impact of COVID-19 on economic well-being and quality of life of the Vietnamese during the national social distancing. *Frontiers in Psychology, 11*, 565153. https://doi.org/10.3389/fpsyg.2020.565153

Trnka, R., & Lorencova, R. (2020). Fear, anger, and media-induced trauma during the outbreak of COVID-19 in the Czech Republic. *Psychological Trauma: Theory, Research, Practice, and Policy, 12*(5), 546–549. https://doi.org/10.1037/tra0000675

Trust for Social Achievement Foundation. (n.d.). *Support united against COVID-19 fund in Bulgaria*. https://www.globalgiving.org/projects/united-against-covid-19-bulgaria/

Tuan, N. Q., Phuong, N. D., Co, D. X., Son, D. N., Chinh, L. Q., Dung, N. H., Thach, P. T., Thai, N. Q., Thu, T. A., Tuan, N. A., San, B. V., Tung, V. S., An, N. V., Khanh, D. N., Long, V. H., Tai, N., Muoi, T., Vinh, N. D., Thien, N. T., Nhan, L. D., & Tuan, N. V. (2021). Prevalence and factors associated with psychological problems of healthcare workforce in Vietnam: Findings from COVID-19 hotspots in the national second wave. *Healthcare, 9*(6), 718. https://www.mdpi.com/2227-9032/9/6/718

UCL COVID-19 Social Study. (2022). *Understanding the psychological and social impact of the pandemic*. https://www.covidsocialstudy.org/

UCLA Law. (2021). *COVID behind bars data project*. https://uclacovidbehindbars.org/

UNICEF. (2021). *South Sudan COVID-19 emergency response and health systems preparedness project: Providing health care for some of the most vulnerable people in South Sudan*. https://www.unicef.org/southsudan/reports/covid-19-emergency-response-and-health-systems-project

UNICEF. (n.d.). *Project Gawa*. https://www.unicef.org/bhutan/project-gawa

United Nations Country Team. (2020). *ONE UN supporting Libya to tackle COVID-19*. https://reliefweb.int/report/libya/one-un-supporting-libya-tackle-covid-19-enar

University of Cambridge. (2022). *Cognition and Motivated Behaviour Lab*. https://www.camblab.psychol.cam.ac.uk/participate-in-research

University of Connecticut. (n.d.). *The pandemic journaling project*. https://pandemic-journaling-project.chip.uconn.edu/

University of Iceland. (n.d.). *COVID-19 projects*. https://english.hi.is/university/covid_19_projects

University of Miami. (2021). *The Pandemic Stress Index (PSI)*. https://elcentro.sonhs.miami.edu/research/measures-library/psi/index.html

University of Sussex. (2022). *SITUATE project: Students in transition at aniversity: Aiming to enhance mental and social health and wellbeing*. http://www.sussex.ac.uk/wellbeing/mentalhealth/situate

UNM Health Sciences. (2022). *Project echo: COVID-19 response*. https://hsc.unm.edu/echo/institute-programs/covid-19-response/

Valiente, C., Contreras, A., Peinado, V., Trucharte, A., Martínez, A. P., & Vázquez, C. (2021). Psychological adjustment in Spain during the COVID-19 pandemic: Positive and negative mental health outcomes in the population. *The Spanish Journal of Psychology, 24*, e8. https://doi.org/10.1017/SJP.2021.7

Van de Velde, S., Buffel, V., Bracke, P., Van Hal, G., Somogyi, N. M., Willems, B., Wouters, E., & C19 ISWS Consortium#. (2021). The COVID-19 international student well-being study. *Scandinavian Journal of Public Health, 49*, 114–122. https://doi.org/10.1177/1403494820981186

van de Vijver, F. J. R. (2019). Cross-cultural research. In J. Edlund & A. Nichols (Eds.), Advanced research methods and statistics for the behavioral and social sciences (pp. 274-286). *Cambridge University Press*. https://doi.org/10.1017/9781108349383.021

Van Rheenen, T. E., Meyer, D., Neill, E., Phillipou, A., Tan, E. J., Toh, W. L., & Rossell, S. L. (2020). Mental health status of individuals with a mood-disorder during the COVID-19 pandemic in Australia: Initial results from the COLLATE project. *Journal of Affective Disorders, 275*, 69–77. https://doi.org/10.1016/j.jad.2020.06.037

Van Tilburg, T. G., Steinmetz, S., Stolte, E., van der Roest, H., & de Vries, D. H. (2020). Loneliness and mental health during the COVID-19 pandemic: A study among dutch older adults. *The Journals of Gerontology: Series B, 76*(7), e249–e255. https://doi.org/10.1093/geronb/gbaa111

Verger, P., Scronias, D., Dauby, N., Adedzi, K. A., Gobert, C., Bergeat, M., Gagneur, A., & Dubé, E. (2021). Attitudes of healthcare workers towards COVID-19 vaccination: a survey in France and French-speaking parts of Belgium and Canada, 2020. *Eurosurveillance, 26*(3), 2002047. https://doi.org/10.2807/1560-7917.ES.2021.26.3.2002047

Villalba-Arias, J., Estigarribia, G., Bogado, J. A., Mendez, J., Toledo, S., Gonzalez, I., Castaldelli-Maia, J. M., Ventriglio, A., & Torales, J. (2020). Psychological impact of COVID-19 pandemic among healthcare workers in Paraguay: A descriptive and preliminary study. *Medicina Clinica y Social, 4*. https://doi.org/10.52379/mcs.v4i3.156

Vinaccia, S., Bahamón, M. J., Trejos-Herrera, A. M., Lee, S. A., Quiceno, J. M., Gómez, C. A., Vega DoLugar, S., & Pelaez, E. C. (2021). Validating the coronavirus anxiety scale in a Colombian sample. *Death Studies*, 1–10. https://doi.org/10.1080/07481187.2021.1944401

Voronin, I. A., Manrique-Millones, D., Vasin, G. D., Millones-Rivalles, R. B., Fernández-Ríos, N., Marakshina, Y. A., Lobaskova, M. M., Symanyuk, E. E., Pecherkina, A. A., Ageeva, I. A., Lysenkova, I. A., Ismatullina, V. I., Sitnikova, M. A., Malykh, S. B., & Manrique-Pino, O. (2020). Coping responses during the COVID-19 pandemic: A cross-cultural comparison of Russia, Kyrgyzstan, and Peru. *Psychology in Russia: State of the Art, 13*, 55–74. https://doi.org/10.11621/pir.2020.0404

Vujčić, I., Safiye, T., Milikić, B., Popović, E., Dubljanin, D., Dubljanin, E., Dubljanin, J., & Čabarkapa, M. (2021). Coronavirus disease 2019 (COVID-19) epidemic and mental health status in the general adult population of Serbia: A cross-sectional study. *International Journal of Environmental Research and Public Health, 18*(4), 1957. https://www.mdpi.com/1660-4601/18/4/1957

Wadoo, O., Latoo, J., Reagu, S. M., Amro, R. A. A., Masoodi, N. A., & Alabdulla, M. (2020). Mental health during COVID-19 in Qatar. *General Psychiatry, 33*(6), e100313. https://doi.org/10.1136/gpsych-2020-100313

Wadoo, O., Latoo, J., Iqbal, Y., Chandrappa, N. S. K., Chandra, P., Masoodi, N. A., Al-Maslamani, M. A. R. S., & Alabdulla, M. (2021). Mental wellbeing of frontline healthcare workers during COVID-19 pandemic in Qatar. *Asian Journal of Psychiatry, 55*, 102517. https://doi.org/10.1016/j.ajp.2020.102517

Wallace, D., & Wallace, R. (Eds.). (2020). *COVID-19 in New York City: An ecology of race and class oppression*. Springer.

Wang, C., Fardin, M. A., Shirazi, M., Pan, R., Wan, X., Tan, Y., Xu, L., McIntyre, R. S., Tran, B., Quek, T. T. C., Husain, S. F., Wang, J., Ho, C., & Ho, R. (2021a). Mental health of the general population during the 2019 Coronavirus Disease (COVID-19) pandemic: A tale of two developing countries. *Psychiatry International, 2*(1), 71–84. https://www.mdpi.com/2673-5318/2/1/6

Wang, C., Tee, M., Roy, A. E., Fardin, M. A., Srichokchatchawan, W., Habib, H. A., Tran, B. X., Hussain, S., Hoang, M. T., Le, X. T., Ma, W., Pham, H. Q., Shirazi, M., Taneepanichskul, N., Tan, Y., Tee, C., Xu, L., Xu, Z., Vu, G. T., Zhou, D., Koh, B. J., McIntyre, R. S., Ho, C., Ho, R. C., & Kuruchittham, V. (2021b). The impact of COVID-19 pandemic on physical and mental health of asians: A study of seven middle-income countries in Asia. *PLoS One, 16*(2), e0246824. https://doi.org/10.1371/journal.pone.0246824

Wang, Y., Shi, L., Que, J., Lu, Q., Liu, L., Lu, Z., Xu, Y., Liu, J., Sun, Y., Meng, S., Yuan, K., Ran, M., Lu, L., Bao, Y., & Shi, J. (2021c). The impact of quarantine on mental health status among general population in China during the COVID-19 pandemic. *Molecular Psychiatry, 26*(9), 4813–4822. https://doi.org/10.1038/s41380-021-01019-y

Wathelet, M., Duhem, S., Vaiva, G., Baubet, T., Habran, E., Veerapa, E., Debien, C., Molenda, S., Horn, M., Grandgenèvre, P., Notredame, C.-E., & D'Hondt, F. (2020). Factors associated with mental health disorders among university students in France confined during the COVID-19 pandemic. *JAMA Network Open, 3*(10), e2025591. https://doi.org/10.1001/jamanetworkopen.2020.25591

Weilenmann, S., Ernst, J., Petry, H., Pfaltz, M. C., Sazpinar, O., Gehrke, S., Paolercio, F., von Känel, R., & Spiller, T. R. (2021). Health care workers' mental health during the first weeks of the SARS-CoV-2 pandemic in Switzerland—A cross-sectional study [Brief Research Report]. *Frontiers in Psychiatry, 12*. https://doi.org/10.3389/fpsyt.2021.594340

Welfare State Research and Reform. (2020). *The impact of the COVID-19 crisis on gender equality in Finland*. https://thl.fi/en/web/thlfi-en/research-and-development/research-and-projects/the-impact-of-the-covid-19-crisis-on-gender-equality-in-finland

Welzel, C., Boehnke, K., Delhey, J., Deutsch, F., & Eichhorn, J. (2020). *Values in crisis – a crisis of values? Moral values under the imprint of the corona pandemic*. https://wapor.org/values-in-crisis-a-crisis-of-values-moral-values-under-the-imprint-of-the-corona-pandemic/

Westrupp, E. M., Karantzas, G., Macdonald, J. A., Olive, L., Youssef, G., Greenwood, C. J., Sciberras, E., Fuller-Tyszkiewicz, M., Evans, S., Mikocka-Walus, A., Ling, M., Cummins, R., Hutchinson, D., Melvin, G., Fernando, J. W., Teague, S., Wood, A. G., Toumbourou, J. W., Berkowitz, T., Linardon, J., Enticott, P. G., Stokes, M. A., McGillivray, J., & Olsson, C. A. (2020). Study protocol for the COVID-19 Pandemic Adjustment Survey (CPAS): A longitudinal study of Australian parents of a child 0–18 years [Study Protocol]. *Frontiers in Psychiatry, 11*. https://doi.org/10.3389/fpsyt.2020.555750

Wieczorek, T., Kołodziejczyk, A., Ciułkowicz, M., Maciaszek, J., Misiak, B., Rymaszewska, J., & Szcześniak, D. (2021). Class of 2020 in Poland: Students' mental health during the COVID-19 outbreak in an academic setting. *International Journal of Environmental Research and Public Health, 18*(6), 2884. https://www.mdpi.com/1660-4601/18/6/2884

Wiguna, T., Anindyajati, G., Kaligis, F., Ismail, R. I., Minayati, K., Hanafi, E., Murtani, B. J., Wigantara, N. A., Putra, A. A., & Pradana, K. (2020). Brief research report on adolescent mental well-being and school closures during the COVID-19 pandemic in Indonesia. *Frontiers in Psychiatry, 11*, 598756–598756. https://doi.org/10.3389/fpsyt.2020.598756

Windarwati, H. D., Ati, N. A. L., Paraswati, M. D., Ilmy, S. K., Supianto, A. A., Rizzal, A. F., Sulaksono, A. D., Lestari, R., & Supriati, L. (2021). Stressor, coping mechanism, and motivation among health care workers in dealing with stress due to the COVID-19 pandemic in Indonesia. *Asian Journal of Psychiatry, 56*, 102470–102470. https://doi.org/10.1016/j.ajp.2020.102470

Winthrop, R., Ershadi, M., Angrist, N., Bortsie, E., & Matsheng, M. (2020). *A historic shock to parental engagement in education: Parent perspectives in Botswana during COVID-19*. The Brookings Institution.

World Bank. (2020a). *Belarus emergency COVID-19 response project*. https://www.worldbank.org/en/news/loans-credits/2020/05/22/belarus-emergency-covid19-response-project

World Bank. (2020b). *Comoros emergency DPO for COVID-19 response*. https://projects.worldbank.org/en/projects-operations/project-detail/P174260

World Bank. (2020c). *Dominican Republic COVID-19 crisis response support*. https://projects.worldbank.org/en/projects-operations/project-detail/P174145

World Bank. (2020d). *Pakistan – COVID-19 pandemic response effectiveness project (English)*. https://documents.worldbank.org/en/publication/documents-reports/documentdetail/651371585953227830/pakistan-covid-19-pandemic-response-effectiveness-project

World Bank. (2020e). *Project information document –India COVID-19 emergency response and health systems preparedness project – P173836 (English)*. https://documents.worldbank.org/en/publication/documents-reports/documentdetail/606831584974996652/project-information-document-india-covid-19-emergency-response-and-health-systems-preparedness-project-p173836

World Bank. (2020f). *Project information document – Liberia COVID-19 emergency response project – P173812 (Inglês)*. https://documents.worldbank.org/pt/publication/documents-reports/documentdetail/702391585256985149/project-information-document-liberia-covid-19-emergency-response-project-p173812

World Bank. (2020g). *Project information document – Mauritania COVID-19 strategic preparedness and response project (SPRP) – P173837 (English)*. https://documents.worldbank.org/en/publication/documents-reports/documentdetail/242481585139834110/project-information-document-mauritania-covid-19-strategic-preparedness-and-response-project-sprp-p173837

World Bank. (2021a). *Afghanistan COVID-19 emergency response and health systems preparedness project*. https://projects.worldbank.org/en/projects-operations/project-detail/P173775

World Bank. (2021b). *Albania emergency COVID-19 response project*. https://projects.worldbank.org/en/projects-operations/project-detail/P174101

World Bank. (2021c). *Azerbaijan COVID-19 emergency response project*. https://projects.worldbank.org/en/projects-operations/project-detail/P176503

World Bank. (2021d). *The Bahamas COVID-19 response and recovery DPF*. https://projects.worldbank.org/en/projects-operations/project-detail/P175490?lang=en

World Bank. (2021e). *Bangladesh: COVID-19 emergency response and pandemic preparedness project*. https://projects.worldbank.org/en/projects-operations/project-detail/P173757

World Bank. (2021f). *Barbados COVID-19 response and recovery DPF*. https://projects.worldbank.org/en/projects-operations/project-detail/P175492

World Bank. (2021g). *Bhutan: COVID-19 emergency response and health systems preparedness project*. https://projects.worldbank.org/en/projects-operations/project-detail/P173787

World Bank. (2021h). *Bosnia and Herzegovina emergency COVID-19 project*. https://projects.worldbank.org/en/projects-operations/project-detail/P173809

World Bank. (2021i). *Burkina Faso COVID-19 preparedness and response project*. https://projects.worldbank.org/en/projects-operations/project-detail/P173858

World Bank. (2021j). *Burundi COVID-19 preparedness and response project*. https://projects.worldbank.org/en/projects-operations/project-detail/P173845

World Bank. (2021k). *Cabo Verde: COVID-19 emergency response project*. https://projects.worldbank.org/en/projects-operations/project-detail/P173857

World Bank. (2021l). *Cambodia COVID-19 emergency response project.* https://projects.worldbank.org/en/projects-operations/project-detail/P173815

World Bank. (2021m). *Cote d'Ivoire COVID-19 strategic preparedness and response project (SPRP).* https://projects.worldbank.org/en/projects-operations/project-detail/P173813

World Bank. (2021n). *Djibouti COVID-19 response.* https://projects.worldbank.org/en/projects-operations/project-detail/P173807

World Bank. (2021o). *Dominica first COVID-19 response and recovery programmatic DPC.* https://projects.worldbank.org/en/projects-operations/project-detail/P174927

World Bank. (2021p). *Ecuador COVID-19 emergency response and vaccination project.* https://projects.worldbank.org/en/projects-operations/project-detail/P173773

World Bank. (2021q). *Egypt COVID-19 emergency response.* https://projects.worldbank.org/en/projects-operations/project-detail/P173912

World Bank. (2021r). *El Salvador COVID-19 emergency response project.* https://projects.worldbank.org/en/projects-operations/project-detail/P173872

World Bank. (2021s). *Eswatini COVID-19 emergency response project.* https://projects.worldbank.org/en/projects-operations/project-detail/P173883

World Bank. (2021t). *Fiji COVID-19 emergency response project.* https://projects.worldbank.org/en/projects-operations/project-detail/P173903

World Bank. (2021u). *Gabon COVID-19 strategic preparedness and response project (SPRP).* https://projects.worldbank.org/en/projects-operations/project-detail/P173927

World Bank. (2021v). *The Gambia COVID-19 preparedness and response project.* https://projects.worldbank.org/en/projects-operations/project-detail/P173798

World Bank. (2021w). *Georgia emergency COVID-19 response project.* https://projects.worldbank.org/en/projects-operations/project-detail/P173911

World Bank. (2021x). *Grenada COVID-19 crisis response and fiscal management DPC.* https://projects.worldbank.org/en/projects-operations/project-detail/P174527

World Bank. (2021y). *Guatemala COVID-19 response.* https://projects.worldbank.org/en/projects-operations/project-detail/P173854

World Bank. (2021z). *Haiti COVID-19 response.* https://projects.worldbank.org/en/projects-operations/project-detail/P173811

World Bank. (2021aa). *Indonesia: Emergency response to COVID-19.* https://projects.worldbank.org/en/projects-operations/project-detail/P173843

World Bank. (2021ab). *Jamaica COVID-19 response and recovery development policy financing.* https://projects.worldbank.org/en/projects-operations/project-detail/P174531?lang=en

World Bank. (2021ac). *Jordan COVID-19 emergency response.* https://projects.worldbank.org/en/projects-operations/project-detail/P173972

World Bank. (2021ad). *Kenya COVID-19 health emergency response project.* https://projects.worldbank.org/en/projects-operations/project-detail/P173820

World Bank. (2021ae). *Kiribati COVID-19 emergency response project.* https://projects.worldbank.org/en/projects-operations/project-detail/P174219

World Bank. (2021af). *Lao PDR COVID-19 response project.* https://projects.worldbank.org/en/projects-operations/project-detail/P173817

World Bank. (2021ag). *Madagascar COVID-19 response DPO.* https://projects.worldbank.org/en/projects-operations/project-detail/P174388

World Bank. (2021ah). *Malawi COVID-19 emergency response and health systems preparedness project.* https://projects.worldbank.org/en/projects-operations/project-detail/P173806

World Bank. (2021ai). *Moldova emergency COVID-19 response project.* https://projects.worldbank.org/en/projects-operations/project-detail/P173776

World Bank. (2021aj). *Mongolia COVID-19 emergency response and health system preparedness project.* https://projects.worldbank.org/en/projects-operations/project-detail/P173799

World Bank. (2021ak). *Myanmar COVID-19 emergency response project.* https://projects.worldbank.org/en/projects-operations/project-detail/P173902

World Bank. (2021al). *Nepal: COVID-19 emergency response and health systems preparedness project*. https://projects.worldbank.org/en/projects-operations/project-detail/P173760
World Bank. (2021am). *Paraguay – Latin America and Caribbean – P173805 – PY: COVID-19 emergency response project – Procurement plan (English)*. https://documents.worldbank.org/en/publication/documents-reports/documentdetail/863911612354529421/paraguay-latin-america-and-caribbean-p173805-py-covid-19-emergency-response-project-procurement-plan
World Bank. (2021an). *Republic of Congo COVID-19 emergency response project*. https://projects.worldbank.org/en/projects-operations/project-detail/P173851
World Bank. (2021ao). *Republic of Congo Lisungi emergency COVID-19 response project*. https://projects.worldbank.org/en/projects-operations/project-detail/P174178
World Bank. (2021ap). *Samoa COVID-19 emergency response project*. https://projects.worldbank.org/en/projects-operations/project-detail/P173920
World Bank. (2021aq). *Senegal COVID-19 response project*. https://projects.worldbank.org/en/projects-operations/project-detail/P173838
World Bank. (2021ar). *Serbia emergency COVID-19 response project*. https://projects.worldbank.org/en/projects-operations/project-detail/P173892
World Bank. (2021as). *Sierra Leone COVID-19 emergency preparedness and response project*. https://projects.worldbank.org/en/projects-operations/project-detail/P173803
World Bank. (2021at). *South Africa COVID-19 response development policy operation*. https://projects.worldbank.org/en/projects-operations/project-detail/P174246
World Bank. (2021au). *Sri Lanka COVID-19 emergency response and health systems preparedness project*. https://projects.worldbank.org/en/projects-operations/project-detail/P173867
World Bank. (2021av). *Sudan COVID-19 emergency response project*. https://projects.worldbank.org/en/projects-operations/project-detail/P174352
World Bank. (2021aw). *Supporting Colombia's COVID-19 crisis response*. https://www.worldbank.org/en/results/2021/04/09/supporting-columbia-s-covid-19-crisis-response
World Bank. (2021ax). *Tajikistan emergency COVID-19 project*. https://projects.worldbank.org/en/projects-operations/project-detail/P173765
World Bank. (2021ay). *Timor-Leste COVID-19 emergency support project*. https://projects.worldbank.org/en/projects-operations/project-detail/P174404
World Bank. (2021az). *Uruguay COVID-19 emergency response project*. https://projects.worldbank.org/en/projects-operations/project-detail/P173876
World Bank. (2021ba). *Uzbekistan emergency COVID-19 response project*. https://projects.worldbank.org/en/projects-operations/project-detail/P173827
World Bank. (2021bb). *Vietnam COVID-19 emergency response project*. https://projects.worldbank.org/en/projects-operations/project-detail/P174389
World Bank. (2022a). *Benin COVID-19 preparedness and response project*. https://projects.worldbank.org/en/projects-operations/project-detail/P173839
World Bank. (2022b). *Cameroon COVID-19 preparedness and response project*. https://projects.worldbank.org/en/projects-operations/project-detail/P174108
World Bank. (2022c). *Central African Republic COVID-19 preparedness and response project*. https://projects.worldbank.org/en/projects-operations/project-detail/P173832
World Bank. (2022d). *Chad COVID-19 strategic preparedness and response project*. https://projects.worldbank.org/en/projects-operations/project-detail/P173894
World Bank. (2022e). *Ethiopia COVID-19 emergency response*. https://projects.worldbank.org/en/projects-operations/project-detail/P173750
World Bank. (2022f). *Ghana COVID-19 emergency preparedness and response project*. https://projects.worldbank.org/en/projects-operations/project-detail/P173788
World Bank. (2022g). *Guinea COVID-19 preparedness and response project*. https://projects.worldbank.org/en/projects-operations/project-detail/P174032
World Bank. (2022h). *Honduras COVID-19 emergency response project*. https://projects.worldbank.org/en/projects-operations/project-detail/P173861
World Bank. (2022i). *Iran COVID-19 emergency response project*. https://projects.worldbank.org/en/projects-operations/project-detail/P173994

World Bank. (2022j). *Kyrgyz Republic – Emergency COVID-19 project*. https://projects.worldbank.org/en/projects-operations/project-detail/P173766

World Bank. (2022k). *Lesotho COVID-19 emergency preparedness and response project*. https://projects.worldbank.org/en/projects-operations/project-detail/P173939

World Bank. (2022l). *Maldives COVID-19 emergency response and health systems preparedness project*. https://projects.worldbank.org/en/projects-operations/project-detail/P173801

World Bank. (2022m). *Mali COVID-19 emergency response project*. https://projects.worldbank.org/en/projects-operations/project-detail/P173816

World Bank. (2022n). *Nicaragua COVID-19 education sector response project*. https://projects.worldbank.org/en/projects-operations/project-detail/P174677

World Bank. (2022o). *Niger COVID-19 emergency response project*. https://projects.worldbank.org/en/projects-operations/project-detail/P173846

World Bank. (2022p). *Nigeria COVID-19 preparedness and response project*. https://projects.worldbank.org/en/projects-operations/project-detail/P173980

World Bank. (2022q). *North Macedonia emergency COVID-19 response project*. https://projects.worldbank.org/en/projects-operations/project-detail/P173916

World Bank. (2022r). *Panama COVID-19 emergency response*. https://projects.worldbank.org/en/projects-operations/project-detail/P173881

World Bank. (2022s). *Papua New Guinea COVID-19 emergency response project*. https://projects.worldbank.org/en/projects-operations/project-detail/P173834

World Bank. (2022t). *Philippines COVID-19 emergency response project*. https://projects.worldbank.org/en/projects-operations/project-detail/P173877

World Bank. (2022u). *Republic of Trinidad and Tobago: COVID-19 emergency response project*. https://projects.worldbank.org/en/projects-operations/project-detail/P173989

World Bank. (2022v). *Rwanda COVID-19 emergency response project*. https://projects.worldbank.org/en/projects-operations/project-detail/P173855

World Bank. (2022w). *Solomon Islands COVID-19 emergency response project*. https://projects.worldbank.org/en/projects-operations/project-detail/P173933

World Bank. (2022x). *Togo emergency COVID-19 DPO 2021*. https://projects.worldbank.org/en/projects-operations/project-detail/P174376

World Bank. (2022y). *Tunisia COVID-19 response project*. https://projects.worldbank.org/en/projects-operations/project-detail/P173945

World Bank. (2022z). *Turkey emergency COVID-19 health project*. https://projects.worldbank.org/en/projects-operations/project-detail/P173988

World Bank. (2022aa). *Uganda COVID-19 response and emergency preparedness project*. https://projects.worldbank.org/en/projects-operations/project-detail/P174041

World Bank. (2022ab). *Zambia COVID-19 emergency response and health systems preparedness project*. https://projects.worldbank.org/en/projects-operations/project-detail/P174185

World Health Organization. (2020). *REACT-C19 project: WHO brings doctors to Azerbaijan in bid to revamp hospitals' COVID-19 response*. https://www.euro.who.int/en/countries/azerbaijan/news/news/2020/7/react-c19-project-who-brings-doctors-to-azerbaijan-in-bid-to-revamp-hospitals-covid-19-response

World Vision Albania. (2020). *Impact assessment of the COVID-19 outbreak on wellbeing of children and families in Albania*. https://www.wvi.org/sites/default/files/2020-06/COVID_Assesment_Report_WVA_final.pdf

Yang, Y., Chua, J. J. E., Khng, K. H., & Yu, Y. (2020). How did COVID-19 impact the lives and perceived well-being of parents? Using the case of Singapore to investigate the mechanisms. *PsyArXiv*. https://doi.org/10.31234/osf.io/b3cua

Yang, B., Chen, B.-B., Qu, Y., & Zhu, Y. (2021). Impacts of parental burnout on Chinese youth's mental health: The role of parents' autonomy support and emotion regulation. *Journal of Youth and Adolescence, 50*(8), 1679–1692. https://doi.org/10.1007/s10964-021-01450-y

Yeasmin, S., Banik, R., Hossain, S., Hossain, M. N., Mahumud, R., Salma, N., & Hossain, M. M. (2020). Impact of COVID-19 pandemic on the mental health of children in Bangladesh:

A cross-sectional study. *Children and Youth Services Review, 117*, 105277. https://doi.org/10.1016/j.childyouth.2020.105277

Yehudai, M., Bender, S., Gritsenko, V., Konstantinov, V., Reznik, A., & Isralowitz, R. (2020). COVID-19 fear, mental health, and substance misuse conditions among university social work students in Israel and Russia. *International Journal of Mental Health and Addiction*. https://doi.org/10.1007/s11469-020-00360-7

Yıldırım, M., & Güler, A. (2020). COVID-19 severity, self-efficacy, knowledge, preventive behaviors, and mental health in Turkey. *Death Studies*, 1–8. https://doi.org/10.1080/07481187.2020.1793434

Yitayih, Y., Mekonen, S., Zeynudin, A., Mengistie, E., & Ambelu, A. (2020). Mental health of healthcare professionals during the early stage of the COVID-19 pandemic in Ethiopia. *British Journal of Psychology Open, 7*(1), e1. https://doi.org/10.1192/bjo.2020.130

Yu, Y., Zheng, Y., Chua, J. J. E., & Yang, Y. (2021). Familial mechanisms linking COVID-19 lockdown with mental health problems in Singaporean children and adolescents. *PsyArXiv*. https://doi.org/10.31234/osf.io/js9c6

Zeballos Rivas, D. R., Lopez Jaldin, M. L., Nina Canaviri, B., Portugal Escalante, L. F., Alanes Fernández, A. M. C., & Aguilar Ticona, J. P. (2021). Social media exposure, risk perception, preventive behaviors and attitudes during the COVID-19 epidemic in La Paz, Bolivia: A cross sectional study. *PLoS One, 16*(1), e0245859. https://doi.org/10.1371/journal.pone.0245859

Zhang, S. X., Sun, S., Afshar Jahanshahi, A., Alvarez-Risco, A., Ibarra, V. G., Li, J., & Patty-Tito, R. M. (2020). Developing and testing a measure of COVID-19 organizational support of healthcare workers – Results from Peru, Ecuador, and Bolivia. *Psychiatry Research, 291*, 113174. https://doi.org/10.1016/j.psychres.2020.113174

Zhu, D., Mishra, S. R., Han, X., & Santo, K. (2020). Social distancing in Latin America during the COVID-19 pandemic: An analysis using the Stringency Index and Google Community Mobility Reports. *Journal of Travel Medicine, 27*(8). https://doi.org/10.1093/jtm/taaa125

ZonMw. (2022). *COVID-19 programme*. https://www.zonmw.nl/en/research-and-results/infectious-diseases-and-antimicrobial-resistance/programmas/programme-detail/covid-19-programme/

Chapter 12
Toward the Practice of Pandemic Patience and Persistence

Charles R. Figley, Lenore E. A. Walker, and Ilene A. Serlin

The world is forever changed. Supply chains, closed stores, children unable to go to school, skyrocketing rates of fear and depression, etc. We thought COVID-19 was going to be over. Instead, we have new variants, predictions of ongoing virus threats, and new contagions from animals. We experience isolation, losses, and inability to grieve. We feel financial instability, health disparities, and a new sense of vulnerability and insecurity. Our sense of time and reality is distorted; we are fed fake news and live in increasingly technological bubbles. We are disconnected from community and each other. Our lives become a blur; we lose months and years. We become disoriented and traumatized. With added threats of climate change, social instability, and violence, we go from pandemic to systemic endemic; people are trying to find a "new normal." How to find the courage to persevere? To trust and love again? To find our inner balance and stability while the world is turning upside down?

We now reach the final chapter of this book. In some ways the pandemic, as it surpasses 3 years, will serve as a marker of the shift from then to now. From this point of view, looking back over the year it took to write it, we find a sense of satisfaction and appreciation. We are more aware of what has happened to us all after living with the pandemic, aware of the enormous toll, and aware of the successful adaptations discovered that were reported from our various authors. We found kindness and collaboration, became a caring support system for each other as we wrote, reached our objectives, and addressed the questions posed in Chap. 1. We have gained enormous appreciation and satisfaction with being practitioners who are

C. R. Figley (✉)
Tulane University, School of Social Work, New Orleans, LA, USA
e-mail: Figley@tulane.edu

L. E. A. Walker
College of Psychology, Nova Southeastern University, Fort Lauderdale, FL, USA

I. A. Serlin
Independent Practice, San Francisco, CA, USA

C. R. Figley et al. (eds.), *Pandemic Providers*,
https://doi.org/10.1007/978-3-031-27580-7_12

trained to focus on the welfare of others, not only the clinical outcomes. We believe that this appreciation shows through the origin stories from each member of the Task Force. Each group was able to find its own justifications for working together, focusing on what is important during these times of adaptation and changing standards, expectations, directions, shifting politics, and protocols. We learned a great deal about collaboration, especially with cultural, professional, and generational differences.

The pandemic was a shock to the system that helped us recognize, as our chapters report, how we were missing clients in our practice or in our research, who were being ignored, despite their need for help. The political strife and its wake are troubling and draw attention and resources away from where it is critically needed. Among what are vitally needed, far more attention to trauma resilience programs and resources were discussed throughout the book but with special attention in Chaps. 2 (the 1918 pandemic), 3 (interpersonal violence), 4 (parents), 5 (vibrant older adults), 6 (medical and addiction), 7 (professional support), 8 (somatic and creative), 9 (international students), and Chaps. 10 (telehealth) and 11 (research initiatives).

Since the purpose of the book, it was noted in the first chapter, is to provide a conceptual and intellectual bridge linking where we are today to where we were months prior to the pandemic, the purpose of this chapter is to bring together all the lines of inquiry and discovery, with the accompanying theories, definitions, and applicational uses in the future. We began with a history of our efforts to learn from historical markers such as a pandemic and its accompanying manifestations and moved on to summarize challenges faced and lessons learned.

The Five Central Questions

This chapter will also suggest answers to the five central questions posed in Chap. 1:

1. *What happened to the world and the USA during the first 3 years of the pandemic?*
   The authors of the nine work group chapters offer the most insight and original perspectives about how the nation and how our fields of practice, especially psychology, have come out of the pandemic. Our colleagues have performed their work personally and professionally while in the midst of their own family or community pandemic crisis. In addition to the pandemic, we were also faced with extreme situations caused by climate change, violence, and political upheavals. It was said that the pandemic became a syndemic and then endemic, with each challenge compounding the others. Each work group with the Task Force faced all these challenges, gathered and shared resources, and found unique ways to innovate.
2. *What were mental health professional challenges faced during the pandemic?*
   The first response to the challenges was to gather and try to help, an altruistic response to trauma that can be a genuine gift. Wonderful human beings showed

up and found ways to move forward. It was essential to identify trauma responses to the pandemic and anticipate the depth of loss, isolation, suicidality, and other experiences. What helped was an unusual collaboration between generations, across disciplines (APA divisions) and even countries. With the help of the younger members, groups learned how to use telehealth and understood that a whole new set of ethical guidelines will be needed during urgent times of psychological distress. We understood again that resources help, but the most important ingredient is the human connection.

3. *What were the innovations and breakthroughs in pandemic-related mental health assessment and services?*

   The pandemic with its shifting instructions to citizens from their governments' authorities regarding safety protocols but also other shifting information caused great confusion and mounting anxiety. We had to learn whole new ways of relating to each other, gauging 6 feet distance and wearing masks. Many of us had to give up our offices and use only telehealth, getting a new perspective on client's lives and changing their perspective on seeing us in our lives. Our modes of service delivery had to change, and those changes were noted by members of the Task Force. Therapists received panicked calls from people who felt confused and scared, distrusting the government and other people. There were so many mental health needs that individual therapists could not cover that need. The insurance companies, Medicare, and the individual therapy model are not built to handle crises of such magnitude. New technologies helped, and many apps and even artificial intelligence programs are being developed, but we are also seeing the problematic consequences of relying on technology. We see now an explosion of fake news and further distortion of what was formerly consensus reality. The politics is becoming personal as more and more communities, families, and countries are polarized. We see an increasing number of people preferring to live alone; and the break down and impact of the emotional development of children. These children were deprived of classroom, in-person learning. We need technology and the scaling of mental health services, but we also see the need for careful human choices.

4. *What did we learn about gender, race, human relations, and helping our fellow humans?*

   Several chapters addressed the beneficial influence of the pandemic in terms of the greater awareness regarding gender and race in particular. Chapter 3, for example, discussed the many initiatives related to gender inequities, comparing data concerning men and women of color to white women. Other chapters reported findings around ageism, differential access to healthcare, and death rates. Yes, there were public expressions of appreciation. But we have learned that there needs to emerge entire departments devoted to the welfare and mental health of hospital staff and others who are pressed to work more than they have before, under extraordinary conditions and pressures. We were reminded of the importance of each healthcare worker in the system, and to show that appreciation to the cleaning people as well as the doctors in the hospital. We learned as healthcare providers that sharing our vulnerability, as we too were hit by losses, was a powerful part of the healing.

5. *How can we play forward what we have learned toward increased social services and greater care for others as well as ourselves?*

   The self-care and the delivery of social services became important to more people, beyond practitioners. During the pandemic when most of us were consigned to our homes, our own and others' care became a central concern. Practitioners are notoriously blind to our own personal needs. The pandemic forced us to place our safety first. We learned about the value of working out more, with a greater focus on what we eat and when and how and where. We rediscovered our own personal and existential needs and used this time as an opportunity to assess and re-prioritize our lives. We survived plague-like conditions with overcrowded hospitals with dying patients and overworked nurses and doctors. The care for staff and others is important, but so is the commitment to 24/7 self-care routines and support systems to offset the highly combustible burnout regime. Self-care also means greater care for family of the caregivers, as well as greater benefits for the practitioner's clients.

What We Have Learned About the Practice of Psychology

The practice of psychology survived and thrived during the pandemic despite all the changes and adaptation that had to occur. First and foremost, we learned that we could provide good psychotherapy without having to see a client in our office. This is not how most of us were trained, but we were forced in our homes just as our clients were remanded to their homes. The rules and regulations that had to be suspended turned out to be unnecessary cautions. Not only were our fears unwarranted, but most of us found we really liked working from home especially if the alternative was being in an office wearing a mask. We also learned that it was possible to add filters and other ways to keep air circulating when we did have to go into the office. Many of those in private independent practice of psychology gave up their offices permanently. Some retired earlier than they had planned, but most psychotherapists found that they adapted to working from home easier than they thought.

The positive side of the ability to effectively treat people using digital technologies is that we were able to see many more people since the time and often inconvenience of travel was eliminated. Many people discovered the importance of psychotherapy being available especially when anxiety and stress soared, and most mental health professionals were working more hours than before. At the same time, it became clear that some people were more likely to not have access to psychotherapy, especially people of color and people with fewer financial resources. When the racial tensions erupted into riots during the first year of the pandemic, they have shown a bright light on these health inequities, and digital therapeutics were developed as one way to overcome them.

There is a negative side of the ability to treat people using digital technologies from our homes to their homes. This has permitted the growth of companies delivering services by part- time or full-time mental health practitioners with little supervision or experienced colleagues on site for consultation on difficult cases. Another problem has been the large numbers of psychotherapists without training in trauma-informed or trauma-specific treatment working with multiple traumatized clients with few or no resources. We did our best to provide resources as widely around the globe as you have read in the stories in this book, but we aware of how inadequate our efforts were compared to the need. The business of providing psychology services to those who need us has been changed, probably forever.

We have begun to define what causes trauma more broadly than the typical PTSD definition of symptoms. As we have described, trauma impacts our brains, bodies, and nervous system as well as our cognitive and affective abilities. Trauma impacts our relationships with others. Hopefully, future graduate students will get to spend more time studying trauma and its impact to meet the continued need for those who assess and provide psychotherapy.

The long-term psychological effects from the ongoing pandemic are still unknown, especially since it has not ended. We can expect that there will continue to be heightened levels of anxiety and stress as is common with trauma. We also can expect that some people will continue to experience fear as the coronavirus continues to mutate and infect people despite the boosters of vaccine and treatment with antibodies. There is less isolation, but major support systems have broken down. What we have learned since the 1918 flu is the need for people to talk about their fears and their experiences. The old messages to forget and not mention the harrowing experiences will not help people get beyond trauma. Psychology is one way to deal with these experiences as we've shown here.

We worry about the impact on the children. It was clear that the attempt to home-school children with parents also having to work at home was a failure. Teachers were unprepared to teach over the internet even when they and the children had access to technology. The lack of contact with peers and extended family that is so critical for development suggests that many were negatively impacted. Reports of traumatized children are common in the psychology literature.

Finally, we have learned that our country and others around the world were totally unprepared to deal with a pandemic such as COVID-19 provided. We did not have trained personnel, the resources, nor effective leaders that trusted our scientists and healthcare specialists. This costs us millions of lives unnecessarily, especially those of our elders and vulnerable at first but then our seemingly healthy youth later on. Those of us who work in the healthcare business decry its mismanagement. Hopefully, we have learned from the mistakes made and will be better prepared both to deal with this pandemic as it continues and others should they occur.

Conclusion

This final chapter, titled *Toward the Practice of Patience and Persistence*, captures the overall lesson of this book. Given the extraordinary era we work within and its unknown and dangerous circumstances, the futures of physical and mental health in the world are emerging daily. Taken and studied like an experiment, this initiative that started with an invitation to collaborate celebrates the report of its work as a Task Force. Expecting this to be a long-term project, this takes us well into the pandemic and beyond. The Task Force has been effective in mobilizing professional and scholarly support among colleagues. We hope that this book, by reflecting on challenges faced and lessons learned from a variety of perspectives, will help you face some of the inevitable challenges from future pandemics, give you more resources to cope, and contribute to your health and well-being.

Author Note The authors thank the American Psychological Association's Interdivisional Task Force on the pandemic for the framework, divisional collaboration, and extraordinary membership that made this book possible.

Index

C. R. Figley et al. (eds.), *Pandemic Providers*,
https://doi.org/10.1007/978-3-031-27580-7

P

R

S

T

CPSIA information can be obtained
at www.ICGtesting.com
Printed in the USA
LVHW051225250623
750721LV00005B/272

9 783031 275791